SELF-ASSESSMENT IN
DERMATOLOGY

Questions & Answers

To my wife and best friend, Jessica, thank you for your unconditional love and support, and your daily inspiration. To my loving parents, Arnold and Elena, thank you for teaching me the importance of hard work and dedication.

—Jonathan S. Leventhal

To my husband, Simon, and beautiful daughter, Ariella, thank you for your support and lending me time to make this possible. To my nontwin twin sister, Racine, thanks for always being by my side. To my amazing and fabulous mother Denise, thank you for always believing in me and giving me everything I ever needed to succeed—I couldn't have done it without you.

—Lauren L. Levy

SELF-ASSESSMENT IN
DERMATOLOGY

Questions & Answers

Jonathan S. Leventhal, MD
Assistant Professor
Associate Residency Program Director
Director of Oncodermatology Clinic
Department of Dermatology
Yale University School of Medicine
New Haven, CT, USA

Lauren L. Levy, MD
Dermatologist, Private practice
Clinical Instructor
Department of Dermatology
Icahn School of Medicine at Mount Sinai
New York City, NY, USA

ELSEVIER

Elsevier
1600 John F. Kennedy Blvd.
Ste 1800
Philadelphia, PA 19103-2899

SELF-ASSESSMENT IN DERMATOLOGY   ISBN: 978-0-323-66200-0

ISBN: 978-0-323-66200-0

Content Strategist: Charlotta Kryhl
Content Development Specialist: Meghan Andress
Publishing Services Manager: Shereen Jameel
Project Manager: Nadhiya Sekar
Design Direction: Brian Salisbury

Printed in China

Last digit is the print number: 9 8 7 6 5 4 3 2 1

CONTRIBUTORS

Christopher G. Bunick, MD, PhD

Assistant Professor
Department of Dermatology
Yale University School of Medicine
New Haven, CT, USA

Sean R. Christensen, MD, PhD

Assistant Professor
Director of Resident Education in Dermatologic Surgery
Department of Dermatology, Section of Dermatologic Surgery
and Cutaneous Oncology
Department of Surgery (Plastic and Reconstructive)
Yale University School of Medicine
New Haven, CT, USA

Brittany Craiglow, MD

Adjunct Assistant Professor
Department of Dermatology
Yale University School of Medicine
New Haven, CT, USA

William Damsky, MD, PhD

Instructor
Department of Dermatology
Yale University School of Medicine
New Haven, CT, USA

Amanda A. Dunec, MD

Assistant Professor of Dermatology
Director of Cosmetic Dermatology
Albert Einstein College of Medicine
Montefiore Medical Center
Division of Dermatology
Bronx, NY, USA

Marianna Freudzon, MD

Clinical Instructor
Department of Dermatology
Yale University School of Medicine
New Haven, CT, USA

Lauren Claire Smith Kole, MD

Assistant Professor
Department of Dermatology
University of Alabama School of Medicine
Birmingham, AL, USA

Ilya Lim, MD

Assistant Professor
Department of Dermatology
Yale University School of Medicine
New Haven, CT, USA

Alicia J. Little, MD, PhD

Instructor
Department of Dermatology
Yale University School of Medicine
New Haven, CT, USA

Gauri Panse, MBBS

Assistant Professor
Departments of Dermatology and Pathology
Yale University School of Medicine
New Haven, CT, USA

Sara H. Perkins, MD

Clinical Instructor
Department of Dermatology
Yale University School of Medicine
New Haven, CT, USA

Sarika M. Ramachandran, MD

Assistant Professor
Medical Director of Yale Branford Dermatology
Department of Dermatology
Yale University School of Medicine
New Haven, CT, USA

Melissa Serravallo, MD

Yardley Dermatology Associates
Yardley, PA

Kathleen Cook Suozzi, MD

Assistant Professor
Director of the Aesthetic Dermatology Program
Department of Dermatology, Section of Dermatologic Surgery
and Cutaneous Oncology
Yale University School of Medicine
New Haven, CT, USA

Mariam B. Totonchy, MD

Clinical Instructor
Department of Dermatology
Yale University School of Medicine
New Haven, CT, USA

Matthew D. Vesely, MD, PhD

Instructor
Department of Dermatology
Yale University School of Medicine
New Haven, CT, USA

Amanda E. Zubek, MD, PhD

Assistant Professor
Medical Director of Yale Middlebury Dermatology
Department of Dermatology
Yale University School of Medicine
New Haven, CT, USA

PREFACE

The American Board of Dermatology's certification and maintenance of certification examinations are challenging tests that evaluate clinical knowledge gained after the culmination of years of training, studying, and dedication. Preparation for these examinations can be daunting given the vast subject matter. While there are many textbooks, journals, study guides, and online practice questions available, there have been no comprehensive, question-based board review books in the style of the contemporary examination—until now.

As recent graduates of the dermatology residency program at Yale School of Medicine, we sought to create a question-based review book for dermatologists at all levels of experience, ranging from first-year residents to those in practice for decades. This text encompasses the most up-to-date and clinically relevant information across the spectrum of dermatology, including general, medical, pediatric, surgical, cosmetic, and basic science/research. This book is designed to prepare dermatologists for the new structure of the certification examination, which now emphasizes patient-centered care and application of knowledge using clinically relevant case scenarios. Organized as mini-tests, the book features 560 questions with succinct explanations of the correct and incorrect choices as well as clinically relevant pearls. The explanations reference corresponding sections of major dermatology textbooks, primary literature, and evidenced-based practice guidelines. The questions are designed to emulate actual patient encounters and challenge the dermatologist to consider what they would do in these scenarios.

Our goal in creating this book was to provide dermatologists with relevant, easy-to-follow, and clinically useful information. It should serve as a useful tool for all dermatologists given the wide array of clinical photos, detailed explanations, and clinical pearls that may directly impact practice. Question-based learning through clinicopathological correlation will help dermatologists synthesize information, review differential diagnoses, and hone in on the application of knowledge to best prepare for the certification and recertification examinations. We hope you have as much fun reading this book as we did creating it.

ACKNOWLEDGMENTS

We would like to acknowledge and extend our sincere gratitude to Drs. Jean Bolognia, Christine Ko, Michael Girardi, and Richard Edelson for providing continued support and mentorship throughout our careers as well as for sharing their fund of knowledge, clinical skills, and expertise. We are greatly indebted to the Yale dermatology residents for their contribution to the numerous photographs used in the book. It is a privilege to work with them and learn from them. We are also grateful to the contributing authors whose hard work and dedication made this book possible.

CONTENTS

GENERAL DERMATOLOGY

1. A 58-year-old woman presented with the following pruritic eruption. There was no response to intramuscular triamcinolone. What medication may be associated with this condition?

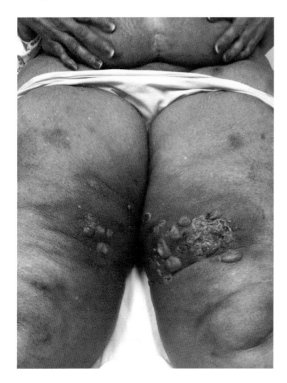

A. Furosemide
B. Valacyclovir
C. Doxycycline
D. Cetuximab

2. The patient presents with violaceous papules with white scale on the upper and lower extremities and these lesions in the oral mucosa. What is the most appropriate lab test to evaluate for an associated infectious agent?

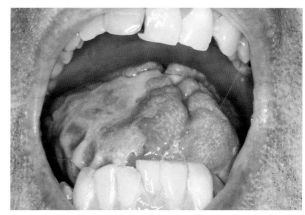

With permission from Olson M, et al. (eds.), in *Clinics in Dermatology*, 2nd edition, Volume 34, Issue 4, 2016, Elsevier, 495–504 (fig. 3).

A. Mycoplasma polymerase chain reaction
B. Hepatitis C antibody
C. Rapid plasma reagin
D. Fungal culture
E. Human immunodeficiency virus antibody

3. What is the best treatment option for this 15-year-old boy?

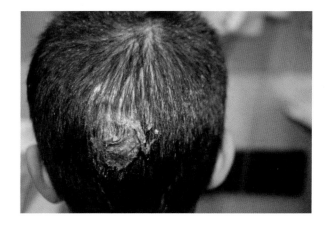

A. Griseofulvin 20–25 mg/kg/day
B. Doxycycline 100 mg twice daily
C. Intralesional triamcinolone injections
D. Ketoconazole shampoo three times weekly

4. You diagnose your 23-year-old female patient with an allergic contact dermatitis to her temporary tattoo. What else is she at risk of reacting to?
   A. Poison ivy
   B. Mango
   C. Hair dye
   D. Nail polish

5. The patient also presents with fevers and myalgias—what other finding may be present?

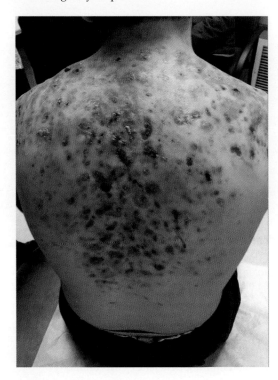

   A. Diarrhea
   B. Headaches
   C. Pilonidal cyst
   D. Clavicular bone lesions

6. The patient most likely has what associated condition?

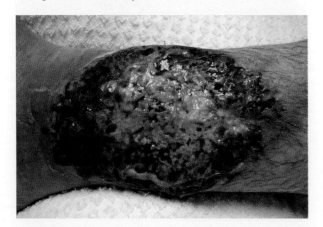

   A. Rheumatoid arthritis
   B. HIV
   C. Venous hypertension
   D. Systemic lupus erythematous

7. Intravenous immunoglobulin (IVIG) can cause which of the following cutaneous reactions?
   A. Leukocytoclastic vasculitis
   B. Immunobullous disease
   C. Dyshidrotic eczema
   D. Fixed drug eruption

8. A 28-year-old postdoctoral fellow presents with the following pruritic lesion on the wrist. He reports that the lesion started while he was in Costa Rica doing fieldwork 4 weeks ago and started after a mosquito bite. He denies any other lesions. What is the most likely diagnosis?

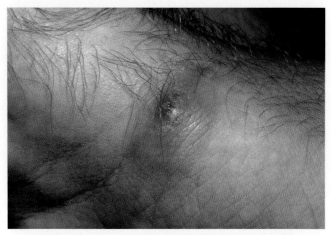

Courtesy Steven Binnick, MD. With permission from James WD, et al. (eds.), in *Andrews' Diseases of the Skin Clinical Atlas*, 2018, Elsevier, 291–307 (ch 20, fig. 20.62).

   A. Furunculosis
   B. Sporotrichosis
   C. Exaggerated arthropod bite reaction
   D. Inflamed epidermoid cyst
   E. Myiasis

9. A 33-year-old immigrant from Columbia presents with the following lesion. A tissue sample sent to the Centers for Disease Control and Prevention confirmed the diagnosis by PCR. The patient does not improve with sodium stibogluconate intramuscular administered for 4 weeks. What is the next best step in management?

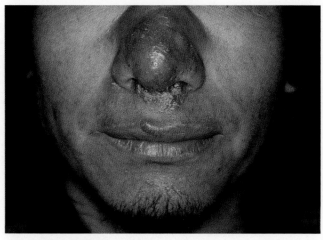

With permission from James WD, et al. (eds.), in *Andrews' Diseases of the Skin*, 12th edition, 2016, Elsevier, 418–450 (fig. 20-6).

A. Intravenous amphotericin B
B. Topical imiquimod
C. Change sodium stibogluconate route of administration to intralesional
D. Oral itraconazole
E. Combination of oral rifampin and dapsone

10. What is the patient's most likely diagnosis?

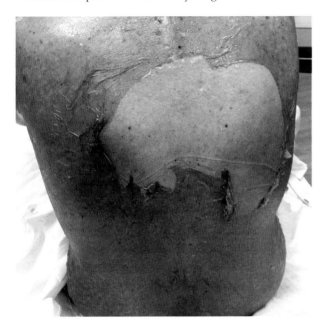

A. Graft-versus-host disease
B. Dermatomyositis
C. Cutaneous lymphoma
D. Staphylococcal scalded skin syndrome

11. Of the various forms of cutaneous lupus listed below, which of the following is LEAST likely to be associated with systemic disease?
A. Subacute cutaneous lupus erythematosus
B. Acute cutaneous lupus erythematosus
C. Discoid lupus erythematosus
D. Bullous lupus erythematosus

12. This patient is 28 weeks pregnant. What is the treatment of choice?

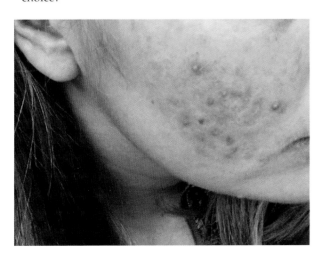

A. Tazarotene gel
B. Azelaic acid
C. Doxycycline
D. Isotretinoin

13. What is the preferred treatment for a 6-year-old female who presents with this eruption?

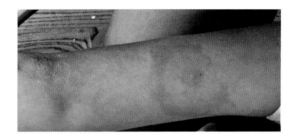

A. Doxycycline
B. Amoxicillin
C. Valacyclovir
D. Clindamycin

14. A 75-year-old man developed the following lesions after babysitting his grandson, who had a diarrheal illness. What is the best diagnosis?

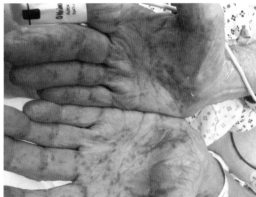

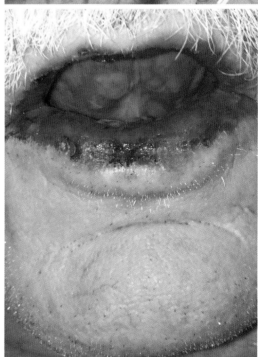

A. Secondary syphilis
B. Erythema multiforme
C. Atypical hand-foot-mouth disease
D. Acrodermatitis enteropathica

15. What is the associated fetal risk with this condition?

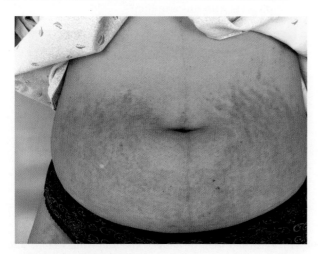

A. Small for gestational age
B. Craniosynostosis
C. No associated risk
D. Placental insufficiency

16. What class of medication is associated with this eruption?

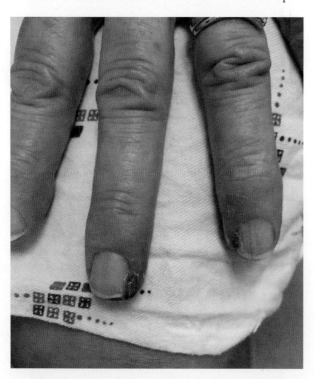

A. Programmed death 1 inhibitor
B. Epidermal growth factor receptor inhibitor
C. BRAF inhibitor
D. Tumor necrosis factor alpha inhibitor

17. What is the most common extra-cutaneous manifestation in this condition?

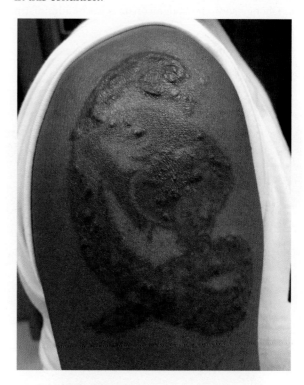

A. Cardiomyopathy
B. Hilar lymphadenopathy
C. Arthritis
D. Thyroiditis

18. What antibody is most specific for this condition?

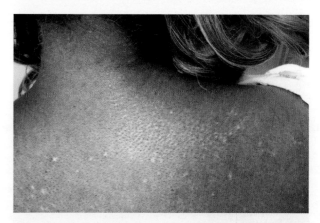

A. ANA
B. Jo-1
C. SCL-70
D. Thyroid peroxidase

19. What gene is associated with this condition?

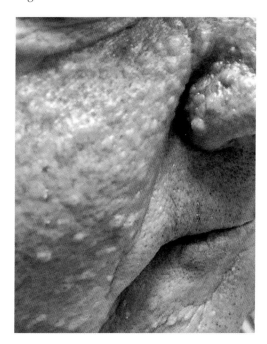

A. FLCN
B. CYLD
C. MSH2
D. PTEN

20. The patient reports having an unprotected sexual encounter 2 months prior and developed a lesion on his penis that resolved with time. The patient then presented with the following rash. Which of the following is NOT true regarding this infection?

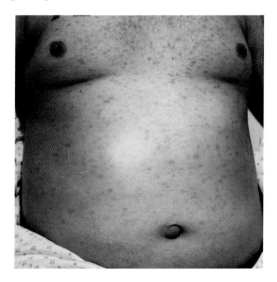

A. These lesions will disappear spontaneously in 3–12 weeks.
B. A majority of untreated individuals will have latent disease without progression.
C. The treatment of choice for penicillin-allergic patients is sulfamethoxazole/trimethoprim.
D. Congenital disease may present with bullae.
E. A neonate without signs of disease and with a negative RPR whose mother was appropriately treated does not require treatment.

21. What are the associated nail findings in this condition?

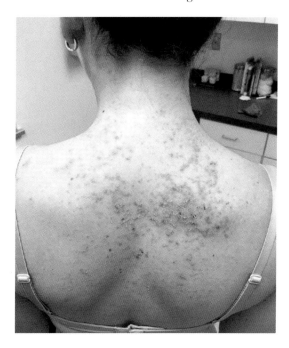

A. Oil spots and onycholysis
B. Red-white longitudinal bands and v-shaped distal nicks
C. Dolichonychia
D. Trachyonychia

22. A patient presents with a severe allergic contact dermatitis to perfumes/fragrances. Patch testing is strongly positive for Balsam of Peru allergen. Which of the following foods is most likely to cause a systemic contact dermatitis in this patient?

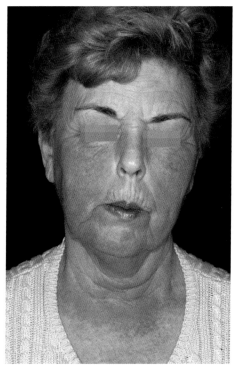

With permission from Habif TP, in *Clinical Dermatology*, 12th edition, 2016, Elsevier, 126–149.

A. Propolis
B. Cashews
C. Mangos
D. Kiwis
E. Tomatoes

23. The patient developed these pruritic lesions that become edematous and inflamed upon rubbing. What immuno-histochemical stain is most likely to be positive?

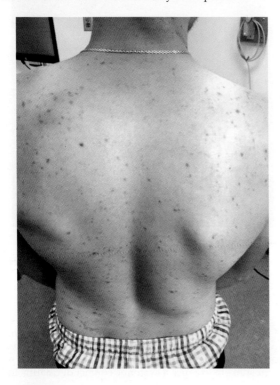

A. HHV-8
B. PAS
C. S100
D. Tryptase

24. A 25-year-old African American female presents with asymptomatic, hyperpigmented nodules localized to the left lower leg; fevers; and large, painless, bilateral cervical lymph-adenopathy. A biopsy of a nodule revealed a dense histiocytic dermal infiltrate. What is the most likely diagnosis?

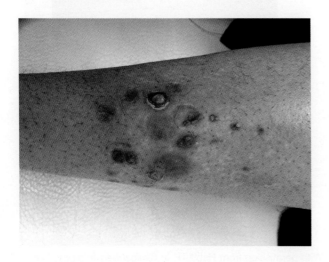

A. Sarcoidosis
B. Juvenile xanthogranuloma
C. Rosai-Dorfman disease
D. Foreign body reaction
E. Reticulohistiocytosis

25. A 60-year-old Caucasian female presents for evaluation. On close inspection there is perifollicular erythema and scale. What is the most likely diagnosis?

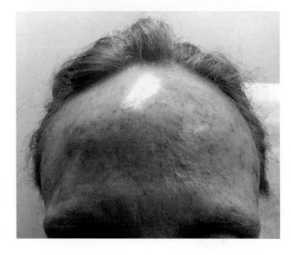

A. Traction alopecia
B. Alopecia areata
C. Discoid lupus erythematosus
D. Central centrifugal cicatricial alopecia
E. Frontal fibrosing alopecia

26. A 50-year-old female patient presents with erythematous papules and pustules on her bilateral cheeks. She reports no improvement with several weeks of an oral tetracycline and topical metronidazole. She also complains of burning and stinging of the skin. What is the best next step?
    A. Have the patient continue her current therapy.
    B. Prescribe an alternative antibiotic.
    C. Perform a scraping of the pustules.
    D. Prescribe a topical corticosteroid.
    E. Prescribe a topical calcineurin inhibitor.

27. A 29-year-old female reports a several-year history of re-current oral, genital, and cutaneous ulcerations. What is the most common nonmucocutaneous finding in patients with this disease?

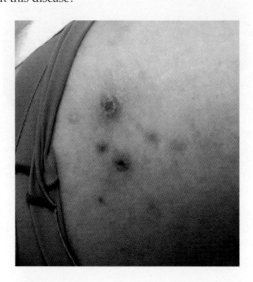

A. Posterior uveitis
B. Arthritis
C. Cranial nerve palsies
D. Glomerulonephritis
E. Cardiac arrhythmias

28. What other findings may be present on exam?

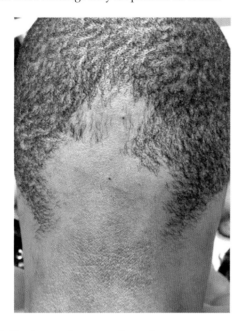

A. Follicular erythema, scale, and scarring alopecia
B. Posterior auricular and occipital lymphadenopathy
C. Scaly pink plaques in the antecubital fossa
D. Obsessive-compulsive behavior

29. A patient presents to your office with these growths found only over the left upper extremity. What are the patient's offspring at risk for?

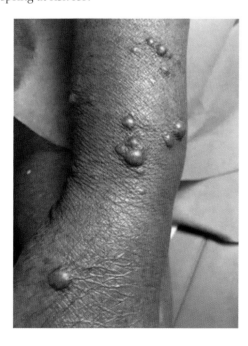

A. Hypertension
B. Kidney stones
C. Gastrointestinal hemorrhage
D. Cardiac rhabdomyoma

30. What is the diagnosis?

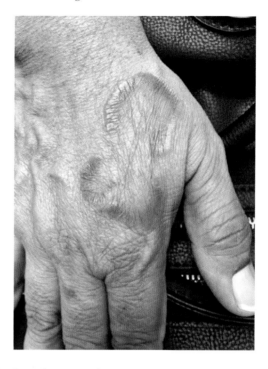

A. Granuloma annulare
B. Subacute cutaneous lupus erythematosus
C. Cutaneous blastomycosis
D. Annular elastolytic giant cell granuloma

31. A patient presents with this pruritic eruption. Which of the following is unlikely to be associated?

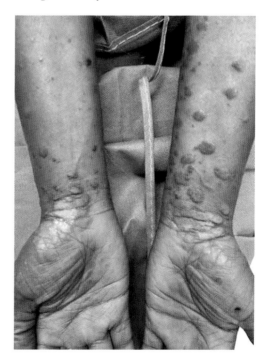

A. Captopril
B. Hepatitis C
C. HIV
D. Diabetes mellitus

32. A patient presents with a 1-year history of these skin findings. She has a history of pelvic surgery 7 years ago. New lesions continue to arise. What is the most common associated finding?

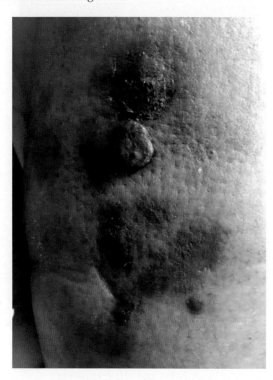

A. Chronic lymphedema
B. Hepatitis C infection
C. Dyspnea
D. HIV infection

33. An 85-year-old woman walks into the office with this skin finding. What is the next best step?

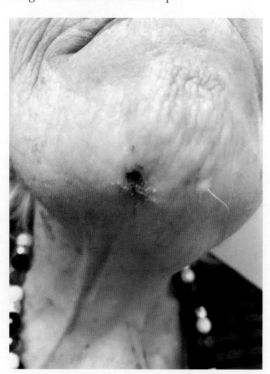

A. Obtain bacterial culture.
B. Perform an oral examination.
C. Perform a skin biopsy.
D. Obtain a viral culture.

34. A 45-year-old obese woman presents with this axillary rash. Which finding is most likely?

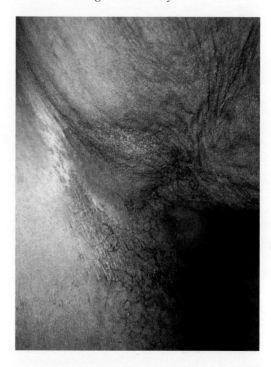

A. Hyphae on KOH examination
B. Coral-red fluorescence on Wood's lamp examination
C. Response to topical steroids
D. Notable pruritus

35. A patient presents with this groin rash for 6 months. What is the most likely diagnosis?

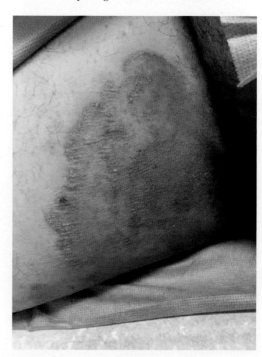

A. Cutaneous candidiasis
B. Lichen simplex chronicus
C. Tinea cruris
D. Psoriasis

A. Central hypothyroidism
B. Tremors
C. Depression
D. Leukopenia

36. A 70-year-old healthy man presents with the following vesicular eruption. He endorses burning pain is the same distribution. What complication may be associated with this condition?

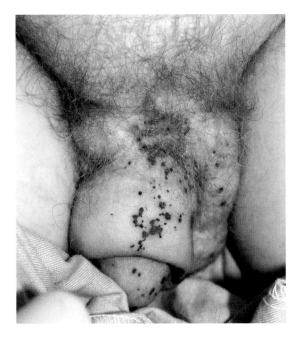

A. Diarrhea
B. Peripheral neuropathy
C. Urinary retention
D. Tethered cord
E. Ipsilateral excessive limb growth

37. This patient was placed on bexarotene 150 mg daily for generalized patch/plaque (stage 1B) cutaneous T-cell lymphoma. The patient developed hypertriglyceridemia while on this medication. What is another common side effect?

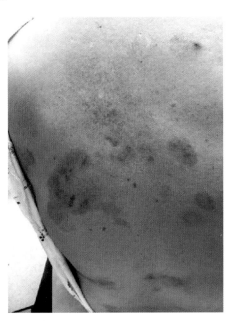

38. A 53-year-old woman presents to your clinic with a 3-month history of asymptomatic papules and plaques as seen below. An HIV test is negative. Which laboratory test is NOT indicated?

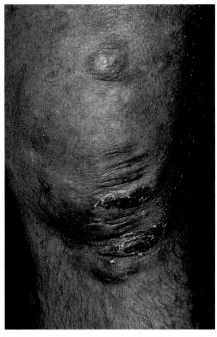

With permission from James W, et al. (eds.), in *Andrews' Disease of the Skin*, 4th edition, 2016, Elsevier, 807–855 (fig. 35-22).

A. Lipid panel
B. RPR
C. Serum immunofixation electrophoresis
D. Hepatitis panel
E. QuantiFERON-TB gold

39. What is the most common associated genetic mutation found in this lesion?

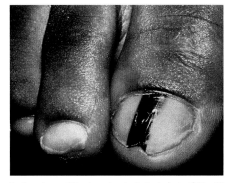

With permission from Dinulos J, et al. (eds.), in *Skin Disease: Diagnosis and Treatment*, 4th edition, 2018, Elsevier, 495–530 (fig. 18-37C).

A. c-KIT
B. NRAS
C. GNAQ
D. BRAF

40. A 48-year-old man with HIV presents with this skin eruption. He was recently started on antiviral therapy. What is the most likely culprit medication?

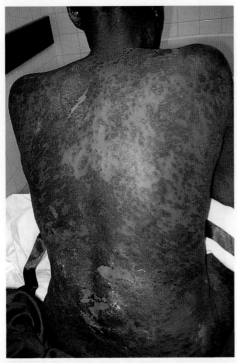

With permission from Introcaso CE, et al., *Journal of the American Academy of Dermatology*, 2010, Elsevier, 563–569 (fig. 3).

A. Abacavir
B. Zidovudine
C. Lamivudine
D. Nevirapine

PEDIATRIC DERMATOLOGY

41. A concerned mother brings her 8-year-old son to your office for evaluation of a new, pruritic eruption on his ears and dorsal hands. He spent the past weekend pitching for his baseball team. He otherwise feels well and has no dermatologic or medical history. What is the most appropriate next step in management of this patient?

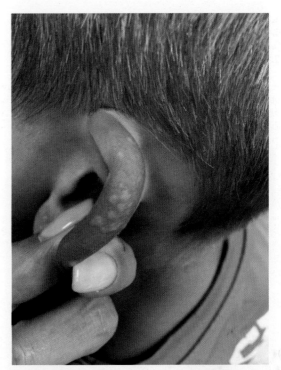

Photo courtesy Anna Guanche, MD, Calabasas, California.

A. Recommend patch testing.
B. Thoroughly review the medication list.
C. Recommend sun avoidance and continued use of sunscreen.
D. Recommend a biopsy for Hematoxylin and eosin and immunofluorescence.

42. You are called to the NICU to evaluate a newborn girl with the following facial lesion. What is the most likely associated finding given this clinical presentation?

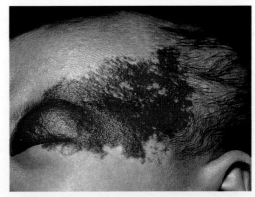

With permission from Haggstrom AN and Garzon MC, Infantile hemangiomas, in Bolognia J, et al. (eds), *Dermatology*, 4th edition, 2018, Elsevier, 1786–1804 (fig. 103.2).

A. Posterior fossa anomalies
B. Intracranial capillary malformations
C. Glaucoma
D. Atrial septal defect
E. No associated abnormalities

43. A distraught mother brings her 4-year-old son to your office for evaluation. Examination is shown below. Which of the following is the next best step in the workup of this patient?

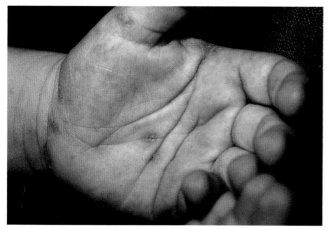

With permission from Paller AS and Mancini AJ (eds.), Infestations, bites, and stings, in *Hurwitz Clinical Pediatric Dermatology*, 5th edition, 2016, Elsevier, 428–447 (fig. 18-2).

A. Wright stain
B. Mineral oil preparation
C. Gram stain
D. KOH preparation
E. Skin biopsy

44. You are called to evaluate a healthy 3-day-old boy with a new rash as shown below. He was born via normal spontaneous vaginal delivery at term, and there were no complications. His mother is healthy with no skin findings. During examination, you appropriately sample the contents of a few of the lesions. Microscopy is most likely to show which of the following?

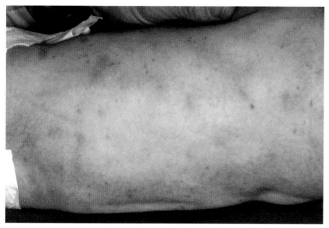

With permission from Paller AS and Mancini AJ (eds.), Cutaneous disorders of the newborn, in *Hurwitz Clinical Pediatric Dermatology*, 5th edition, 2016, Elsevier, 11–37 (fig. 2-13)

A. Mites, eggs, and scybala
B. Sterile contents with numerous eosinophils
C. Sterile contents with numerous neutrophils
D. Gram-positive cocci in clusters
E. Pseudohyphae and yeast forms
F. Multinucleated giant cells

45. The parents of this 4-year-old girl are concerned that her hair is thin and unruly. Upon further history you learn that she has never gotten a haircut. Microscopic examination of hair shafts is most likely to show which of the following?

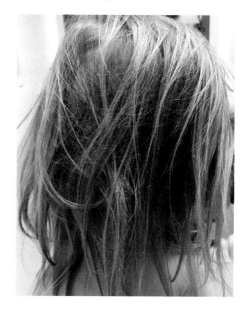

A. Alternating light and dark bands under polarized light
B. Irregularly spaced bubbles within the hair shaft
C. Ruffled proximal cuticle
D. Breakage points with ball-and-socket appearance
E. No abnormalities

46. A teenage girl is brought to your office by her parents for widespread "freckling." Her parents note lesions on her face, trunk, and extremities. Her history is notable for a congenital heart defect. Clinical photograph is shown below, and there is relative sparing of the mucosal surfaces. The remainder of her examination is most likely to reveal which of the following?

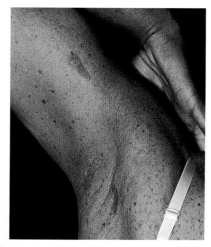

With permission from Paller AS and Mancini AJ (eds.), Disorders of pigmentation, in *Hurwitz Clinical Pediatric Dermatology*, 5th edition, 2016, Elsevier, 245–278 (fig. 11-42).

A. Cutaneous neurofibromas
B. Ocular hypertelorism
C. Nail dystrophy
D. Longitudinal melanonychia

47. For which of the following ichthyoses is a skin biopsy always diagnostic?
A. Lamellar ichthyosis
B. Epidermolytic ichthyosis
C. X-linked ichthyosis
D. Netherton syndrome
E. Sjögren–Larsson syndrome

48. A 14-year-old girl is brought in for evaluation of red spots on her lips and tongue as shown. A review of systems is notable for frequent nosebleeds. Which of the following is the most likely association with this condition?

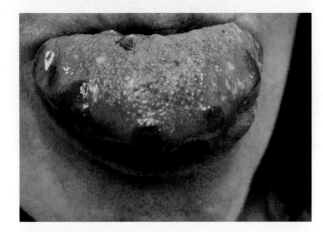

A. No associated abnormalities
B. Truncal ataxia
C. Pulmonary arteriovenous malformations
D. Noninfectious granulomas
E. Increased risk of hematologic malignancy

49. A teenager is brought in by his parents for progressive nail changes, as shown below. Genetic testing confirms the diagnosis and reveals a mutation in KRT6A. What additional findings are most likely to be seen on examination?

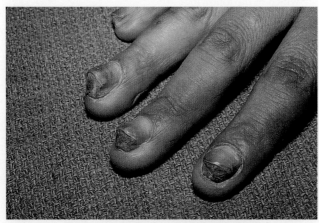

With permission from James WD, Berger TG, and Elston DM (eds.), Genodermatoses and congenital anomalies, in *Andrews' Diseases of the Skin*, 12th edition, 2016, Elsevier, 542–578 (fig. 27-34)

A. Hypohidrosis
B. Natal teeth
C. Steatocystomas
D. Benign oral leukoplakia
E. Premalignant oral leukoplakia

50. The patient below has an abnormal liver ultrasound. The next most appropriate diagnostic test is:

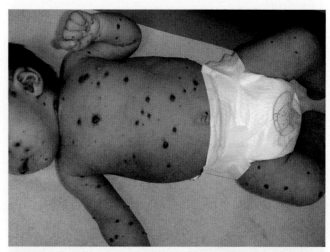

With permission from James W, et al. (eds.), *Andrews' Disease of the Skin Clinical Atlas*, 2018, Elsevier, 405–435 (fig. 28.57).

A. Laryngoscopy
B. Magnetic resonance imaging/Magnetic resonance angiogram of the head and neck
C. Thyroid function tests
D. Platelets, Pothrombin Time/International Normalized Ratio, Partial Thromboplastin Time

DERMATOPATHOLOGY

51. A 30-year-old healthy male presents with pruritic lesions on the elbows. Based on the physical examination, two biopsies, one for H&E and one for Direct immunofluorescence, are collected. What are the most likely patterns to be seen on the biopsies?

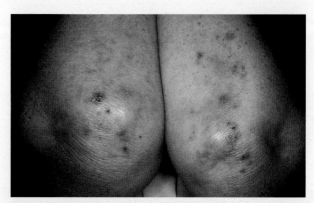

With permission from Karpati, S, *Clinics in Dermatology*, 2012, 30:56–69 (fig. 1, p. 57).

A. Neutrophils and eosinophils in the dermal papillae with linear Immunoglobulin IgA along the basement membrane zone
B. Eosinophils in the dermal papillae with linear IgA along the BMZ
C. Neutrophils in the dermal papillae with linear IgA along the BMZ
D. Eosinophils in the dermal papillae with granular IgA in the dermal papillae
E. Neutrophils in the dermal papillae with granular IgA in the dermal papillae

52. What is the best diagnosis?

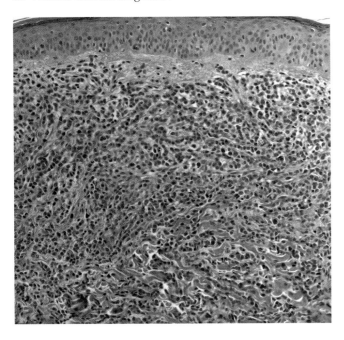

A. Dermatofibroma
B. Interstitial granuloma annulare
C. Interstitial granulomatous dermatitis
D. Leukemia cutis

53. What is the best diagnosis for this oral lesion?

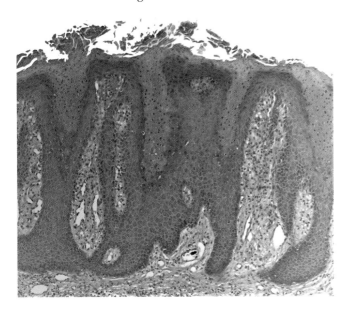

A. Bowenoid papulosis
B. Psoriasis
C. Verruca vulgaris
D. Verruciform xanthoma

54. Which drug might be associated with this condition?

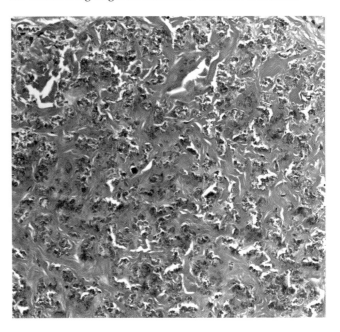

A. Anticonvulsants
B. Nonsteroidal antiinflammatory drugs
C. Penicillamine
D. Sulfonamides

55. Which of the following is the most likely causative organism for this lesion?

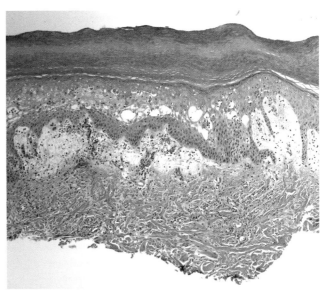

A. Coxsackievirus
B. Epstein-Barr virus
C. Herpes simplex virus
D. Polyoma virus

56. What is the best diagnosis?

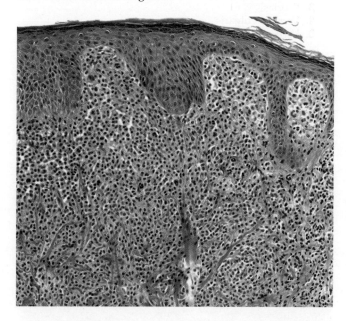

A. Glomus tumor
B. Langerhan cell histiocytosis
C. Mastocytosis
D. Spitz nevus

57. What is the best diagnosis?

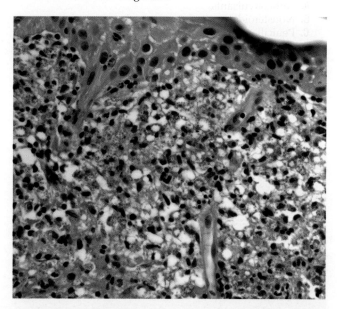

A. Blastomycosis
B. Chromoblastomycosis
C. Cryptococcosis
D. Leishmaniasis

58. What is the best diagnosis for this lesion in a neonate?

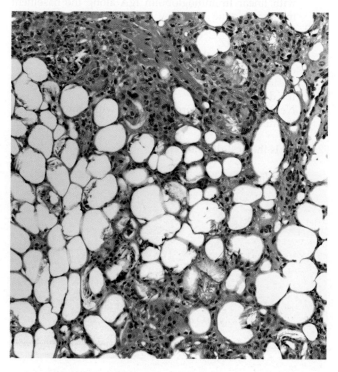

A. Erythema nodosum
B. Pancreatic panniculitis
C. Sclerema neonatorum
D. Subcutaneous fat necrosis of the newborn

59. What is the most common location for this lesion?

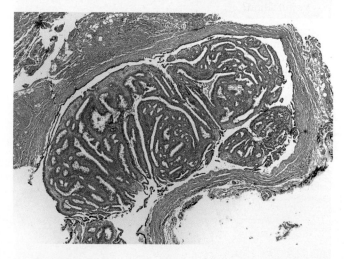

A. Oral mucosa
B. Scalp
C. Trunk
D. Vulva

60. What is the best diagnosis for this plantar lesion?

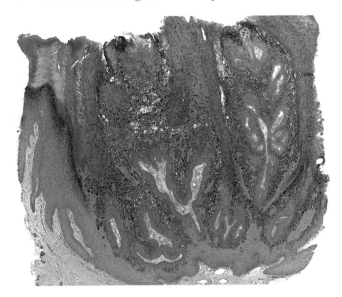

A. Myrmecia
B. Pitted keratolysis
C. Psoriasis
D. Verrucous carcinoma

PROCEDURAL DERMATOLOGY

61. A patient presents with drooping of her upper eyelid after having botulinum toxin injections performed by another practitioner. What is the best treatment for this complication?
A. Botulinum toxin injected into the frontalis muscle
B. Iopidine drops into the affected eye
C. Iopidine drops into the contralateral eye
D. No treatment
E. An alpha-adrenergic antagonist

62. Which medication below can potentially diminish the effect of neuromodulators?
A. Cyclosporine
B. Tobramycin
C. Verapamil
D. Donepezil
E. Lisinopril

63. A 72-year-old man presented with a 2.5-centimeter cutaneous squamous cell carcinoma of the left mandibular cheek. The cancer was treated with excisional surgery, revealing infiltration of the parotid gland. Adjuvant radiation treatment was then performed, with the treatment field including the left cheek, parotid, and neck. One year later, CT scan identified the mass shown, and fine-needle biopsy revealed keratinizing carcinoma. Which of the following medications has shown the greatest efficacy in treatment of this condition in investigational studies?

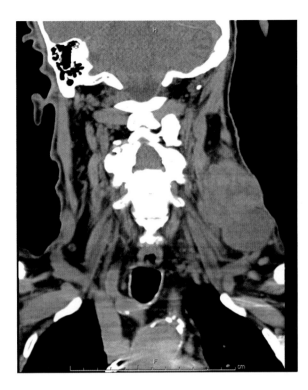

A. Ipilimumab
B. Carboplatin
C. Cetuximab
D. Cemiplimab
E. Bevacizumab

64. A 68-year-old man presents with an asymptomatic 1.4-cm nodule on the scalp that has been increasing in size over 2 months. The patient has a history of two prior basal cell carcinomas and one squamous cell carcinoma on other cutaneous sites of the head and neck. Biopsy of the lesion reveals a dense proliferation of small blue cells with minimal cytoplasm and numerous mitoses. Immunohistochemical staining is negative for S100 and shows punctate perinuclear staining with CK20. What is the best initial management for this lesion?

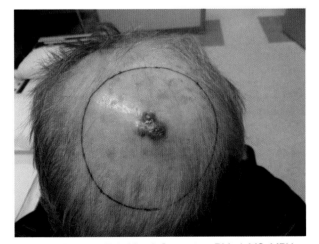

With permission from Dakshika A Gunaratne, BMed, MS, MPH, Definitive radiotherapy for Merkel cell carcinoma confers clinically meaningful in-field locoregional control: A review and analysis of the literature, *Journal of the American Academy of Dermatology*, 77(1):142–148.e1 (© 2017 American Academy of Dermatology, Inc.).

A. Conservative local excision
B. Wide local excision alone
C. Wide local excision plus sentinel node biopsy or nodal imaging, followed by adjuvant radiation therapy
D. Intralesional corticosteroid therapy
E. Systemic immunomodulatory therapy

65. A patient presents to your office complaining of blurry vision 1 day after receiving laser diode 800-nm therapy for photo-epilation of eyebrow hair. During the procedure she had complained of pain above and behind the eye. A photo of the gross eye exam is shown below, demonstrating distortion of the pupil. What type of eye injury is she most at risk for?

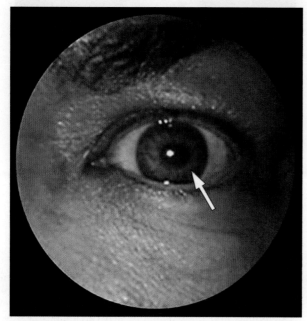

With permission from Mikis K, Whittington A, and Alam M, in *Journal of the American Academy of Dermatology*, 2016, Elsevier, 265–284 (fig. 4).

A. Cataract formation and iris atrophy
B. Ptosis
C. Vitreous floaters
D. Corneal burn

66. A patient presents for treatment of a large squamous cell carcinoma on the lip. He weighs 50 kg. The area is anesthetized with 1% lidocaine with epinephrine. Adequate anesthesia is difficult to obtain, and over 35 mL are injected into the area. The patient begins to vomit and complains of blurry vision and tinnitus. Management for this patient includes:
A. Oxygen supplementation
B. Emergency medical services activation
C. Diazepam
D. Airway maintenance
E. A–C
F. A–D

67. A patient with a basal cell carcinoma on the lower eyelid undergoes Mohs surgery, and tumor-free margins are obtained after two stages. Repair of the defect is performed with a full thickness skin graft. Which of the following statements are true regarding the design of this repair?
A. Graft survival is low in this location.
B. Graft should be designed as the same size of the defect.

C. If the defect involved the tarsus then a graft should be avoided.
D. The graft should be at least 25% larger than the defect.

68. Which of the patients listed below does NOT require antibiotic prophylaxis prior to dermatologic surgery for a squamous cell carcinoma in the pretibial region?
A. 78-year-old male with history of infective endocarditis
B. 65-year-old female with total knee replacement performed 1 year ago
C. 83-year-old male with bovine aortic valve
D. 67-year-old female immunosuppressed secondary to history of cardiac transplant

69. Which of the following lesions is NOT appropriate for treatment with Mohs micrographic surgery?
A. A 5-mm nodular basal cell carcinoma on the neck of an immunocompetent host
B. A 2.5-cm recurrent superficial basal cell carcinoma on the back of a healthy male
C. A 1.2-cm keratoacanthoma-type SCC on the lower leg of an elderly female
D. A 1.5-cm squamous cell carcinoma in situ on the trunk of an immunocompromised host
E. A 6-mm desmoplastic trichoepithelioma on the cheek of a healthy 30-year-old female

70. A patient presents for follow-up after treatment with medium-depth chemical peel. Which of the following complications puts the patient at greatest risk for scarring?
A. Persistent erythema
B. Pain
C. Impetiginization
D. Hypopigmentation

BASIC SCIENCE

71. Which of the following active sunscreen ingredients has the broadest spectrum?
A. Oxybenzone
B. Zinc oxide
C. Avobenzone
D. PABA

72. Autoantibodies to which of the following may be found in the pictured condition?

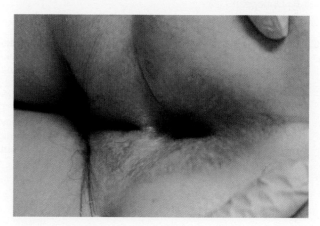

A. Desmoglein 3
B. Collagen VII

C. Extracellular matrix protein 1
D. Bullous pemphigoid antigen 2
E. Desmoplakin

73. Why do patients with anti-desmoglein 1 antibodies NOT have oral ulcerations as part of their clinical presentation?
    A. Not enough of the antibody is present to affect the mucosa.
    B. The mucosa is immunologically protected.
    C. Desmoglein 1 is not expressed in the mucosa.
    D. Compensation of desmoglein 3 in the mucosa.

74. A 12-year-old girl presents for evaluation a rash that began in early infancy—with sharply demarcated pink scaly patches involving the cheeks, chin, and ears, and a psoriasiform eruption on the trunk and extremities. She has tried numerous therapies in the past with only minimal improvement, including topical steroids, isotretinoin, and methotrexate. Genetic testing reveals a heterozygous mutation in CARD14. What is the target of the biologic medication that is most likely to be effective for this patient?
    A. Tumor necrosis factor-alpha
    B. Interleukin-23
    C. IL-17
    D. Interleukin-13
    E. IL-33

75. Rituximab's mechanism of action is:
    A. Depletion of plasma cells
    B. Depletion of CD20+ B cells
    C. Depletion of stem cells
    D. Binding of antibodies and marking them for apoptosis

76. A patient with a history of chronic sun exposure presents with the lesion shown. Biopsy shows aggregates of basaloid cells. Which cancer-associated gene is most commonly mutated?

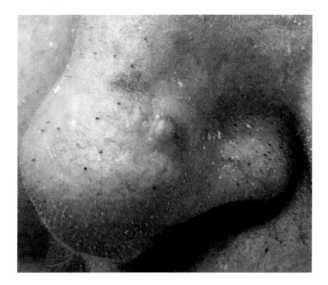

   A. BRAF
   B. GNAQ
   C. TP53
   D. PTCH1
   E. c-KIT

77. The patient presents with a blistering rash on the torso. H&E demonstrates acantholysis and DIF is positive for intercellular IgG and C3 deposition. What is the function of the protein targeted by autoantibodies in this disease?

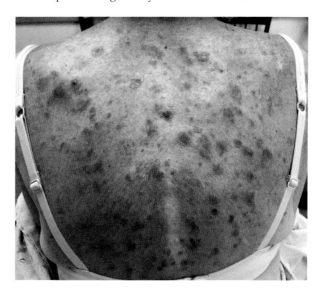

   A. Selective barrier between the epidermis and dermis
   B. Calcium-dependent cell-cell adhesion molecules
   C. Transmembrane channels functioning in cell-cell communication
   D. Formation of ceramides for corneocytes

78. A patient on a BRAF inhibitor presents with phototoxic eruption on the dorsal hands. He reported wearing sun-protective clothing and a hat, but his hands were exposed to the sun during prolonged driving. What is the primary mechanism of this UV-related phototoxicity?
    A. Oxidative damage
    B. Cyclobutane-pyrimidine dimers
    C. Nucleotide excision repair
    D. P53 mutations

79. The patient presents with inflammatory pustules on the face and reports intermittent flares after heavy drinking of alcohol, spicy food, or exposure to sun. Which of the following does NOT contribute to the pathogenesis of this condition?
    A. Gram-positive, nonmotile rods found within the sebaceous follicle
    B. Induction of angiogenesis by UV radiation
    C. Upregulation of cathelicidin
    D. Increased levels of Demodex mites

80. A patient with a history of melanoma presents with pigmented nodules adjacent to the prior melanoma site, consistent histopathologically with in-transit metastases. CT/PET imaging demonstrates no visceral involvement. This patient is not a candidate for systemic therapy because of poorly controlled inflammatory bowel disease and declines surgical treatment. Which of the following injectable agents is an oncolytic virus that is Food and Drug Administration (FDA)–approved for inoperable disease?
    A. Talimogene laherparepvec (T-VEC)
    B. Interleukin-2
    C. Granulocyte-macrophage colony-stimulating factor
    D. Rose bengal

GENERAL DERMATOLOGY

1. A. Furosemide
Bullous pemphigoid is an immunobullous eruption that has a predilection for elderly patients. It classically presents with pruritic urticarial plaques with tense vesicles or bullae. Several drugs have been implicated in drug-induced bullous pemphigoid, with furosemide being a common culprit. Other culprits include nonsteroidal antiinflammatory drugs, dipeptidyl peptidase-4 (DPP-4) inhibitors, spironolactone, anti-program cell death-1/ anti-program death-ligand 1 and antibiotics. Drug-induced bullous pemphigoid should be considered in younger patients. The workup is the same as for idiopathic bullous pemphigoid, including biopsy for hematoxylin and eosin and direct immunofluorescence and titers for BP180, BP230, on enzyme-linked immunosorbent assay.
Valacyclovir is an antiherpetic agent that does not typically cause an immunobullous drug eruption but may be used to treat erythema multiforme associated with herpes simplex virus.
Doxycycline may cause a phototoxic eruption and has been used as a conservative treatment for bullous pemphigoid in conjunction with niacinamide. Other side effects include esophagitis, headaches, nausea and abdominal pain, and pseudotumor cerebri.
Cetuximab is an epidermal growth factor receptor (EGFR) inhibitor that causes a variety of dermatologic toxicities, including papulopustular eruption, paronychia, phototoxicity, and other hair/nail changes.
Bolognia J, Schaffer J, Cerroni L, eds. *Dermatology.* [Philadelphia]: Elsevier, 2018 (ch. 30).

2. B. Hepatitis C antibody
Lichen planus is a papulosquamous eruption consisting of pruritic, flat-topped violaceous papules with scale that typically manifests on the extremities. Mucosal involvement may occur in the mouth, genitalia, eyes, and esophagus. The classic presentation of oral lichen planus is lacy-white Wickham striae on the buccal mucosa, but an ulcerative form may present with painful ulcers and erosions on the labial mucosa, gingiva, tongue, and buccal mucosa.
There is a correlation between oral lichen planus and hepatitis C viral infection.
Mycoplasma infection is a reported trigger for erythema multiforme and more specifically can cause mycoplasma-induced rash and mucositis (MIRM), with ulcers and erosions on the lips that may have overlying crust. The sclera may be injected, and cutaneous lesions of erythema multiforme may be present elsewhere (palms/soles/trunk).
Syphilis can cause a myriad of oral manifestations, including a chancre (painless ulcer), condyloma lata, and split papules at the angular commissures.
Fungal culture would be used to evaluate for candida stomatitis and thrush.
Human immunodeficiency virus is less likely to be associated with erosive lichen planus. Mucosal findings in acute HIV include aphthous ulcers.
Bolognia J, Schaffer J, Cerroni L, eds. *Dermatology.* [Philadelphia]: Elsevier, 2018 (ch. 11).

3. A. Griseofulvin 20–25 mg/kg/day
Oral antifungal medications (A) are required for the treatment of kerion, a severe pustular form of tinea capitis. Causative pathogens include *M. canis*, *T. verrucosum*, *T. mentagrophytes*, and *T. tonsurans*. Kerions present with painful, inflammatory boggy plaques often associated with alopecia and regional lymphadenopathy. Treatment is with oral antifungals, and oral prednisone may be added for severe inflammatory reactions.

Doxycycline (B) can be used in the treatment of dissecting cellulitis of the scalp, a type of scarring alopecia part of the follicular occlusion tetrad (acne conglobata, hidradenitis suppurativa, dissecting cellulitis, and pilonidal sinus). African American males between the ages of 20 and 40 are most often affected, although it can also occur in other races, women, and children on occasion. Patients present with multiple, interconnected, boggy nodules on the scalp that may have purulent drainage. Other treatment options include oral isotretinoin, clindamycin/rifampin, and intralesional triamcinolone. Intralesional triamcinolone injections (C) can be used in the treatment of acne keloidalis nuchae or other cicatricial alopecias. Ketoconazole shampoo (D) can be used to supplement tinea capitis treatment, but oral antifungals are required for inflammatory lesions that affect the hair follicles. It is commonly used to treat seborrheic dermatitis.
Bolognia J, Schaffer J, Cerroni L, eds. *Dermatology.* [Philadelphia]: Elsevier, 2018 (ch. 77).

4. C. Hair dye
Paraphenylenediamine (PPD) is an allergen found in temporary tattoos as well as hair dyes. There may be cross-reactivity with para-aminobenzoic acid, sulfonamides, ester anesthetics, and azo dyes.
Mango and poison ivy contain urushiol which does not cross-react with PPD.
Tosylamide sulfonamide formaldehyde resin is an allergen commonly associated with nail polish.
Bolognia J, Schaffer J, Cerroni L, eds. *Dermatology.* [Philadelphia]: Elsevier, 2018 (ch. 14).

5. D. Clavicular bone lesions
Acne fulminans is a severe eruptive form of acne associated with fevers, joint pains, hepatomegaly, malaise, myalgias, and arthralgias that most commonly occur in teenage males. The initial lesions are comedones that become rapidly inflamed and evolve into tender cysts that coalesce into painful plaques, which can lead to scarring. There may be osteolytic bone lesions, with the clavicle and sternum being the most common sites. Treatment is with prednisone and low-dose isotretinoin. Dapsone or other immunosuppressants (tumor necrosis factor-alpha inhibitors) may be necessary. Isotretinoin may trigger acne fulminans during the first few weeks of treatment.
Headaches are not commonly associated with acne fulminans. The follicular occlusion triad consists of acne conglobata, dissecting cellulitis of the scalp, hidradenitis suppurativa, and pilonidal cysts. Acne conglobata is eruptive nodulocystic acne without systemic symptoms.
Bolognia J, Schaffer J, Cerroni L, eds. *Dermatology.* [Philadelphia]: Elsevier, 2018 (ch. 36).

6. A. Rheumatoid arthritis
Pyoderma gangrenosum is a neutrophilic dermatosis that begins as a pustule, which then evolves into an ulcer with rolled undermined borders and central cribriform scarring. One-half to one-third of patients have a systemic disease, and common associations include inflammatory bowel disease; rheumatoid arthritis; and hematologic malignancy, such as leukemia, myelodysplasia, and monoclonal gammopathy (Immunoglobulin A most commonly).
Bolognia J, Schaffer J, Cerroni L, eds. *Dermatology.* [Philadelphia]: Elsevier, 2018 (ch. 21).

7. C. Dyshidrotic eczema
Intravenous immunoglobulin (IVIG) is used in dermatology in the treatment of various inflammatory conditions,

including immunobullous disease, toxic epidermal necrolysis, and neutrophilic dermatoses. Adverse reactions include anaphylaxis, thromboembolic events, hyperviscosity syndromes, headaches, and pulmonary edema. Dyshidrotic dermatitis is a reported cutaneous effect.

8. **E.** Myiasis
Myiasis is a cutaneous infestation of fly larvae, most commonly *Dermatobia hominis* (human botfly) and *Cordylobia anthropophaga* (tumbu fly). Mode of transmission to the human host varies between fly species. *D. hominis* deposits its eggs on mosquitoes, which then hatch on human skin following a mosquito bite. *C. anthropophaga* deposits its eggs on moist clothing, blankets, and in sand, which then invade skin with contact. Cutaneous lesions are often furuncle-like papules or nodules that may be pruritic, tender, or painful. Some patients report the sensation of movement. On occasion, close examination of the nodule will reveal a distinct central punctum that the larvae use for breathing. Although self-limited in nature, treatment options include surgical excision and ivermectin. Antibiotics may be necessary for secondary bacterial infections.
Lesions of furunculosis are more disseminated (A), while sporotrichoid lesions tend to follow a lymphocutaneous linear configuration (B). Exaggerated arthropod bite reaction would likely improve after a month (C), and an inflamed epidermoid cyst would not develop after a mosquito bite (D).
Bolognia J, Schaffer J, Cerroni L, eds. *Dermatology.* [Philadelphia]: Elsevier, 2018 (ch. 84).

9. **A.** Intravenous amphotericin B
Leishmaniasis is a parasitic infection spread by sandflies, *Phlebotomus* (Old World) and *Lutzomyia* (New World). There are three distinct clinical manifestations of disease that depend on the *Leishmania* species and host immune response:
1. **Cutaneous**: *L. major, L. tropica;* typically a solitary expanding ulcerated or verrucous plaque that is restricted to the skin on exposed sites such as the face, neck, and extremities; may exhibit sporotrichoid spread; often resolves spontaneously within several months and heals with scarring. In rare cases that are often associated with a poor cell-mediated immune response, patients may develop disseminated disease with multiple secondary lesions. These disseminated or diffuse forms of cutaneous leishmaniasis are commonly caused by *L. braziliensis* (in the Americas) or *L. aethiopica* (in Africa).
2. **Mucocutaneous**: *L. (Viannia)* spp, including *L. braziliensis, L. panamensis, L. guyanensis;* often occur concurrently or several years after cutaneous leishmaniasis; affects mucous membranes predominantly on the face, nose, lips, and pharynx, which may lead to nasal septum perforation, oropharyngeal destruction, and airway obstruction if left untreated.
3. **Visceral (kala-azar)**: *L. donovani, L. infantum, L. chagasi* (predominantly Old World) causes a systemic infection of the bone marrow, liver, and spleen with significantly high morbidity and mortality if left untreated. The clinical presentation includes fever, wasting, lymphadenopathy, and hepatosplenomegaly.
Diagnosis can be made by tissue biopsy demonstrating parasitized histiocytes, culture, polymerase chain reaction, or serologic testing. In the United States, the Centers for Disease Control and Prevention (CDC) provides reference diagnostic services for leishmaniasis. Numerous local and systemic treatments have been reported. Indications for systemic treatment include an immunocompromised host; large or multiple lesions; and involvement of face, mucosa, hands, feet, or genitalia. For cutaneous and mucocutaneous

leishmaniasis, treatments of choice include intralesional and parental pentavalent antimony. There is increasing resistance, however, to antimonial medications. Patients who show poor response to antimonials or who have visceral leishmaniasis should be treated with amphotericin B (A). Case reports of topical imiquimod (B) and intralesional antimonial drugs (C) have shown some efficacy in the treatment in nonfacial Old World cutaneous leishmaniasis. These, however, are not the treatment of choice for New World mucocutaneous leishmaniasis. Oral itraconazole (D) is used in the treatment of systemic mycoses, such as blastomycosis, histoplasmosis, and paracoccidioidomycosis. Oral rifampin and dapsone (E) are recommended by the World Health Organization for paucibacillary leprosy. Clofazimine is added to this combined therapy for multibacillary leprosy.
Bolognia J, Schaffer J, Cerroni L, eds. *Dermatology.* [Philadelphia]: Elsevier, 2018 (ch. 83).

10. **A.** Graft-versus-host disease
Large sheets of denuded skin is a dermatologic emergency and requires a thorough workup. Few skin diseases manifest with such desquamation, including toxic epidermal necrolysis/Stevens-Johnson syndrome, acute graft-versus-host disease (GVHD; grade 4, which presents as toxic epidermal necrolysis (TEN)-like clinically), pemphigus vulgaris, bullous pemphigoid, paraneoplastic pemphigus, linear IgA bullous dermatosis, and systemic lupus erythematosus (TEN-like acute cutaneous lupus or acute syndrome of apoptotic pan-epidermolysis [ASAP]). As TEN is not an answer choice, GVHD is the best answer.
Dermatomyositis does not classically present with epidermal necrolysis (extremely rare TEN-like manifestations may occur). Staphylococcal scalded skin syndrome (SSSS) is also in the differential diagnosis of denuded skin, but the blistering is typically accentuated in intertriginous skin, with other classic findings including perioral furrowing and crusting, and intertriginous erythema and pain, with a primary site of staphylococcal infection.
Bolognia J, Schaffer J, Cerroni L, eds. *Dermatology.* [Philadelphia]: Elsevier, 2018 (ch. 52).

11. **C.** Discoid lupus erythematosus
Patients with any form of cutaneous lupus have the potential to develop systemic lupus erythematosus (SLE). Acute cutaneous lupus erythematosus and bullous lupus (antibodies to collagen VII may be present) are strongly associated with systemic disease. Subacute cutaneous lupus erythematosus (antibodies to Sjögren's-syndrome-related antigen A/Ro are present in a majority) is more strongly associated with SLE than discoid lupus erythematosus, for which 5%–15% of patients may develop systemic disease. In general, those with more widespread lesions of discoid lupus erythematosus have a greater risk of developing SLE.
Bolognia J, Schaffer J, Cerroni L, eds. *Dermatology.* [Philadelphia]: Elsevier, 2018 (ch. 41).

12. **B.** Azelaic acid
Azelaic acid is safe to use in pregnancy for acne vulgaris. The other listed medications should be avoided and are teratogenic.
Bolognia J, Schaffer J, Cerroni L, eds. *Dermatology.* [Philadelphia]: Elsevier, 2018 (ch. 36).

13. **B.** Amoxicillin
The clinical picture is that of erythema chronicum migrans due to Lyme disease. First-line treatment in children (<8 years of age) is amoxicillin for 14–21 days. In adults and children older than 8 years of age, first-line treatment is doxycycline for 14–21 days.

Bolognia J, Schaffer J, Cerroni L, eds. *Dermatology*. [Philadelphia]: Elsevier, 2018 (ch. 74).

14. **C.** Atypical hand-foot-mouth disease
Hand-foot-mouth disease (HFMD) is an eruption caused by Coxsackie enterovirus, a single-stranded RNA virus. HFMD manifests as oval papulovesicles on the palms and soles, and erosions and ulcers in the oral mucosa. Coxsackie virus A16 is the most common cause of HFMD, while the A6 strain may cause atypical Coxsackie infections, which may manifest with widespread cutaneous lesions and accentuation in areas of existing dermatitis (eczema coxsackium). Coxsackie viral infection also causes herpangina, which manifests as erosions and ulcerations on the posterior pharynx. A clinical clue to HFMD are that papulovesicles often follow dermatoglyphics.
Secondary syphilis classically presents with copper penny-like lesions on the palms and soles. The lesions usually have scale and there may be papulosquamous oval-shaped papules and plaques on the trunk. Erythema multiforme may also manifest with an acral and oral eruption but typically with targetoid cutaneous lesions. Acrodermatitis enteropathica is the cutaneous manifestation of zinc deficiency and usually manifests with periorificial, intertriginous, and acral dermatitis. Repletion of zinc leads to resolution of the eruption.
Bolognia J, Schaffer J, Cerroni L, eds. *Dermatology*. [Philadelphia]: Elsevier, 2018 (ch. 81).

15. **C.** No associated risk
The figure illustrates polymorphic eruption of pregnancy (PUPPP) with erythematous papules and plaques within striae. PUPPP may be associated with twin gestation, primigravidas, maternal obesity, and third trimester pregnancy. Patients may be reassured that there is no associated maternal or fetal risk.
Bolognia J, Schaffer J, Cerroni L, eds. *Dermatology*. [Philadelphia]: Elsevier, 2018 (ch. 27).

16. **B.** Epidermal growth factor receptor inhibitor
Epidermal growth factor receptor (EGFR) inhibitors cause a variety of cutaneous adverse reactions, including paronychia, papulopustular (acneiform) eruption, photosensitivity, skin fragility, and hair changes, in addition to periungual pyogenic granulomas (seen here).
Program cell death-1 inhibitors are associated with maculopapular eruptions, pruritus, lichenoid reactions, eczema, Stevens-Johnson syndrome, bullous disorders, and vitiligo. BRAF inhibitors are associated with maculopapular eruptions, photosensitivity, seborrheic dermatitis-like eruptions, keratosis pilaris-like eruptions, and squamoproliferative growths. TNF inhibitors may be associated with injection site reactions and paradoxical psoriasiform eruptions.
Bolognia J, Schaffer J, Cerroni L, eds. *Dermatology*. [Philadelphia]: Elsevier, 2018 (ch. 21).

17. **B.** Hilar lymphadenopathy
Sarcoidosis is a multisystem granulomatous disease that commonly involves the skin in up to one-third of patients. Cutaneous lesions often present as red-brown papules and plaques that favor the face, lips, neck, upper trunk, and extremities. A classic finding is involvement of tattoo sites or areas of trauma. Subcutaneous lesions, hypopigmentation, ulceration, acquired ichthyosis, and alopecia are other findings, while erythema nodosum is a nonspecific cutaneous manifestation. Pulmonary involvement is the most common form of systemic disease, classically

manifesting with hilar lymphadenopathy. Granulomatous inflammation may also develop in the liver, kidney, GI tract, heart, lymph nodes, eyes, endocrine glands, and reproductive organs.
Bolognia J, Schaffer J, Cerroni L, eds. *Dermatology*. [Philadelphia]: Elsevier, 2018 (ch. 93).

18. **C.** Scleroderma-70 (SCL-70)
Systemic sclerosis is an autoimmune connective tissue disease that is characterized by symmetric hardening of the skin of the fingers, hands, and face that may generalize. Raynaud phenomenon is common, and digital ulcers may develop. Other features include edema of the hands in the acute phase, mat telangiectasias, and leukoderma with retention of perifollicular pigmentation. Antibodies against SCL-70 or topoisomerase are associated with systemic sclerosis. Antinuclear antibody is less specific and may be found in other autoimmune diseases, including lupus, dermatomyositis, and scleroderma. Anti-Jo-1 antibodies are typically associated with dermatomyositis, and antibodies against thyroid peroxidase are associated with autoimmune thyroid disease such as Hashimoto thyroiditis.
Bolognia J, Schaffer J, Cerroni L, eds. *Dermatology*. [Philadelphia]: Elsevier, 2018 (ch. 43).

19. **A.** FLCN
The figure illustrates fibrofolliculomas as seen in Birt-Hogg-Dube syndrome. The syndrome features autosomal dominant inheritance, multiple fibrofolliculomas, trichodiscomas, lipomas, oral fibromas, renal cell carcinoma, medullary thyroid carcinoma, and colon cancer. Patients are at risk for pulmonary cysts and spontaneous pneumothoraces. The associated mutation is FLCN (folliculin gene). The other mutations are found in familial cylindromatosis (CYLD), Muir-Torre (MSH2), Cowden/PTEN hamartoma syndrome, and Bannayan-Riley-Ruvalcaba syndrome (PTEN).
Bolognia J, Schaffer J, Cerroni L, eds. *Dermatology*. [Philadelphia]: Elsevier, 2018 (ch. 53).

20. **C.** The treatment of choice for penicillin-allergic patients is sulfamethoxazole/trimethoprim.
The Kodachrome illustrates secondary syphilis, with papulosquamous lesions that may appear similar to pityriasis rosea. Lesions may vary in color from pink to violaceous to red-brown, and mucosa involvement may occur (may resemble aphthous ulcers or condylomata lata in the anogenital skin). Lymph node enlargement is present in the majority of patients. Additional presentations may include annular or figurate plaques with central hyperpigmentation on the face, nonscarring "moth-eaten" alopecia, split papules at the oral commissures, granulomatous nodules and plaques, and crusted necrotic ulcerative lesions (lues maligna). It is true that early congenital syphilis may present with bullous and erosive lesions (pemphigus syphiliticus). Additional findings include "snuffles" (bloody or purulent mucinous nasal discharge), perioral and perianal fissures, lymphadenopathy, and hepatosplenomegaly, and skeletal involvement (i.e., osteochondritis) may result in pseudoparalysis of Parrot. A variety of cutaneous, dental, skeletal, and ocular findings may occur. Without treatment, lesions of secondary syphilis resolve over several weeks to months (3–12 weeks on average). However, relapse may occur in approximately 20% of cases within 1 year. In a majority of patients, untreated secondary syphilis will resolve spontaneously. About two-thirds will develop latent disease that will not progress to symptomatic tertiary syphilis.

The treatment of choice for syphilis is penicillin G. For those allergic to penicillin, doxycycline, tetracycline, ceftriaxone, or azithromycin are recommended (not sulfamethoxazole/trimethoprim). For pregnant women who are penicillin-allergic, desensitization or treatment with azithromycin or ceftriaxone is recommended. For a neonate born to a mother with treated disease without signs of syphilis and with a negative serum nontreponemal antibody titer less than fourfold the maternal titer, treatment is optional. Alternatively, a single dose of benzathine penicillin, 50,000 U/kg is acceptable.
Bolognia J, Schaffer J, Cerroni L, eds. *Dermatology.* [Philadelphia]: Elsevier, 2018 (ch. 82).

21. **B.** Red-white longitudinal bands and v-shaped distal nicks
Darier disease presents with hyperkeratotic papules in seborrheic areas, acrokeratosis verruciformis of Hopf, palmar keratosis and pits, and nail findings including red-white longitudinal bands and v-shaped distal nicks. Oil spots and onycholysis may occur in psoriasis. Dolichonychia may occur in Ehlers-Danlos and Marfan syndrome, and trachyonychia may occur in lichen planus.
Bolognia J, Schaffer J, Cerroni L, eds. *Dermatology.* [Philadelphia]: Elsevier, 2018 (ch. 59).

22. **E.** Tomatoes
Balsam of Peru, or *Myroxylon pereirae*, is obtained from the bark of a Central American tree. It is added to topical formulations for its pleasant smell and antimicrobial effects. Some patients with severe Balsam of Peru allergy benefit from dietary restriction of citrus fruit, tomatoes, cinnamon, cloves, vanilla, curry, nutmeg, allspice, anise, ginger, colas, wine, beer, gin, and vermouth. Cashews and mangos may cause a systemic contact dermatitis in those allergic to urushiol (i.e., poison ivy). Kiwi can cause a protein contact dermatitis, as well as oral allergy syndrome, with itching of the oral cavity as well as edema of the lips, tongue, and palate. Propolis allergy can cause allergic contact dermatitis of the lips, as it is found in natural lip balms.
Bolognia J, Schaffer J, Cerroni L, eds. *Dermatology.* [Philadelphia]: Elsevier, 2018 (ch. 14).

23. **D.** Tryptase
The figure illustrates lesions of urticaria pigmentosa, which stain positively for tryptase or c-KIT as well as Giemsa, Leder, or toluidine blue. Patients typically present with red-brown macules or slightly raised papules, which may demonstrate a positive Darier sign (urtication with rubbing). HHV-8 is positive in Kaposi sarcoma; Periodic acid–Schiff is positive in a variety of conditions and is helpful in visualizing dermatophytes in the epidermis; and S100 is found in a variety of conditions, including melanoma.
Bolognia J, Schaffer J, Cerroni L, eds. *Dermatology.* [Philadelphia]: Elsevier, 2018 (ch. 118).

24. **C.** Rosai-Dorfman disease
Rosai-Dorfman disease is an uncommon histiocytic proliferative disorder that may present with massive painless bilateral cervical lymphadenopathy, a polyclonal hypergammaglobulinemia, elevated erythrocyte sedimentation rate neutrophilia, and anemia. Approximately 10% of patients with systemic disease have cutaneous findings. However, patients may have isolated skin findings. Cutaneous lesions have a dense dermal infiltrate of histiocytes with large vesicular nuclei; small nucleoli, and abundant foamy, eosinophilic cytoplasm with feathery borders. Emperipolesis is a consistent finding. Many lesions are asymptomatic and heal spontaneously. When treatment is indicated, surgical excision, radiotherapy, systemic corticosteroids, alkylating agents, and thalidomide have been used with some success.
Although sarcoidosis may present with cutaneous nodules, a biopsy would reveal dermal "naked" granulomas. Juvenile xanthogranuloma is the most common histiocytosis, which usually presents in infants and young children with lesions on the head, neck, and upper body. The classic histologic finding is a Touton giant cell. A foreign body reaction should not cause large, bilateral, cervical lymphadenopathy. Reticulohistiocytosis can present as papules and nodules that favor the head, hands, and elbows. On biopsy, the histiocytes have a characteristic "ground glass" appearance.
Bolognia J, Schaffer J, Cerroni L, eds. *Dermatology.* [Philadelphia]: Elsevier, 2018 (ch. 91).

25. **E.** Frontal fibrosing alopecia
Frontal fibrosing alopecia (FFA) is a form of cicatricial alopecia characterized by progressive hair loss along the frontal hair line, as well as loss of the eyebrows. The histopathologic features are similar to lichen planopilaris. Thinning of the patient's eyebrows would not be seen in traction alopecia or central cicatricial alopecia. The perifollicular erythema and scale would be absent in alopecia areata. Alopecia areata is a noncicatricial alopecia with patch hair loss with exclamation point hairs, and yellow dots may be seen on dermoscopy. DLE and central centrifugal cicatricial alopecia are both cicatricial alopecias but do not present like FFA. DLE usually manifests as round to oval, red to hyperpigmented plaques with loss of follicular ostia. CCCA is most common in darker skin types and presents as an expanding plaque on the crown of the scalp with loss of follicular ostia. The cause is unknown. Traction alopecia can affect the frontal hair line and can result in scarring but would not have loss of eyebrows and a diffuse band of alopecia.
Bolognia J, Schaffer J, Cerroni L, eds. *Dermatology.* [Philadelphia]: Elsevier, 2018 (ch. 69).

26. **C.** Perform a scraping of the pustules
This diagnostic test should be performed to evaluate for *Demodex folliculorum* mites. A patient who reports no improvement with traditional treatments for rosacea is unlikely to improve with continuing those treatments. Topical corticosteroids or calcineurin inhibitors will likely worsen the patient's symptoms.
Bolognia J, Schaffer J, Cerroni L, eds. *Dermatology.* [Philadelphia]: Elsevier, 2018 (ch. 37).

27. **A.** Posterior uveitis
Behçet disease is a multisystem inflammatory disorder. Recurrent oral ulceration is the hallmark of the disease and is required for diagnosis as a major criterion. Minor criteria include recurrent genital ulceration, eye lesions (anterior and posterior uveitis), and cutaneous lesions (papulopustules, erythema nodosum–like lesions, or pseudofolliculitis). Ocular disease is found in 90% of patients, with posterior uveitis being the most characteristic finding; however, retinal vasculitis, anterior uveitis, conjunctivitis, and optic neuritis may occur. All other answer choices are possible systemic manifestations of Behçet disease, but these are less common.
Bolognia J, Schaffer J, Cerroni L, eds. *Dermatology.* [Philadelphia]: Elsevier, 2018 (ch. 26).

28. C. Scaly pink plaques in the antecubital fossa

Alopecia areata is a nonscarring, patterned alopecia most commonly presenting as circular areas of alopecia. It is thought to be a hair-specific autoimmune disease. Associated diseases include atopy (allergic rhinitis, atopic dermatitis, and asthma), autoimmune thyroid disease (e.g., Hashimoto thyroiditis), vitiligo, inflammatory bowel disease, and autoimmune polyendocrinopathy syndrome type 1. This picture shows circular, smooth alopecia consistent with alopecia areata. Patients may have associated atopic dermatitis, which can manifest with scaly pink plaques on the antecubital fossa. Follicular erythema, scale and scarring alopecia may be seen in lichen planopilaris/frontal fibrosing alopecia (FFA) spectrum. In the FFA variant, there is band-like fibrosis and alopecia. Tinea capitis is a fungal infection of the scalp/hair and can present with alopecia, broken hairs, erythema, and scale. A clinical clue may be pustules, and lymphadenopathy may be present. Trichotillomania presents with irregular patches of alopecia and broken hairs. There is often concomitant psychiatric disease, such as obsessive-compulsive disorder.
Bolognia J, Schaffer J, Cerroni L, eds. *Dermatology.* [Philadelphia]: Elsevier, 2018 (ch. 69).

29. A. Hypertension

Segmental neurofibromatosis type 1 (NF1) is a form of NF1 that is a reflection of somatic mosaicism due to a postzygotic mutation in the NF1 gene. If the mutation involves the gonads (germline mutation) as well as the skin, there is a chance of neurofibromatosis in the patient's offspring. NF1 is inherited in an autosomal dominant manner, although ~30%–50% of patients have no affected relatives and thus likely harbor new spontaneous mutations. Extracutaneous findings include hypertension (essential and secondary to renal artery stenosis), seizures, pheochromocytoma, and malignancy (breast, gastrointestinal stromal tumor malignant peripheral nerve sheath tumor). The other options are not associated with NF. Gastrointestinal hemorrhage may occur in pseudoxanthoma elasticum. Cardiac rhabdomyomas are found in tuberous sclerosis.
Bolognia J, Schaffer J, Cerroni L, eds. *Dermatology.* [Philadelphia]: Elsevier, 2018 (ch. 61 and 62).

30. A. Granuloma annulare

Granuloma annulare (GA) is a benign and usually self-limiting condition of unknown etiology. It classically presents as arciform or annular plaques located on extremities, often with a papular edge. Less commonly, patch, disseminated, and subcutaneous forms may occur. In 60% of cases, lesions are isolated to the hands and arms. On pathology, it is characterized by focal degeneration of collagen and elastic fibers, mucin deposition, and a perivascular and interstitial lymphohistiocytic infiltrate in the upper and mid dermis. The differential includes annular sarcoidosis, leprosy, and reactive granulomatous dermatitis (i.e., interstitial granulomatous dermatitis). The kodachrome here is a fairly classic presentation for GA. Subacute cutaneous lupus erythematosus (SCLE) usually has more scale, a predilection for the trunk, and is photodistributed. Cutaneous blastomycosis presents as a vegetative or crusted plaque. Annular elastolytic giant cell granuloma usually favors the head and neck with annular plaques with an erythematous border and classically an atrophic/hypopigmented center.
Bolognia J, Schaffer J, Cerroni L, eds. *Dermatology.* [Philadelphia]: Elsevier, 2018 (ch. 93).

31. D. Diabetes mellitus

Lichen planus (LP) is an idiopathic inflammatory disease (T-cell-mediated autoimmune disorder) of the skin, hair, nails, and mucous membranes, most commonly developing in middle-aged adults. It classically manifests with flat-topped violaceous papules and plaques that favor the wrists, forearms, genitalia, distal lower extremities, and presacral area. The lesions are generally pruritic. Some lichenoid drug eruptions have a photodistribution, while others are clinically and histologically indistinguishable from idiopathic lichen planus. The most commonly implicated drugs include angiotensin-converting enzyme inhibitors, thiazide diuretics, antimalarials, quinidine, gold, and NSAIDs. Hepatitis C (typically oral-erosive), hepatitis B vaccination, and HIV have been associated with LP. Diabetes mellitus is not typically associated with lichen planus.
Bolognia J, Schaffer J, Cerroni L, eds. *Dermatology.* [Philadelphia]: Elsevier, 2018 (ch. 11).

32. A. Chronic lymphedema

The kodachrome depicts angiosarcoma in the setting of chronic lymphedema (pelvic surgery is a risk factor for the development of lymphedema). Angiosarcoma is an uncommon malignant neoplasm of the endothelium with a predilection for the skin and superficial soft tissues. It may arise primarily (typically manifesting as bruise-like lesions on the face and scalp of elderly patients) or secondarily (e.g., chronic lymphedema, postirradiation, immunosuppression). Hepatitis C infection may be associated with lichen planus (typically oral), and HIV infection may be associated with AIDS-related Kaposi sarcoma. Dyspnea is not a feature.
Bolognia J, Schaffer J, Cerroni L, eds. *Dermatology.* [Philadelphia]: Elsevier, 2018 (ch. 114).

33. B. Perform an oral examination.

Cutaneous sinus of dental origin occurs when a dental infection is untreated and spreads. Infections of incisors and cuspids may result in this cutaneous finding on the chin and submental region. Treatment involves elimination of the focus of infection, which often requires extraction of the involved tooth, and antibiotics are often required. Referral to a dentist is of paramount importance. Bacterial culture is a reasonable step, but awareness of the bound-down lesion and its location should prompt a thorough physical examination first of the oral mucosa.
Bolognia J, Schaffer J, Cerroni L, eds. *Dermatology.* [Philadelphia]: Elsevier, 2018 (ch. 72).

34. B. Coral-red fluorescence on Wood's lamp examination

Erythrasma is a superficial and often chronic skin infection caused by Corynebacterium minutissimum (gram-positive rods). It manifests with pink to red patches with fine scale that eventually leads to hyperpigmentation. There is a predilection for the folds and interdigital toe web space. Corynebacterium minutissimum will fluoresce bright coral-red on Wood's lamp examination as a result of porphyrin produced by the bacteria. Lesions are most often asymptomatic, although some patients report pruritus. Tinea would result in a positive KOH and clinically presents with a well-defined scaly border, which may affect the buttocks. Intertrigo due to irritant contact dermatitis or seborrheic dermatitis, inverse psoriasis, or inverse lichen planus typically respond to topical steroids.
Bolognia J, Schaffer J, Cerroni L, eds. *Dermatology.* [Philadelphia]: Elsevier, 2018 (ch. 74).

35. C. Tinea cruris
Tinea cruris is a dermatophyte infection of the skin. The three most common organisms include *Epidermophyton floccosum*, *Trichophyton rubrum*, and *Trichophyton mentagrophytes*. The eruption spreads centrifugally with central clearing, typically resulting in annular lesions of varying sizes. Other shapes can be seen (arcuate, circinate, oval). Clues that aid in the diagnosis include a papular/pustular and scaly edge. Scale can be attenuated if topical steroids have been used (tinea incognito). Associated symptoms may include pruritus and burning. Cutaneous candidiasis presents as bright red plaques, which may be studded with papules and pustules, classically with satellite lesions. Inverse psoriasis most often presents in the inguinal folds, with shiny, pink-red, moist well-demarcated plaques with or without scale. Lichen simplex chronicus results from chronic scratching and demonstrates lichenification. There would be no well-demarcated border or leading scale. Note: in men with tinea cruris, the scrotum is typically spared. Consider other diagnoses if the scrotum is involved, such as candida, irritant or contact dermatitis, or lichen simplex chronicus.
Bolognia J, Schaffer J, Cerroni L, eds. *Dermatology*. [Philadelphia]: Elsevier, 2018 (ch. 77).

36. C. Urinary retention
Herpes zoster occurs following dermatomal reactivation of latent varicella-zoster virus. It presents with prodromal pruritus, tingling, tenderness, and/or hyperesthesia followed by a group vesicular eruption on a red base in a dermatomal distribution. The trunk is most commonly affected, followed by the face, lumbar, and sacral areas. Sacral herpes zoster, affecting S2-S4 dermatomes, can occasionally cause a neurogenic bladder. Acute urinary retention and polyuria are the most common symptoms. Peripheral motor neuropathy of the ipsilateral leg is an uncommon complication associated with lumbar herpes zoster. Peripheral neuropathy and angiokeratomas in a bathing trunk distribution are also a feature of Fabry's disease.
Tethered cord is associated with LUMBAR syndrome. Other clinical findings include **l**ower body hemangioma, **u**rogenital anomalies/**u**lcerations, **m**yelopathy (myelomeningocele), **b**ony deformities, **a**norectal malformation, and **r**enal anomalies.
Ipsilateral limb growth is seen in patients with Klippel-Trenaunay syndrome. It is often diagnosed in infancy with excessive growth of the soft tissues, venous malformations, and capillary malformations of an extremity. Diarrhea is not typically associated with herpes zoster.
Bolognia J, Schaffer J, Cerroni L, eds. *Dermatology*. [Philadelphia]: Elsevier, 2018 (ch. 80).

37. A. Central hypothyroidism
While on bexarotene, it is important to monitor TSH and T4 given the risk of central hypothyroidism. Hypertriglyceridemia is another common side effect. While leukopenia may occur at higher doses of bexarotene, this is less common than hypertriglyceridemia or central hypothyroidism. Bexarotene can also cause alopecia, xerosis, and myalgias. Tremors are not a commonly reported side effect.
Bolognia J, Schaffer J, Cerroni L, eds. *Dermatology*. [Philadelphia]: Elsevier, 2018 (ch. 126).

38. A. Lipid panel
This patient has erythema elevatum diutinum (EED), a rare fibrosing leukocytoclastic vasculitis that typically manifests with red-violet to red-brown papules and plaques that favor extensor surfaces. EED has been associated with infections (including HIV, hepatitis B, syphilis, tuberculosis, and beta hemolytic streptococcus), hematologic disorders (in particular, IgA paraproteinemia), as well as autoimmune and inflammatory disorders. The treatment of choice is oral dapsone. Tuberous xanthomas are in the differential diagnosis and are associated with hyperlipidemia; however, they are typically more yellow in color.
Bolognia J, Schaffer J, Cerroni L, eds. *Dermatology*. [Philadelphia]: Elsevier, 2018 (ch. 24).

39. A. c-KIT
The majority of melanomas (40%–60%) have BRAF mutations. BRAF mutations are most commonly found in melanomas that arise in intermittently sun-exposed and nonchronically sun-damaged skin. Neuroblastoma RAS Viral Oncogene Homolog (NRAS) mutations are most often seen in late age-of-onset melanoma. c-KIT mutations are associated with melanomas arising in acral, mucosal, and in chronically sun-damaged skin. G Protein Subunit Alpha Q (GNAQ) mutations are associated with uveal melanomas.
Bolognia J, Schaffer J, Cerroni L, eds. *Dermatology*. [Philadelphia]: Elsevier, 2018 (ch. 113).

40. D. Nevirapine
There is a wide variety of cutaneous eruptions to HIV medications. While several HIV medications may cause Stevens-Johnson syndrome or toxic epidermal necrolysis, nevirapine is a high-risk medication. Abacavir is more often associated with drug hypersensitivity syndrome (also referred to as DRESS). Zidovudine is associated with lipodystrophy and blue/brown pigmentation of the nails. Lamivudine is associated with pancreatitis, pruritus, and paronychia.
Bolognia J, Schaffer J, Cerroni L, eds. *Dermatology*. [Philadelphia]: Elsevier, 2018 (ch. 78).

PEDIATRIC DERMATOLOGY

41. C. Recommend sun avoidance and continued use of sunscreen
This vignette describes a classic presentation of juvenile spring eruption, which commonly affects boys ages 5–12 in the early spring. Lesions involve both helices but can also involve the dorsal hands and trunk. It is thought to be a variant of polymorphous light eruption (PMLE). Lesions spontaneously resolve within 1 week but may recur during a subsequent spring. Thus recommendation of sun avoidance and use of sun protection is critical.
Patch testing would be useful in the diagnosis of allergic contact dermatitis and photoallergic eruptions. Photoallergy is most commonly induced by topical sensitizers, including sunscreens containing oxybenzone, but the localized nature of the eruption and the history make juvenile spring eruption a more likely diagnosis. Similarly, while oral medications can cause photoallergic reactions, as well as other bullous eruptions, this is less likely given the clinical scenario of a healthy 8-year-old boy.
A skin biopsy for H&E and immunofluorescence would be an important next step in the evaluation of suspected immunobullous disorders.
Bolognia J, Schaffer J, Cerroni L, eds. *Dermatology*. [Philadelphia]: Elsevier, 2018 (ch. 87).

42. A. Posterior fossa anomalies
The photograph demonstrates a segmental infantile hemangioma in a V1 distribution, highly concerning for

PHACE(S) syndrome. The syndrome includes **p**osterior fossa and other structural brain malformations, segmental **h**emangiomas, **a**rterial anomalies (internal carotid and cerebral arteries), **c**ardiac defects (coarctation of the aorta, ventral, and atrial septal defects and patent ductus arteriosus), **e**ye anomalies (microphthalmos, optic atrophy, cataracts, strabismus, and exophthalmos), and **s**ternal cleft or **s**upraumbilical raphe. Of the listed associations, cerebrovascular anomalies are the most common extracutaneous findings, and those with involvement of the frontotemporal segment are at highest risk. While cardiovascular anomalies are a feature of this syndrome, the most common manifestations are an aberrant subclavian artery and coarctation of the aorta.

Intracranial capillary malformations and glaucoma are features of Sturge-Weber syndrome, which involves segmental capillary malformations, not infantile hemangiomas as shown in this vignette. Nonsegmental capillary malformations can be seen in healthy infants without associated abnormalities.

Bolognia J, Schaffer J, Cerroni L, eds. *Dermatology*. [Philadelphia]: Elsevier, 2018 (ch. 103).

43. B. Mineral oil preparation

The clinical image depicts pink papules and linear burrows on the palm, suggesting a diagnosis of scabies. Bedside diagnostics allow for an efficient and inexpensive diagnosis, and a mineral oil preparation is the best next step. Mites, eggs, and feces (scybala) may be seen to confirm the diagnosis.

A Wright stain would be helpful in the diagnosis of erythema toxicum neonatorum (eosinophils) and transient neonatal pustular melanosis (neutrophils), but these occur in the neonatal period. A gram stain would be helpful in the diagnosis of bullous impetigo. A KOH preparation is helpful to diagnose dermatophyte infections, which can often involve the hand but typically with more scale. A skin biopsy could also be diagnostic but is unnecessary in this case.

Bolognia J, Schaffer J, Cerroni L, eds. *Dermatology*. [Philadelphia]: Elsevier, 2018 (ch. 84).

44. B. Sterile contents with numerous eosinophils

The vignette and clinical image are suggestive of erythema toxicum neonatorum—an asymptomatic, benign, and self-limited eruption seen most often in full-term newborns, manifesting with highly inflammatory papules, pustules, and/or vesicles surrounded by blotchy erythema. It most often appears on day 3–4 of life but can be seen at birth or may develop as late as 10 days of life. A Wright stain of pustular contents will reveal numerous eosinophils.

Mites, eggs, and scybala would be seen in scabies. Numerous neutrophils would be seen in transient neonatal pustular melanosis, which often presents as hyperpigmented macules and collarettes of scale in infants with darker skin types. Gram-positive cocci in clusters would be seen in bullous impetigo. Pseudohyphae and yeast forms would suggest neonatal or congenital candidiasis, while multinucleated giant cells would suggest a diagnosis of neonatal herpes infection.

Bolognia J, Schaffer J, Cerroni L, eds. *Dermatology*. [Philadelphia]: Elsevier, 2018 (ch. 34; Table 34.1 for a complete differential diagnosis of vesiculopustular eruptions in newborns).

45. C. Ruffled proximal cuticle

This patient has loose anagen hair syndrome. In this condition, microscopic examination of hair shafts reveals a ruffled proximal cuticle that is often said to resemble a fallen sock. Alternating light and dark bands under polarized light are seen in trichothiodystrophy (A); bubbles within the hair shaft are seen in bubble hair, which is caused by damage from heat (B); breakage points with ball-and-socket appearance describe trichorrhexis invaginata or "bamboo hair," which is commonly seen in association with Netherton syndrome (D).

46. B. Ocular hypertelorism

The clinical image shows multiple lentigines, and the vignette describes a young person with widespread lesions, suggesting a diagnosis of LEOPARD syndrome, a mnemonic that stands for **l**entigines, **e**lectrocardiogram abnormalities (hypertrophic cardiomyopathy), **o**cular hypertelorism, **p**ulmonic stenosis, **a**bnormal genitalia, **r**etardation of growth, and **d**eafness. Numerous café-au-lait macules (CALM) are often seen. The disorder is within the spectrum of RASopathies, and mutations in PTPN11 have been found in 90% patients; genotyping may be required to confirm the diagnosis.

CALM and axillary freckling are features of neurofibromatosis, but this vignette describes widespread lentigines. Nail dystrophy and longitudinal melanonychia are seen in Cronkhite-Canada and Laugier-Hunziker syndromes, respectively, which also feature multiple lentigines. However, Cronkhite-Canada syndrome most commonly presents with lentigines of the hands, feet, and buccal mucosa, with associated alopecia and nail dystrophy, and gastrointestinal polyposis. In Laugier-Hunziker, lentigines are most commonly seen on the lips, buccal mucosa, and genital mucosa.

Bolognia J, Schaffer J, Cerroni L, eds. *Dermatology*. [Philadelphia]: Elsevier, 2018 (ch. 53).

47. B. Epidermolytic ichthyosis

Epidermolytic ichthyosis, caused by mutations in KRT1 and KRT10, has highly characteristic histopathologic findings. These include dense hyperkeratosis, hypergranulosis, intracellular vacuolization of keratinocytes, and clumps of keratin filaments and are collectively referred to as "epidermolytic hyperkeratosis." Histopathologic findings are not diagnostic for the other disorders listed (A, C–D).

Bolognia J, Schaffer J, Cerroni L, eds. *Dermatology*. [Philadelphia]: Elsevier, 2018 (ch. 57).

48. C. Pulmonary arteriovenous malformations

The vignette and image support a diagnosis of hereditary hemorrhagic telangiectasia, a condition caused by mutations in endoglin (HHT1) and ALK1 (HHT2). Mucocutaneous telangiectasias appear prominently on the lips and tongue (which represent small arteriovenous malformations), and epistaxis is a common presentation. It is important to screen affected individuals for pulmonary (HHT1), cerebral, and hepatic (HHT2) arteriovenous malformations which can be life threatening.

In a young patient with a history of slowly progressive telangiectasias on the face, trunk, and arms, a diagnosis of hereditary benign telangiectasia, which has no associated abnormalities, can be considered. The predominant tongue and lip involvement, as well as the epistaxis, make this diagnosis less likely. Truncal ataxia, noninfectious granulomas, and increased risk of hematologic malignancies may be seen in ataxia-telangiectasia.

Bolognia J, Schaffer J, Cerroni L, eds. *Dermatology*. [Philadelphia]: Elsevier, 2018 (ch. 104).

49. D. Benign oral leukoplakia

The vignette and clinical image are diagnostic of pachyonychia congenita type I, which is caused by mutations in

KRT6A and KRT16. Pachyonychia congenita type II is characterized by mutations in KRT6B and KRT17. Both subtypes feature onychodystrophy and painful plantar keratoderma. Hyperhidrosis is common. Type I disease is characterized by later onset, benign oral leukoplakia and spiny follicular keratoses.

Pachyonychia congenita type II is characterized by the presence of natal teeth and steatocystoma multiplex. Two additional subtypes, type III and type IV, exist but are less common. Premalignant oral leukoplakia is a feature of dyskeratosis congenita.

50. C. Thyroid function tests

Multifocal infantile hemangiomas, previously referred to as diffuse infantile hemangiomatosis, can occur with or without extracutaneous hemangiomas. The most common site of extracutaneous hemangiomas is the liver, and hepatic hemangiomas are associated with hypothyroidism and high-output cardiac failure. As such, thyroid function tests should be checked in any patient with hepatic hemangiomatosis or large cutaneous hemangiomas.

Laryngoscopy would be indicated for the workup of a patient with a lower facial or "beard" distribution hemangiomas, which can be a marker of laryngeal hemangiomatosis. MRI/MRA of the head and neck would be indicated for a patient with a facial segmental hemangioma in the workup of PHACES syndrome. Platelets, Pothrombin Time/International Normalized Ratio and Partial Thromboplastin Time would be indicated for the workup of Kasabach-Merritt phenomenon, which is associated with the vascular tumors kaposiform hemangioendothelioma and tufted angioma.

Bolognia J, Schaffer J, Cerroni L, eds. *Dermatology.* [Philadelphia]: Elsevier, 2018 (ch. 103).

DERMATOPATHOLOGY

51. E. Neutrophils in the dermal papillae with granular IgA in the dermal papillae

The clinical photograph shows dermatitis herpetiformis (DH), a cutaneous manifestation of celiac disease. DH is pruritic and often manifests with vesicles/erosions on extensor surfaces (scalp, elbows, knees, buttocks). H&E in DH shows papillary dermal edema with neutrophils; there can be a perivascular lymphocytic infiltrate, but this is a nonspecific feature. DIF shows granular IgA in the dermal papillae. Deposition of IgA can also be found along the basement membrane zone (BMZ) in 5%–10% of cases of DH, but should also be present in dermal papillae in these cases. In linear IgA bullous dermatosis (LABD), linear (not granular) IgA staining along the BMZ is characteristic. LABD presents with tense bullae that can resemble BP and often have a herpetiform or annular (beads-on-a-string) arrangement.

Bolognia J, Schaffer J, Cerroni L, eds. *Dermatology.* [Philadelphia]: Elsevier, 2018 (ch. 31).

52. D. Leukemia cutis

Underlying an uninvolved epidermis, there are rows of uniform blasts with hyperchromatic nuclei and minimal cytoplasm, infiltrating between collagen bundles. The morphology of the blasts is variable and depends on the primary leukemic process. Interstitial granuloma annulare and interstitial granulomatous dermatitis demonstrate a relatively less dense interstitial infiltrate composed of histiocytes and lymphocytes. Dermatofibroma (DF) shows a proliferation of spindle and stellate fibrohistiocytes within

the dermis, with collagen trapping at the periphery. DF typically demonstrates epidermal hyperplasia, which is not seen here.

Bolognia J, Schaffer J, Cerroni L, eds. *Dermatology.* [Philadelphia]: Elsevier, 2018 (ch. 121 and 122).

53. D. Verruciform xanthoma

The lesion demonstrates regular acanthosis (uniform bulbous epidermal ridges that extend to the same depth) with parakeratosis that may contain neutrophils. The papillary dermis between the epidermal ridges contains foamy to granular xanthomatous cells. The regular acanthosis with columns of parakeratosis seen at low magnification is a helpful clue that should prompt a search for the xanthomatous cells. Verruciform xanthomas occur most commonly on oral or anogenital skin and are typically not associated with lipid abnormalities.

Hypergranulosis with clumped keratohyaline granules would be seen in verruca vulgaris, whereas bowenoid papulosis would be associated with cytologic atypia and mitotic figures. While acanthosis, hypogranulosis, and parakeratosis with neutrophils are all features of psoriasis, the foamy xanthomatous cells within the papillary dermis are characteristic of verruciform xanthoma.

Bolognia J, Schaffer J, Cerroni L, eds. *Dermatology.* [Philadelphia]: Elsevier, 2018 (ch. 92).

54. C. Penicillamine

The figure illustrates irregular, haphazardly arranged and fragmented basophilic elastic fibers within the dermis typical of pseudoxanthoma elasticum (PXE). The abnormal elastic fibers show calcium deposition that can be illustrated with von Kossa stain. Mutations in ABCC6 gene are implicated in the inherited form of the disease. PXE-like change can be seen as an adverse reaction to penicillamine. The other choices are not associated with PXE.

Bolognia J, Schaffer J, Cerroni L, eds. *Dermatology.* [Philadelphia]: Elsevier, 2018 (ch. 97).

55. A. Coxsackie virus

Hand-foot-mouth disease is most often caused by infection with coxsackievirus A16; however, the A6 strain may cause an atypical coxsackievirus infection. The characteristic histologic features include intraepidermal vesiculation with reticular degeneration and necrotic keratinocytes affecting the upper half of the epidermis, while the lower half of the epidermis is usually spared.

Cutaneous manifestations of Epstein-Barr virus infections typically include a morbilliform eruption, cutaneous lymphomas, and lymphoproliferative disorders. Inclusions associated with herpes simplex are ground glass and multinucleated with margination of nuclear chromatin. Polyoma virus is associated with Merkel cell carcinoma.

Bolognia J, Schaffer J, Cerroni L, eds. *Dermatology.* [Philadelphia]: Elsevier, 2018 (ch. 81).

56. C. Mastocytosis

Cutaneous manifestations of mastocytosis include mastocytoma (solitary or multiple), urticarial pigmentosa, diffuse cutaneous mastocytosis, and telangiectasia macularis eruptive perstans (TMEP). Histologic features include a diffuse proliferation of monomorphous, oval to polygonal cells with eosinophilic granular cytoplasm, and a central round nucleus, giving the "fried-egg" appearance as seen in the figure. The findings in TMEP are more subtle with an increased number of mast cells surrounding dilated vessels in the dermis. Mast cells label with CD117 (c-KIT), mast cell tryptase, and Giemsa and Leder stains.

Cells of Spitz nevi have abundant amphophilic cytoplasm and are usually associated with large nests at the dermal-epidermal junction. In Langerhans cell histiocytosis, there are histiocytes with large reniform nuclei with groves and abundant eosinophilic cytoplasm. Glomus tumor is typically associated with dilated vascular spaces containing red blood cells.

Bolognia J, Schaffer J, Cerroni L, eds. *Dermatology.* [Philadelphia]: Elsevier, 2018 (ch. 118).

57. D. Leishmaniasis
The figure illustrates parasite-laden macrophages containing *Leishmania* organisms. The organisms localize to the periphery of the histiocyte, giving rise to the "marquee sign," which is not typically associated with other infections caused by organisms of similar size (histoplasmosis, granuloma inguinale, and rhinoscleroma).
Cryptococcus presents with yeast forms varying in size from 4–20 microns characteristically associated with a mucoid capsule. Blastomycosis is associated with broad-based budding yeasts, while chromoblastomycosis demonstrates sclerotic bodies ("copper pennies"). Deep fungal infections are often associated with pseudoepitheliomatous hyperplasia.
Bolognia J, Schaffer J, Cerroni L, eds. *Dermatology.* [Philadelphia]: Elsevier, 2018 (ch. 83).

58. D. Subcutaneous fat necrosis of newborn
Subcutaneous fat necrosis of the newborn histologically shows multiple radial crystalline spaces within the adipocytes surrounded by a heavy mixed infiltrate. The prognosis is excellent, unlike sclerema neonatorum, which is associated with high morbidity and mortality. The histologic findings in sclerema neonatorum are similar to those seen in subcutaneous fat necrosis of the newborn but less intense (fewer crystalline structures and sparse infiltrate). Pancreatic panniculitis demonstrates "ghost" cells with basophilic calcifications, while erythema nodosum is a septal panniculitis that may show Miescher radial granulomas.
Bolognia J, Schaffer J, Cerroni L, eds. *Dermatology.* [Philadelphia]: Elsevier, 2018 (ch. 83).

59. D. Vulva
Hidradenoma papilliferum usually affects female patients and presents in the vulvar, perineal, or perianal locations. It is a benign adnexal tumor that presents as a well-demarcated nodule within the dermis, composed of branching papillary processes lined by a two-cell layer. The oral mucosa, trunk, and scalp are not sites commonly associated with hidradenoma papilliferum.
Bolognia J, Schaffer J, Cerroni L, eds. *Dermatology.* [Philadelphia]: Elsevier, 2018 (ch. 111).

60. A. Myrmecia
Myrmecia or palmoplantar wart is an endophytic lesion that demonstrates large cytoplasmic inclusions that may be eosinophilic or basophilic in appearance. Myrmecial warts are usually caused by human papillomavirus-1.
Verrucous carcinoma is a relatively indolent squamous cell carcinoma that infiltrates with a pushing border and occurs on plantar skin and mucosal surfaces. Pitted keratolysis demonstrates organisms of *Corynebacterium* spp within the stratum corneum while psoriasis will show acanthosis, hypogranulosis, and parakeratosis with neutrophils.
Bolognia J, Schaffer J, Cerroni L, eds. *Dermatology.* [Philadelphia]: Elsevier, 2018 (ch. 79).

PROCEDURAL DERMATOLOGY TEST 1

61. B. Iopidine drops applied to the affected eye
Iopidine drops, an alpha-adrenergic agonist, applied three times per day to the affected eye may elevate the eyelid 1–2 mm. Iopidine is an alpha-adrenergic agonist, which stimulates Müller muscle to elevate the ptotic eyelid.
Bolognia J, Schaffer J, Cerroni L, eds. *Dermatology.* [Philadelphia]: Elsevier, 2018 (ch. 159).

62. D. Donepezil
Donepezil is an acetylcholinesterase inhibitor that can potentially diminish the effect of botulinum toxin. Cyclosporine, aminoglycosides (such as tobramycin), and calcium channel blockers (such as verapamil) can all potentiate the effect of botulinum toxin. Lisinopril should have no effect on neuromodulators.
Bolognia J, Schaffer J, Cerroni L, eds. *Dermatology.* [Philadelphia]: Elsevier, 2018 (ch. 159).

63. D. Cemiplimab
Cemiplimab is a monoclonal antibody targeting the receptor programmed death 1 (PD-1) on T lymphocytes. Inhibition of PD-1 with cemiplimab and similar agents stimulates immune recognition of malignant neoplasms. In preliminary phase 1 and 2 trials, cemiplimab has demonstrated an objective response rate of up to 50% for locally advanced or metastatic cutaneous squamous cell carcinoma.
Ipilimumab is an anti-CTLA4 monoclonal antibody approved as immunotherapy for melanoma. Carboplatin is a cytotoxic chemotherapy, and cetuximab is a monoclonal antibody inhibiting the EGFR. Both carboplatin and cetuximab have been used off-label for treatment of advanced cutaneous squamous cell carcinoma, with response rates less than 25%. Bevacizumab is a monoclonal antibody-inhibiting vascular endothelial growth factor A (VEGF-A) that is approved for treatment of internal malignancies, including colorectal and lung cancer.
Bolognia J, Schaffer J, Cerroni L, eds. *Dermatology.* [Philadelphia]: Elsevier, 2018 (ch. 113).

64. C. Wide local excision plus sentinel node biopsy or nodal imaging, followed by adjuvant radiation therapy
This presentation is diagnostic of Merkel cell carcinoma, which has a high risk of local recurrence and regional and distant metastasis. Recommended initial treatment is wide local excision plus lymph node staging and adjuvant radiation to the primary site. Some low-risk lesions may be treated with wide local excision without radiation, but nodal staging is still required, as approximately one-third of patients have nodal disease without clinical lymphadenopathy. Tumors over 2 cm have a significantly worse prognosis. If lymph node or other metastatic disease is identified, systemic immunomodulatory therapy is indicated (e.g., anti-PD-1 or anti-PD-L1 therapy).
Bolognia J, Schaffer J, Cerroni L, eds. *Dermatology.* [Philadelphia]: Elsevier, 2018 (ch. 115).

65. A. Cataract formation and iris atrophy
This patient was treated with diode 800-nm laser for photoepilation of eyebrow hair. The figure demonstrates distortion of her pupil shape into a horizontal ellipse. This resulted in cataract formation and iris atrophy, requiring surgical treatment to repair.
Retinal laser injuries are often characterized by a sudden loss of vision, which generally improves over weeks but occasionally leads to severe complications such as a

scotoma (blind spot in the fovea). Because the iris and retina contain pigment, they are susceptible to selective photothermolysis with laser exposure. Laser light in the visible to near infrared spectrum (400–1400 nm) are part of the "retinal hazard region." Laser light in the ultraviolet B (290–320 nm) spectrum may result in photokeratitis, ultraviolet A (320–400 nm) spectrum may result in cataracts (choice C), and infrared (760–100,000 nm) spectrum may cause a corneal burn.

One of the most commonly reported eye injuries from laser therapy is following epilation with laser hair removal around the eyelid. Injuries after laser hair removal include cataract formation, iris atrophy, posterior synechiae, conjunctival hyperemia, photophobia, and reduced visual acuity. Vitreous floaters can be induced by the pulsed dye laser. Protective eyewear must be chosen that matches the wavelength of emitted light. Eye shields can be internal or external. External eye shields are routinely used, except when target structures are very close to the eye. Internal eye shields may shift after application, and care should be taken to ensure that the iris is fully protected. While generally safe, internal eye shields can cause minor injuries, such as corneal abrasion.

Bolognia J, Schaffer J, Cerroni L, eds. *Dermatology*. [Philadelphia]: Elsevier, 2018 (ch. 137).

66. **F.** A–D

Lidocaine toxicity is a rare but reported complication of dermatologic surgery. Symptoms vary with serum lidocaine concentration. The maximum safe dose of lidocaine (at standard 1% or 2% concentrations) in an adult is 5 mg/kg without epinephrine and 7 mg/kg with epinephrine. For tumescent anesthesia, the safe dose is 35–50 mg/kg. Early symptoms of lidocaine toxicity include circumoral and digital paresthesia, restlessness, and lightheadedness. Central nervous system (CNS) symptoms progress to include tinnitus, visual disturbances, slurred speech, and muscle twitching, and eventually seizures and coma may occur. Management includes all of the above with administration of benzodiazepines and airway maintenance before serious CNS and cardiopulmonary manifestations result.

Bolognia J, Schaffer J, Cerroni L, eds. *Dermatology*. [Philadelphia]: Elsevier, 2018 (ch. 143).

67. **D.** The graft should be at least 25% larger than the defect.

To account for wound contraction and minimize the risk of ectropion, full thickness skin grafts on the lower eyelid should be sized such that the graft is at least 25% larger than the actual size of the wound. In other locations, oversizing by 5%–10% is sufficient. An excellent tissue reservoir for harvesting grafts for the lower eyelids are from the upper eyelids, as there is often tissue redundancy in this area and the skin texture is an excellent match.

Bolognia J, Schaffer J, Cerroni L, eds. *Dermatology*. [Philadelphia]: Elsevier, 2018 (ch. 148).

Jewett BS, Shockley WW. Reconstructive options for periocular defects. *Otolaryngol Clin North Am*. 2001 Jun;34(3):601–25.

68. **D.** 67-year-old female immunosuppressed secondary to history of cardiac transplant

Antibiotic prophylaxis is recommended for certain patients with high-risk cardiac conditions including: (1) prosthetic heart valve; (2) history of infective endocarditis; (3) unrepaired cyanotic congenital heart disease; (4) repaired congenital heart defects with prosthetic materials or repairs with residual defects; and (5) cardiac transplant patients who develop cardiac valvulopathy. Transplant alone does not obligate prophylaxis prior to dermatologic

surgery. For patients with history of total joint replacement, prophylaxis recommendations are less well defined, and can be considered for a joint replacement in the past two years, previous prosthetic joint infection, type 1 diabetes, immunosuppression, malnourishment, or hemophilia.

Bolognia J, Schaffer J, Cerroni L, eds. *Dermatology*. [Philadelphia]: Elsevier, 2018 (ch. 151).

69. **B.** A 2.5-cm recurrent superficial basal cell carcinoma on the back of a healthy male

In 2012, the appropriate use criteria for Mohs micrographic surgery (MMS) was developed. A panel of Mohs surgeons and medical dermatologists analyzed more than 270 clinical scenarios for referral to MMS, including tumor type, location, size, immune status, histologic features, and whether or not the lesion was recurrent. Based on the consensus data, the AUC was defined to provide a guideline for the rational use of MMS. Tumor locations are divided into three regions: H, which includes the mask area and perioral region of the face, hands, feet, genitalia, and nipple/areola complex; M, which includes the rest of the head and neck as well as the distal lower extremities; and L, which includes the rest of the body, that is, trunk and proximal extremities.

A recurrent superficial basal cell carcinoma is not an indication for MMS, even if >2 cm in a healthy adult. If the lesion was located within a field of prior radiation, then MMS would be indicated. The other choices are appropriate for MMS given the location and histopathology (choices A and C), immunocompromised host (choice D), and recommendation for removal of desmoplastic trichoepithelioma because of its potential aggressive growth pattern (choice E), despite being a benign lesion.

70. **A.** Persistent erythema

Complications from chemical peels include dyspigmentation, textural abnormalities, skin atrophy, infections, persistent erythema, and scarring. Persistent erythema beyond 2 months after a medium-depth peel may be precipitated by the use of topical or systemic retinoids, contact with various allergens or irritants, an underlying skin condition, genetic susceptibility, or the presence of active infection. Persistent erythema may indicate the impending development of scar formation, especially when the area is indurated. Management includes use of topical, intralesional, or occasionally systemic corticosteroids, silicone gel sheets, and pulsed dye laser therapy. Infections are a relatively rare complication and can be bacterial, fungal, or viral in origin. Without prompt treatment, infections can result in persistent erythema.

Bolognia J, Schaffer J, Cerroni L, eds. *Dermatology*. [Philadelphia]: Elsevier, 2018 (ch. 154).

BASIC SCIENCE

71. **B.** Zinc oxide

Zinc oxide and titanium dioxide are physical blockers that absorb both ultraviolet A (UVA) and ultraviolet B (UVB). Avobenzone absorbs UVA. PABA absorbs UVB. Oxybenzone absorbs UVB and UVA2.

Bolognia J, Schaffer J, Cerroni L, eds. *Dermatology*. [Philadelphia]: Elsevier, 2018 (ch. 132).

72. **C.** Extracellular matrix protein 1

The clinical picture is of lichen sclerosus, which commonly affects the genital area with shiny white atrophic plaques

with a red/violaceous rim. Purpura may be present in addition to follicular plugging. A figure-eight configuration often occurs in women with perineal involvement. Common symptoms include burning, itching, or pain, and ultimately the development of scarring, atrophy, or fusion of the labia and clitoris may occur with longstanding disease. A bullous form does exist. Rare development of SCC may occur, necessitating surveillance. Autoantibodies against extracellular matrix protein 1 (ECM-1) may be found in 80% of patients. Autoantibodies to desmoglein 3 (Dsg 3) are found in pemphigus vulgaris. Autoantibodies to collagen VII may occur in EBA and bullous lupus erythematosus. BPAG2 (or BP180) antibodies are found in bullous pemphigoid. Desmoplakin antibodies can be found in paraneoplastic pemphigus.
Bolognia J, Schaffer J, Cerroni L, eds. *Dermatology*. [Philadelphia]: Elsevier, 2018 (ch. 44).

73. **D.** Compensation of desmoglein 3 in the mucosa
Patient with anti-Dsg 1 antibodies (pemphigus foliaceous) do not usually manifest with mucosal ulcerations due to the desmoglein compensation theory: Dsg 1 and Dsg 3 compensate for each other when they are coexpressed in the same cell. In the skin, Dsg 1 is expressed throughout the epidermis but more so in the superficial layers, while Dsg 3 has greater expression in the basal layers. Therefore patients with Dsg 1 antibodies have localization of blisters to the superficial epidermis. In the mucosae, on the other hand, Dsg 1 and Dsg 3 are both expressed, although Dsg 3 has a greater expression than Dsg 1. Further, the presence of Dsg 3 compensates for the loss of function of Dsg 1 and is sufficient for cell-cell adhesion.
Bolognia J, Schaffer J, Cerroni L, eds. *Dermatology*. [Philadelphia]: Elsevier, 2018 (ch. 29).

74. **B.** IL-23
This patient has CARD14-associated papulosquamous eruption (CAPE), a recently described condition associated with mutations in CARD14. This eruption is often recalcitrant to traditional psoriasis therapies but improve with treatment with ustekinumab, which targets IL-12/23. Treatment with medications that target the other choices (A and C–D) have not been associated with improvement in this condition.
See Craiglow BG, et al. CARD14-associated papulosquamous eruption: a spectrum including features of psoriasis and pityriasis rubra pilaris. *J Am Acad Dermatol.* 2018 Sep; 79(3):487–494.

75. **B.** Depletion of CD20+ B cells
Rituximab is a monoclonal antibody that binds to the CD20 receptor on mature B cells and induces apoptosis of these cells. It does not affect stem cells or plasma cells. Rituximab is now approved for pemphigus vulgaris, where the medication depletes B cells and decreases anti-desmoglein-3 antibody levels.
Bolognia J, Schaffer J, Cerroni L, eds. *Dermatology*. [Philadelphia]: Elsevier, 2018 (ch. 128).

76. **D.** PTCH1
Patched (PTCH1) is the most commonly mutated gene in basal cell carcinoma (70% of BCCs). Mutations in PTCH1 as well as other genes in the hedgehog signaling pathway are responsible for hereditary basal cell nevus syndrome (Gorlin syndrome). The most commonly mutated protein in squamous cell carcinoma (SCC) is the tumor suppressor p53 (TP53). TP53 is the second most common mutation in BCC and is present in 50% of BCCs. BRAF is commonly mutated in both benign melanocytic nevi as well as cutaneous melanoma. GNAQ is commonly mutated in blue nevi and uveal nevi. In addition, GNAQ is mutated in Sturge-Weber syndrome. c-KIT is commonly mutated in acral and mucosal melanoma.
Bolognia J, Schaffer J, Cerroni L, eds. *Dermatology*. [Philadelphia]: Elsevier, 2018 (ch. 107–108, 113).

77. **B.** Calcium-dependent cell-cell adhesion molecules
Desmosomes are calcium-dependent cell-cell adhesion molecules between epidermal keratinocytes and serve as attachment points for intermediate filaments (cytoskeleton). Desmosomes are composed of desmoglein, desmocollin, and plaque proteins. In pemphigus, antibodies form against Dsg 1 and 3. Additional associated diseases include striate PPK (Dsg 1), bullous impetigo (Dsg 1), staphylococcal scalded skin syndrome (Dsg 1), subcorneal pustular dermatosis (desmocollin 1), monilethrix (Dsg 4), Naxos disease (plakoglobin), and paraneoplastic pemphigus (desmoplakin).
The basement membrane zone (BMZ) is the selective barrier between the epidermis and dermis. The basal keratinocytes interact with hemidesmosomal antigens (BPAG1, BPAG2, plectin, alpha 6 beta4 integrin), providing attachment between basal keratinocytes and extracellular matrix. The lamina lucida, lamina densa, and sublamina densa are deeper layers. Associated diseases include bullous pemphigoid (BPAG1, BPAG2), linear IgA bullous dermatosis (BPAG2), epidermolysis bullosa simplex with muscular dystrophy (plectin), ocular cicatricial pemphigoid (alpha 6 beta 4 integrin), and junctional epidermolysis bullosa with pyloric atresia (alpha 6 beta 4 integrin). Gap junctions are transmembrane channels formed by connexins. Associated diseases include KID (connexin 26), Vohwinkel syndrome (connexin 26), PPK with deafness (connexin 26), hidrotic ectodermal dysplasia (connexin 30), and erythrokeratoderma variabilis (connexin 30.3/31). Lamellar granules are intracellular lipid-carrying granules made in the Golgi apparatus and contain glycoprotein and lipid precursors that form "mortar" or ceramide, contributing to the lipid barrier. In Flegel disease and harlequin ichthyosis, there are decreased lamellar granules.
Bolognia J, Schaffer J, Cerroni L, eds. *Dermatology*. [Philadelphia]: Elsevier, 2018 (ch. 28).

78. **A.** Oxidative damage
UVA travels through glass windows and plays an important role in drug-induced phototoxic reactions (such as to BRAF inhibitors, EGFR inhibitors, and tetracyclines). UVB, on the other hand, is mostly blocked by glass windows. UVA plays a more prominent role in oxidative damage (reactive oxygen species) in the skin, while UVB plays an important role in carcinogenesis through the formation of cyclobutane-pyrimidine dimers. Nucleotide excision repair is a pathway by which bulky mutated DNA photoproducts (pyrimidine dimers) are repaired. In disorders such as xeroderma pigmentosum (XP), there is a disruption of nucleotide excision repair. As a consequence, increased UV sensitivity and UV mutagenesis occurs, resulting in nonmelanoma and melanoma skin cancers. Other inherited disorders with abnormal DNA repair include Cockayne syndrome (CS), XP-CS overlap, trichothiodystrophy, and Muir-Torre syndrome (mismatch DNA repair). Mutations in P53 are important in cutaneous SCCs and actinic keratoses.
Bolognia J, Schaffer J, Cerroni L, eds. *Dermatology*. [Philadelphia]: Elsevier, 2018 (ch. 86).

79. A. Gram-positive, nonmotile rods found within the sebaceous follicle

Propionibacterium acnes contributes to the pathogenesis of acne vulgaris, not rosacea. These gram-positive, nonmotile rods are located deep within the sebaceous follicle and result in the release of enzymes that contribute to comedo rupture, lipases, and chemotactic factors, as well as stimulation of a host response via proinflammatory mediators and reactive oxygen species. The vignette describes papulopustular rosacea rather than classical acne vulgaris.

The remaining choices are all theorized to play a potential role in the pathogenesis of rosacea. In rosacea, there is upregulation of cytokines and antimicrobial molecules, such as cathelicidin and its processing serine protease, suggesting dysfunction of the innate immune system. In addition, UV radiation exposure has been shown to induce angiogenesis and increase production of reactive oxygen species, which then leads to upregulation of matrix metalloproteinases. *Demodex* mites, rather than *P. Acnes*, may be found in greater numbers in rosacea patients, and topical treatments such as permethrin and ivermectin target these mites in addition to their antiinflammatory properties. Neurogenic inflammation and impaired epidermal function may also contribute to the pathogenesis of rosacea.

Bolognia J, Schaffer J, Cerroni L, eds. *Dermatology.* [Philadelphia]: Elsevier, 2018 (ch. 37).

80. A. Talimogene laherparepvec

Talimogene laherparepvec (T-VEC) is an FDA-approved injectable treatment for inoperable melanoma. It is an oncolytic herpes virus bioengineered with Granulocyte-macrophage colony-stimulating factor to invade and destroy melanoma tumor cells. The other agents are not approved by the FDA for intralesional use.

Andtbacka RH, et al. Talimogene laherparepvec improves durable response rate in patients with advanced melanoma. *J Clin Oncol.* 2015; 33(25):2780–8.

GENERAL DERMATOLOGY

1. This 6-year-old male developed ataxia and the clinical findings shown. What other cutaneous finding is he at risk for?

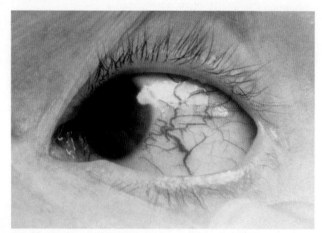

With permission from James W, et al. (eds.), in *Andrews' Disease of the Skin Clinical Atlas*, 4th edition, 2018, Elsevier, 379–404 (fig. 27.37).

   A. Diffuse silvery hair
   B. Early-onset eczematous dermatitis
   C. Noninfectious granulomas
   D. Gingivitis/periodontitis

2. Which is the least likely cause of the patient's eruption?

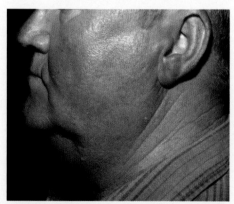

With permission from James W, et al. (eds), in *Andrews' Disease of the Skin Clinical Atlas*, 4th edition, 2018, Elsevier, 65–85 (fig. 6.74).

   A. Chlorpromazine
   B. Diltiazem
   C. Amiodarone
   D. Quinacrine

3. This tumor is associated with what chromosomal translocation?

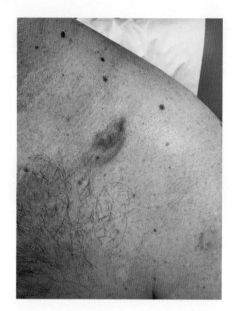

   A. t(9;22)
   B. t(11;22)
   C. t(15;22)
   D. t(17;22)

4. A 56-year-old female presents with this extremely pruritic rash. Which of the following medications is associated with a drug-induced form of this condition?

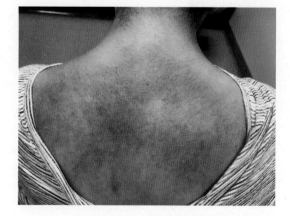

A. Simvastatin
B. Furosemide
C. Hydrochlorothiazide
D. Metoprolol

5. A 62-year-old female presents with fever and acute onset of this eruption on her bilateral lower extremities. Biopsy for direct immunofluorescence shows perivascular C3 and IgA deposits. Which malignancy is most commonly associated with these findings?

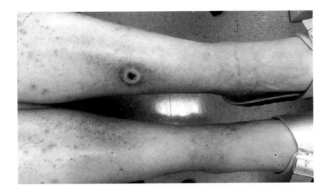

A. Breast cancer
B. Acute myelogenous leukemia
C. Lung cancer
D. Colon cancer

6. A 36-week pregnant female presents with sudden-onset intense pruritus with scattered excoriations on her extremities and abdomen. Laboratory workup reveals elevated bile acids. The patient is at increased risk of which of the following?
A. Intrapartum and postpartum hemorrhage
B. Cardiac abnormalities
C. Permanent liver dysfunction
D. No associated maternal risks

7. An 84-year-old man with history of metastatic carcinoid tumor presents with the following rash on the abdomen. The development of what secondary cutaneous malignancy is the patient most at risk for?

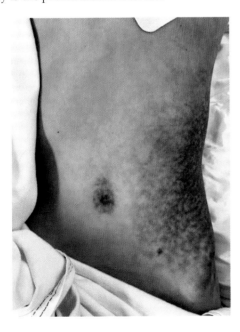

A. Basal cell carcinoma
B. Cutaneous B-cell lymphoma
C. Melanoma
D. Squamous cell carcinoma
E. Extramammary Paget disease

8. A 24-year-old male presents with this long-standing, asymptomatic eruption on his forearms, abdomen, and thighs. Biopsy shows multiple dilated and ectatic telangiectasias with Periodic acid–Schiff (PAS)-positive concentric hyaline deposits around the blood vessels. What is the most likely diagnosis?

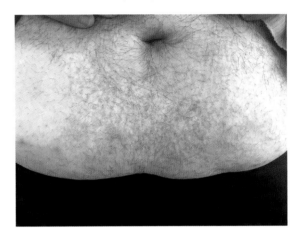

A. Generalized essential telangiectasia
B. Erythropoietic protoporphyria
C. Hereditary hemorrhagic telangiectasia
D. Cutaneous collagenous vasculopathy

9. Which medication is most likely associated with increased production of this growth?

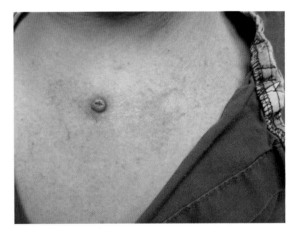

A. Trametinib
B. Vemurafenib
C. Ipilimumab
D. Nivolumab

10. Which of the following regarding Barraquer-Simmons syndrome (acquired partial lipodystrophy) is true?
A. Increased risk of recurrent *Neisseria meningitides* infections.
B. Liver disease is a significant cause of death.
C. Onset is at birth.
D. Excess fat accumulation occurs in the head and neck.

11. Digital squamous cell carcinoma is associated with which of the following human papillomavirus (HPV) types?
    A. HPV 13, 32
    B. HPV 2, 7
    C. HPV 5, 8
    D. HPV 16
    E. HPV 6, 11

12. A 42-year-old man with a history of human immunodeficiency virus (HIV) presents with the following enlarging lesions present for at least 3 months. He reports no improvement with oral acyclovir. What is the best treatment option?

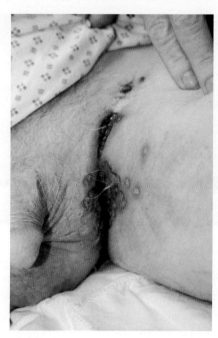

    A. Azithromycin
    B. Foscarnet
    C. Penicillin G
    D. Famciclovir

13. A 16-month-old boy with a history of atopic dermatitis presents with acute fevers, irritability, and the pictured skin eruption. What is the next best step in management?

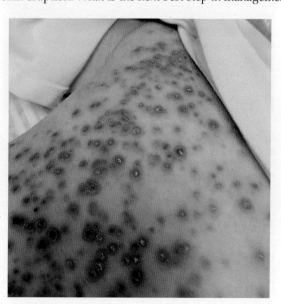

A. Hospitalize and initiate intravenous acyclovir.
B. Obtain a superficial skin culture and start oral cephalexin.
C. Begin topical hydrocortisone cream around the eyes.
D. Begin bleach baths and mupirocin ointment for Methicillin-resistant Staphylococcus aureus (MRSA) decolonization.
E. Apply penciclovir cream.

14. You receive a consult from ophthalmology regarding a patient seen urgently in clinic with the ocular findings pictured. The oral mucosa is clear, and the patient has no evidence of other cutaneous lesions. A biopsy and direct immunofluorescence (DIF) are performed. The biopsy shows subepithelial bulla formation, and DIF is positive for IgG and C3 directed against mucosal basement membrane. What antibody is NOT associated with this condition?

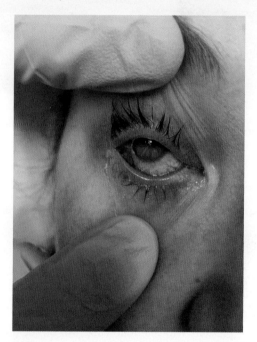

A. BP180
B. Laminin 332
C. Alpha 6 beta 4 integrin
D. Type VII collagen

15. A 65-year-old female with acute myeloid leukemia is started on induction chemotherapy and 10 days later developed the following eruption on the face, hands, and trunk. The patient is febrile and neutropenic. What is the most common drug culprit?

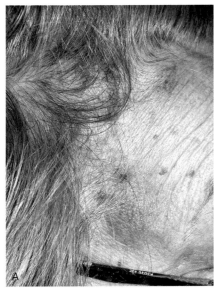

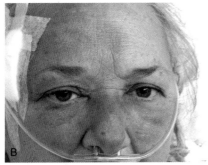

With permission from Srivastava M, *Journal of the American Academy of Dermatology*, 2007, volume 56, issue 4, 693–696.

A. Acyclovir
B. Etoposide
C. Sorafenib
D. Cytarabine

16. An 16-year-old girl presents with these painful lesions. She denies any history of sexual activity. What is the most likely etiology of this condition?

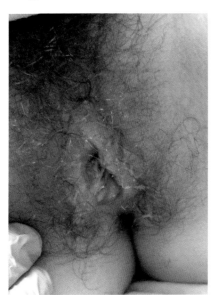

A. Herpes simplex virus 2 infection
B. Primary human immunodeficiency virus infection
C. Cytomegalovirus infection
D. Primary Epstein-Barr virus infection
E. Behçet disease

17. What would you expect to find on histology of these lesions on the leg of a 70-year-old man?

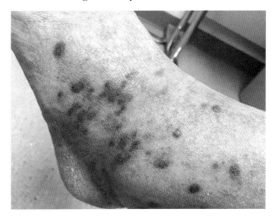

A. Neutrophil nuclear debris surrounding damaged superficial blood vessels
B. Spindle cells with slitlike spaces containing red blood cells
C. Plump hyperchromatic atypical spindle cells with anastomosing blood vessels
D. Infiltrate of atypical immature myeloid cells with "Indian filing"

18. A 32-year-old male presents to clinic with acute onset of subjective fevers, headache, rash, and conjunctivitis. He reports that he and his pregnant girlfriend recently returned from a trip to the Caribbean where they both received numerous mosquito bites. He denies similar symptoms in his girlfriend. What is the next best step?

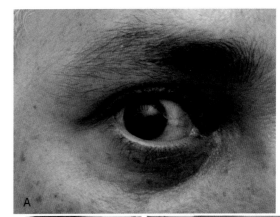

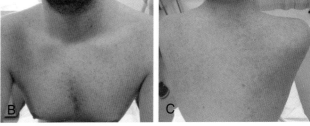

With permission from Cosano-Quero A, Velasco-Tirado V, Seco MPS, Manzanedo-Bueno L, Belhassen-García M, in *Dermatology (Actas Dermo-Sifiliográficas, English Edition)*, 2018, Elsevier, e13-e16 (figs. 1 & 4).

A. Recommend rest, hydration, and acetaminophen for fevers and pain.
B. Recommend Zika diagnostic testing for the patient and monitor his girlfriend for symptoms.
C. Recommend Zika diagnostic testing for the patient and his girlfriend.
D. Recommend Chikungunya diagnostic testing for the patient and monitor his girlfriend for symptoms.
E. Admit for intravenous immunoglobulin treatment.

19. The patient is on dialysis three times a week and presented with exquisitely tender lesions on the right leg 1 week ago, which started to ulcerate. What is the best diagnosis?

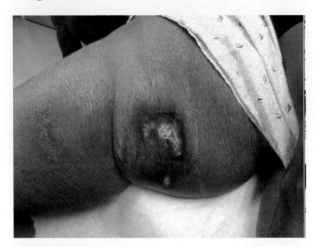

A. Venous ulcer
B. Arterial ulcer
C. Vasculitis
D. Calciphylaxis
E. Ecthyma

20. The diagnosis for the image shown is:

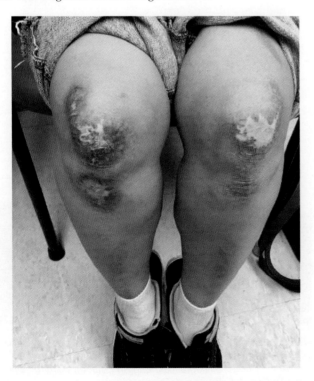

A. Discoid lupus erythematosus
B. Porphyria cutanea tarda
C. Epidermolysis bullosa acquisita
D. Bullous pemphigoid
E. Dermatitis herpetiformis

21. Prior to initiating cyclosporine, all of the following should be checked EXCEPT:
A. Uric acid
B. Blood pressure
C. Triglycerides
D. Glucose-6-phosphate dehydrogenase
E. Potassium

22. The patient pictured here should be monitored for the development of:

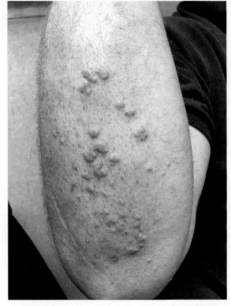

Photo Courtesy of Edward Sarkisian, MD, Fort Wayne, IN.

A. Gluten enteropathy
B. Pancreatitis
C. Monoclonal gammopathy
D. Hypothyroidism

23. The most appropriate diagnostic test for the person pictured is:

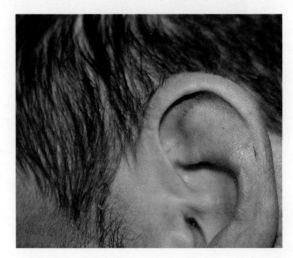

A. Urine toxicology screen for cocaine
B. Sterile tissue culture
C. X-ray
D. Antibodies to type II collagen

24. The patient presented with this eruption on the leg. What is the best diagnosis?

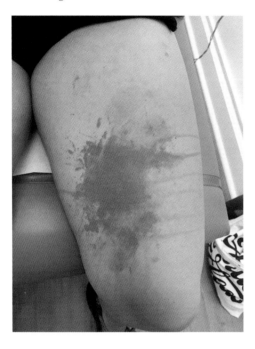

A. Necrotizing fasciitis
B. Loxosceles reclusa bite
C. Calciphylaxis
D. Phytophotodermatitis

25. The patient underwent ear surgery 4 days prior and describes the lesions as pruritic. What is the most likely diagnosis?

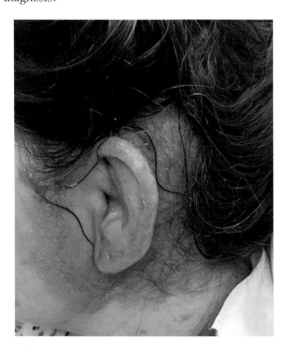

A. Chondritis
B. Pseudomonal cellulitis
C. Allergic contact dermatitis
D. Tinea corporis

26. The patient reports new hypopigmentation over his knee. The likely diagnosis is:

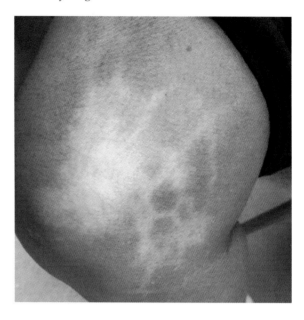

A. Vitiligo
B. Corticosteroid-induced hypopigmentation
C. Hypopigmented mycosis fungoides
D. Morphea
E. Lichen sclerosus

27. The patient reports a strong family history of nodular growths that are painful to touch. What is the patient at risk for?

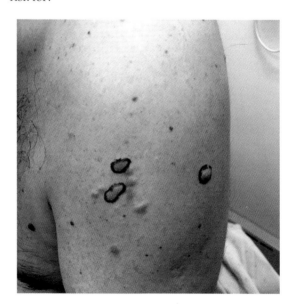

A. Retinoblastoma
B. Spontaneous pneumothoraces
C. Non–small cell lung carcinoma
D. Renal cell carcinoma
E. Colorectal carcinoma

28. This rash may be associated with:

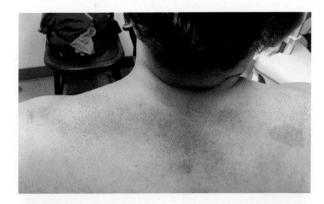

   A. Notalgia paresthetica
   B. Type II diabetes
   C. Multiple endocrine neoplasia type 2A
   D. A & C
   E. A, B, & C

29. The patient developed the lesions pictured after initiating which medication?

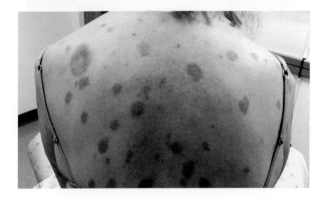

   A. Terbinafine
   B. Penicillin
   C. Penicillamine
   D. Vemurafenib
   E. Prednisone

30. A male patient reported decreased mobility of the hands and thickening of skin on his face. Which laboratory test should be obtained in the evaluation of this condition?

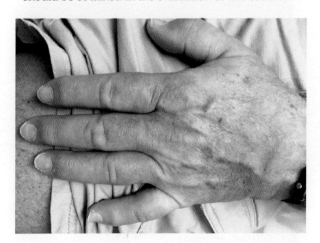

   A. Anti-DNase B
   B. Serum immunofixation electrophoresis
   C. Antinuclear antibody
   D. Hemoglobin A1C
   E. Ferritin

31. The patient presents with the lesion below. Biopsy confirms the diagnosis of verruca plantaris. The patient did not respond to topical salicylic acid, cryotherapy, curettage, electrodessication, or intralesional candida antigen. You decide to proceed with intralesional bleomycin. Which of the following adverse events is most likely?

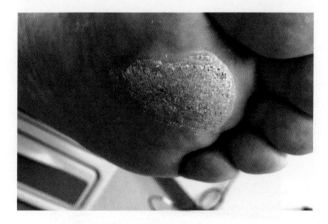

   A. Raynaud phenomenon
   B. Lupus-like reaction
   C. Dermatomyositis
   D. Flagellate erythema

32. An otherwise healthy patient developed the lesion pictured, which continues to progress at a rapid rate onto her forehead. What is the best management plan?

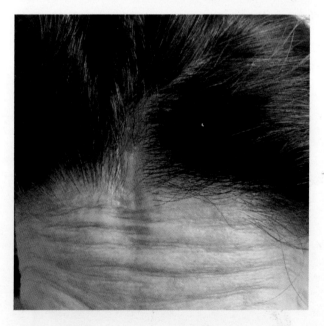

   A. Observation
   B. Prednisone
   C. Methotrexate
   D. Doxycycline
   E. B & C

33. A 70-year-old man with non–small cell lung carcinoma on pembrolizumab (antiprogrammed death 1 inhibitor) presents with this intensely pruritic eruption. He notes lesions in his oral mucosa as well. What changes are most likely to be found on histopathology?

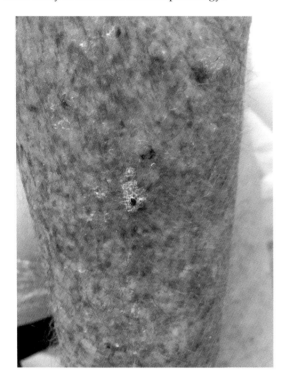

A. Subepidermal bulla with eosinophils
B. Dyskeratosis of keratinocytes and acantholysis
C. Bandlike lichenoid infiltrate and epidermal spongiosis with eosinophils
D. Epidermal hyperplasia with acanthosis and hypogranulosis
E. Naked granulomas within the dermis

34. Which of the following statements regarding this condition is FALSE?

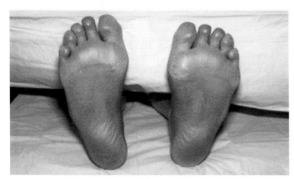

With permission from Jaff MR, Bartholomew JR, in *Goldman-Cecil Medicine*, 2015, Elsevier, 504–511.e2 (ch. 80, fig. 80).

A. Misoprostol has been used to treat this condition.
B. Serotonin reuptake inhibitors have been used to treat this condition.
C. The patient recently started sorafenib.

D. Mutations in the gene that encodes the voltage-gated sodium channel alpha subunit have been implicated in the familial form of this condition.
E. Complete blood count evaluation may show thrombocytosis.

35. The patient was treated with dupilumab for refractory atopic dermatitis, with marked improvement. Which potential adverse event is most commonly associated with this medication?

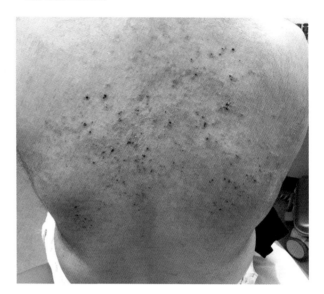

A. Ocular keratitis
B. Herpes labialis
C. Conjunctivitis
D. Stevens-Johnson syndrome

36. An otherwise healthy patient presents to the office with fevers, chills, and the rash pictured. You obtain a superficial wound culture and begin empiric antibiotics. What organism is most likely to be present in the wound culture?

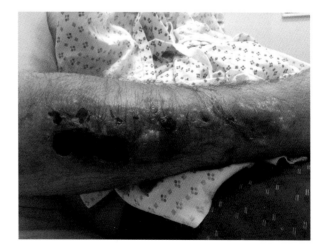

A. Staphylococcus
B. Streptococcus
C. Pseudomonas
D. Vibrio
E. Klebsiella

37. Which of the following is a risk factor for the development of this condition?

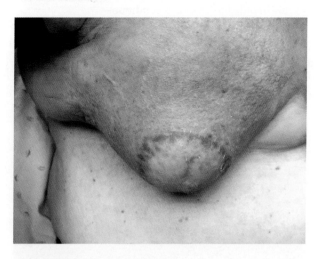

   A. Penicillamine
   B. Radiation
   C. Lymphedema
   D. PUVA
   E. Methotrexate

38. A 55-year-old woman developed the lesions below 4 months after starting which of the following medications?

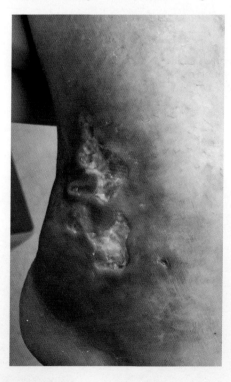

   A. Plaquenil
   B. Hydroxyurea
   C. Minocycline
   D. Penicillamine
   E. Montelukast

39. What is the best diagnosis?

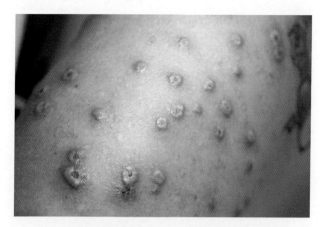

   A. Bullous pemphigoid
   B. Acute allergic contact dermatitis
   C. Leukocytoclastic vasculitis
   D. Exaggerated arthropod reaction
   E. Sweet syndrome

40. A healthy 35-year-old man presents with a new pigmented lesion. Biopsy confirms the diagnosis of melanoma with a Breslow depth of 2.1 mm, without mitoses or ulceration. What is the recommendation for treatment?

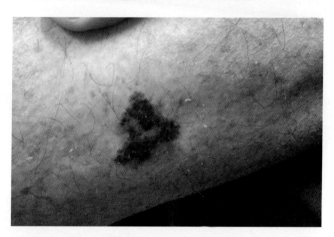

   A. Excision with 1-cm margins
   B. Excision with 2-cm margins
   C. Excision with 2-cm margins and evaluation for sentinel lymph node biopsy
   D. Neoadjuvant ipilimumab
   E. Chest x-ray and serum lactate dehydrogenase

PEDIATRIC DERMATOLOGY

41. Patients with the disease pictured below have an increased incidence of all of the following EXCEPT:

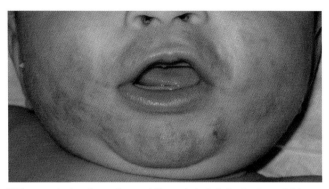

With permission from James W, et al. (eds), in *Andrews' Disease of the Skin Clinical Atlas*, 2018, Elsevier, 53–64 (fig. 5.1).

    A. Keratosis pilaris
    B. Pityriasis versicolor
    C. Palmoplantar hyperlinearity
    D. Ichthyosis vulgaris
    E. Anterior subcapsular cataracts

42. The best initial treatment for the infant pictured is:

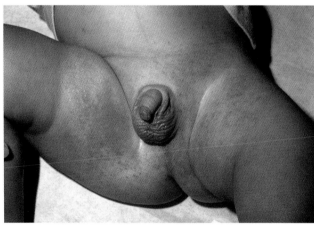

With permission from James W, et al. (eds), in *Andrews' Disease of the Skin Clinical Atlas*, 2018, Elsevier, 53–64 (fig. 5.34).

    A. Oral zinc supplementation
    B. Clotrimazole cream
    C. Hydrocortisone ointment
    D. Zinc oxide cream with frequent diaper changes
    E. Triamcinolone ointment
    F. Mupirocin ointment

43. This otherwise healthy 10-year-old boy presents with the shown clinical and dermoscopic findings. Which of the following would be the best treatment option?

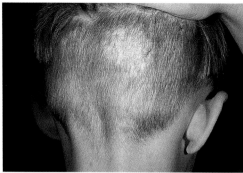

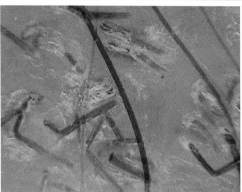

Courtesy Antonella Tosti, MD.

    A. Oral griseofulvin at 10 mg/kg/day
    B. Oral griseofulvin at 20 mg/kg/day
    C. Clomipramine
    D. Doxycycline
    E. Intralesional triamcinolone
    F. Topical clindamycin

44. The pathogenesis of this infant's rash involves which of the following?

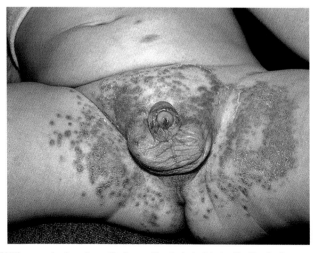

With permission from Puttgen K, et al. (eds), in *Pediatric Dermatology*, 4th edition, 2018, Elsevier, 14–67 (fig. 2.40).

A. Mutation of the *SLC39A4* gene
B. Overabundance of IL-17
C. Exposure to proteases and lipases
D. Clonal proliferation of antigen-presenting cells
E. Superficial fungal infection

45. Which of the following may trigger a systemic reaction in this patient?

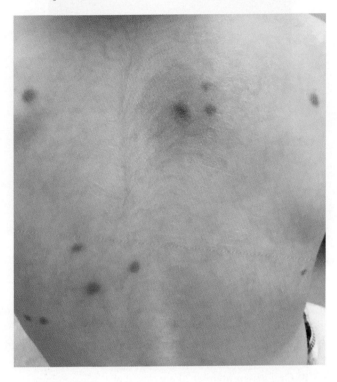

A. Acetaminophen
B. Ibuprofen
C. Cetirizine
D. Cephalexin
E. Levothyroxine

46. A 4-year-old previously healthy boy who was recently adopted and has unknown vaccination history is hospitalized for fever, malaise, runny nose, and the pictured eruption. What is the most appropriate initial treatment?

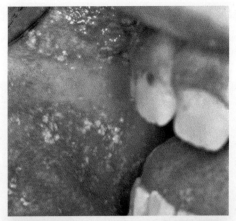

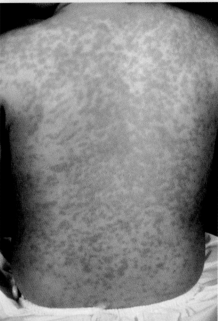

With permission from Paller A, et al. (eds), in *Hurwitz Clinical Pediatric Dermatology*, 2016, Elsevier, 382–401 (fig. 16-7) TOP FIGURE; with permission from James W, et al. (eds), in *Andrews' Disease of the Skin Clinical Atlas*, 2018, Elsevier, 263–289 (fig. 19.87) BOTTOM FIGURE.

A. Measles, mumps and rubella (MMR) vaccine
B. Vitamin A
C. Intravenous immune globulin
D. Vitamin C
E. Penicillin
F. Supportive care only

47. A 3-year-old boy presented with the pictured skin findings. What is the most likely diagnosis?

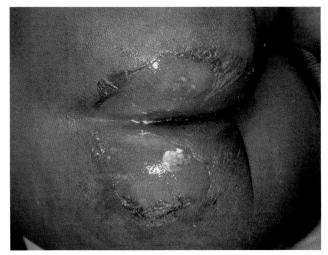

With permission from Cohen BA, in *Pediatric Dermatology*, 2013, Elsevier, 264–277 (fig. 10.9).

A. Staphylococcal scalded skin syndrome
B. Acrodermatitis enteropathica
C. Nonaccidental injury
D. Stevens-Johnson syndrome
E. Irritant contact dermatitis

48. At birth, this patient's skin was most likely notable for which of the following?

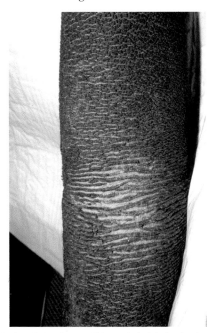

With permission from James W, et al. (eds), in *Andrews' Disease of the Skin Clinical Atlas*, 2018, Elsevier, 379–404 (fig. 27.65).

A. Blistering and erosions
B. Thick yellow-brown plates of scale with extreme eclabium and ectropion
C. Generalized fine white scales
D. Collodion membrane with ectropion and eclabium
E. Normal neonatal skin

49. An 18-month-old boy is brought in by his parents for lesions on his tongue. A representative image is shown. What is the most likely diagnosis?

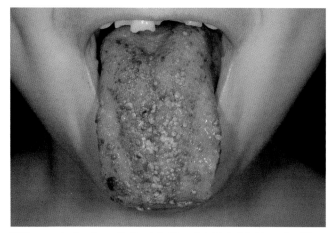

With permission from Paller AS, Mancini AJ (eds), Vascular Disorders of Infancy and Childhood, in *Hurwitz Clinical Pediatric Dermatology*, 5th edition, 2016, Elsevier, 279–316 (fig. 12-75).

A. Mucocutaneous candidiasis
B. Herpes simplex infection
C. Herpangina
D. Infantile hemangioma
E. Lymphangioma circumscriptum

50. An 18-year-old man is seen for skin evaluation, and the depicted lesions are noted. The patient reports onset during puberty. His medical history is notable for hypertension and renal disease. What other condition is this patient likely to have?

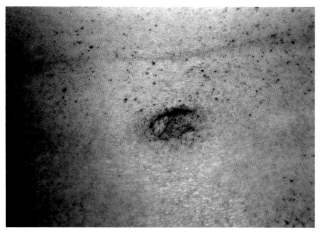

Courtesy Ken Greer, MD.

A. Arteriovenous malformation
B. Truncal ataxia
C. Peripheral neuropathy
D. Liver failure
E. Hematologic malignancy

DERMATOPATHOLOGY

51. What is the best diagnosis for this axillary lesion?

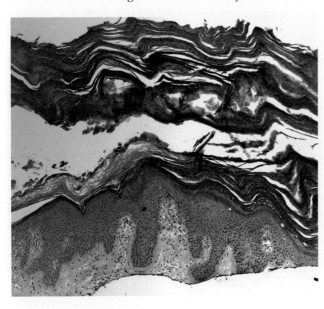

A. Acanthosis nigricans
B. Confluent and reticulate papillomatosis
C. Granular parakeratosis
D. Ichthyosis vulgaris

52. What disease is associated with this lesion?

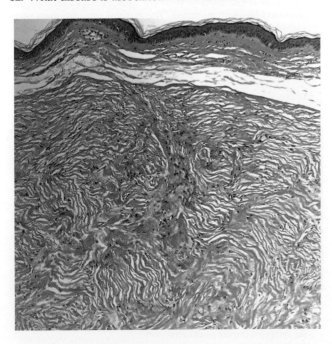

A. IgA monoclonal gammopathy
B. Cowden syndrome
C. Neurofibromatosis
D. Hereditary leiomyomatosis and renal cell cancer syndrome

53. What is the best diagnosis?

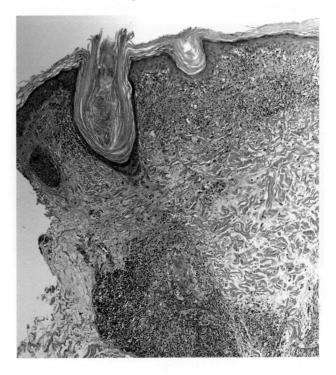

A. Dermatomyositis
B. Discoid lupus erythematosus
C. Flegel disease
D. Lichen sclerosus et atrophicus

54. What is the best diagnosis?

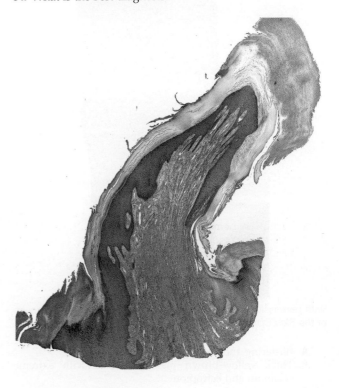

A. Accessory digit
B. Acquired digital fibrokeratoma
C. Punctate keratoderma
D. Verruca vulgaris

55. What is the best diagnosis?

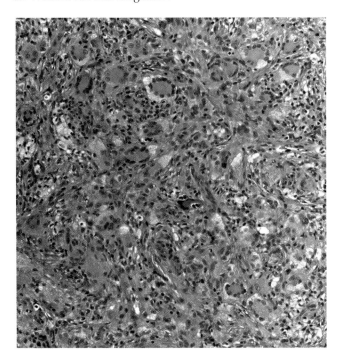

- **A.** Giant cell tumor of tendon sheath
- **B.** Necrobiotic xanthogranuloma
- **C.** Reticulohistiocytoma
- **D.** Xanthogranuloma

56. What syndrome might this lesion be associated with?

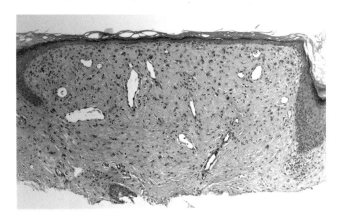

- **A.** Hereditary hemorrhagic telangiectasia
- **B.** Neurofibromatosis type I
- **C.** Reed syndrome
- **D.** Tuberous sclerosis

57. What is the best diagnosis?

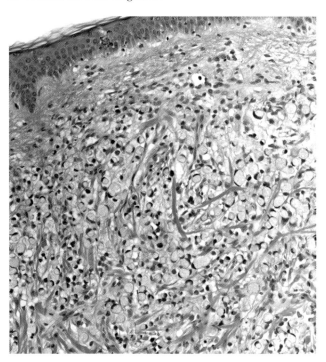

- **A.** Lepromatous leprosy
- **B.** Metastatic signet ring cell carcinoma
- **C.** Reaction to silicone injection
- **D.** Xanthoma

58. This lesion was apparent a few weeks after birth. Mutation in which of the following genes would be involved in the pathogenesis?

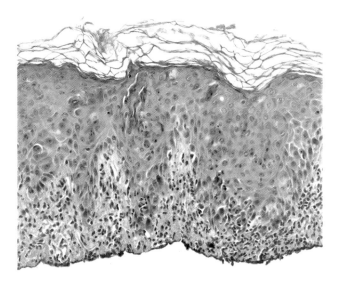

- **A.** *ATP2A2*
- **B.** *KRT1*
- **C.** *NEMO*
- **D.** *TGM1*

59. A 5-year-old boy presents with the following lesions. A shave biopsy is performed as illustrated in the figure. The patient should be counseled when he reaches reproductive age that his offspring will have a small chance of inheriting which of the following disorders:

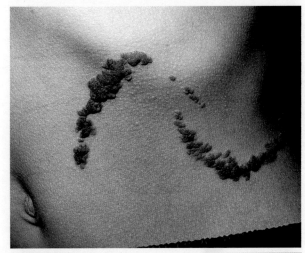

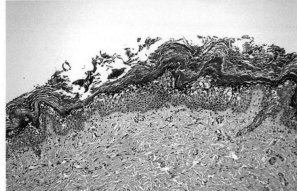

With permission from Habif TP, *Clinical Dermatology*, Elsevier, 2016, 801 (fig. 20-38, ch. 20) (*upper image*); with permission from Ross R, et al. Histopathologic characterization of epidermolytic hyperkeratosis: A systematic review of histology from the National Registry for Ichthyosis and Related Skin Disorders. *J Am Acad Dermatol*. 2008, volume 59, issue 1, 86–90 (fig. 3, p. 5) (*lower image*).

  A. Epidermal nevus syndrome
  B. No increased risk of any genetic anomaly
  C. Epidermolytic ichthyosis
  D. An epidermal nevus

60. A 10-year-old healthy girl presents with a 2-month history of low-grade fever, malaise, and skin rash. Dozens of yellow-brown papules are noted on the trunk and face. Cervical lymphadenopathy is also noted on examination. Leukocytosis is present and triglycerides are normal. A biopsy is performed (a high-power view as shown). This histologic finding is most consistent with which diagnosis:

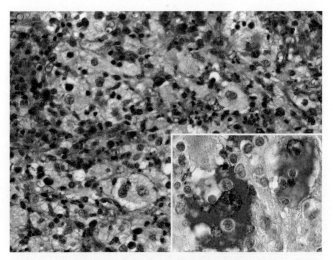

Courtesy Lorenzo Cerroni, MD.

  A. Emperipolesis—Rosai-Dorfman
  B. Hemophagocytosis—hemophagocytic lymphohistiocytosis (HLH)
  C. Parasitized macrophages—leishmaniasis
  D. Multinucleate giant cells—xanthoma disseminatum

PROCEDURAL DERMATOLOGY

61. An 87-year-old male undergoes Mohs for a large recurrent basal cell carcinoma on the posterior scalp. The tumor was cleared in two stages, resulting in an 11-centimeter defect extending to the calvarium (see image). The procedure was performed in the seated position for easier operative access. Shortly after removal of the final stage, the patient was noted to be tachypneic and complained of severe dyspnea. Soon after, he developed a right facial droop and right-sided hemiparesis. What is the most likely cause of the patient's complication?

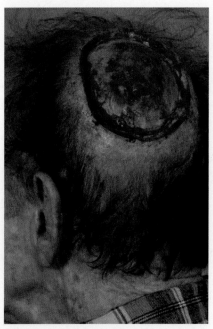

With permission from Minkis K., et al., Dermatologic Surgery Emergencies, in *J Amer Acad Derm*, 2016, Volume 75, issue 2, Elsevier, 243–262 (fig. 1).

A. Air embolism
B. Ischemic stroke
C. Hemorrhagic stroke
D. Sagittal sinus thrombosis

62. A 55-year-old man presents for treatment of the large tumor shown on the back. It has been increasing in size for over 10 years. Which of the following medications is FDA approved for locally advanced basal cell carcinoma not amenable to surgical therapy?

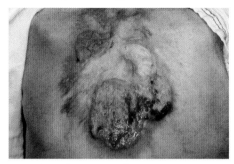

With permission from Chapman MS, Premalignant and malignant nonmelanoma skin tumors, in *Skin Disease: Diagnosis and Treatment*, Fig 17.21, Copyright © 2018, Elsevier Inc., 454–494.

A. Ipilimumab
B. Sonidegib
C. Erlotinib
D. Interferon alpha
E. 5-Fluorouracil

63. A patient had sclerotherapy performed on spider veins on her lower legs. She later developed nausea, vomiting, flushing, dizziness, and a headache. Which sclerosant was used to treat her spider veins?
A. Hypertonic saline
B. Sodium tetradecyl sulfate
C. Polidocanol
D. Glycerin
E. Sodium morrhuate

64. Which of the following is considered a permanent filler?
A. Polymethylmethacrylate
B. Calcium hydroxylapatite
C. Hyaluronic acid
D. Poly-L-lactic acid
E. Bioengineered human collagen

65. A 71-year-old man presents with a biopsy-confirmed infiltrative basal cell carcinoma of the nose. He had recent cardiac bypass surgery and is reluctant to undergo Mohs micrographic surgery or wide local excision of the skin cancer. If the lesion is treated with electrodesiccation and curettage (ED&C), what is the expected recurrence rate within 5 years?
A. Less than 5%
B. 6%–15%
C. 16%–25%
D. 26% –45%
E. Greater than 50%

66. A 45-year-old woman presents with the lesion pictured on the abdomen. It has been asymptomatic but slowly increasing in size over the last 5 years. Biopsy reveals a proliferation of bland spindle cells infiltrating the dermis and subcutaneous adipose. What is the expected prognosis for this lesion?

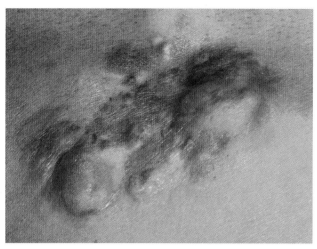

With permission from Kutzner HH, Fibrous and fibrohistiocytic proliferations of the skin and tendons, in *Dermatology*, 116, Copyright © 2018, Elsevier Limited, 2068–2085.e1. All rights reserved.

A. Remains asymptomatic with a high rate of spontaneous resolution
B. Expected progression without treatment, low rate of recurrence with complete excision
C. Expected progression without treatment, greater than 10% rate of local recurrence with complete excision
D. High risk of progression and metastasis despite aggressive treatment

67. A 59-year-old man presents with a nodular basal cell carcinoma of the left cheek. The lesion was treated with Mohs micrographic surgery, and clear surgical margins were achieved in two stages. The resulting surgical defect measured 1.2 centimeters in diameter. What is the optimal reconstructive approach to avoid ectropion of the lower eyelid?

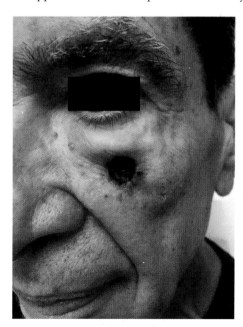

A. Linear repair with long axis of ellipse oriented vertically
B. Linear repair with long axis of ellipse oriented horizontally

C. Healing by second intention (granulation)

D. Wedge repair of the lower eyelid with or without lateral cantholysis

E. Advancement/rotation flap repair with superior advancement of the mid-cheek

68. Which of the following skin cancers is best treated with Mohs micrographic surgery according to the published appropriate use criteria?
    A. Primary nodular basal cell carcinoma on the female breast, 1.2 cm diameter
    B. Primary superficial basal cell carcinoma on the mid forehead, 0.4 cm diameter
    C. Primary nodular basal cell carcinoma arising within prior radiation treatment field on the neck, 0.5 cm diameter
    D. Actinic keratosis with focus of squamous cell carcinoma in situ on the nasal tip, 0.6 cm diameter
    E. Primary invasive squamous cell carcinoma of the shoulder, 1.0 cm diameter

69. What structure of the eye is most at risk with exposure to a Q-switched alexandrite laser?
    A. Cornea
    B. Sclera
    C. Uvea
    D. Iris
    E. Retina

70. Which ingredient in the Baker-Gordon peel is most essential for its efficacy?
    A. Phenol
    B. Croton oil
    C. Mineral oil
    D. Septisol
    E. Water

BASIC SCIENCE

71. A 15-year-old woman comes to the office with the pictured lesions on her scalp. She is asking to be enrolled in a study using ruxolitinib for treatment. What protein is targeted by ruxolitinib?

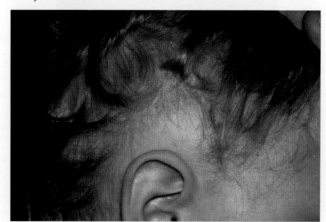

With permission from Lebwohl MG, et al. (eds), in *Treatment of Skin Diseases*, 2018, Elsevier, 29–33.

A. Mammalian target of rapamycin
B. Calcineurin
C. Janus kinase
D. Toll-like receptor 7
E. NF-kB

72. A patient with unresectable, advanced malignant melanoma is treated with talimogene laherparepvec, the first oncolytic virus approved by the FDA. Which human virus has been modified to make talimogene laherparepvec?

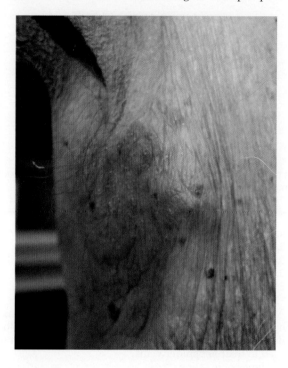

A. Coxsackie virus
B. Adenovirus
C. Coronavirus
D. Herpes simplex virus type I
E. Epstein-Barr virus

73. A 50-year-old man comes to the office with the lesion shown. He was found to have metastatic disease and was later treated with nivolumab, which blocks programmed death 1 receptor (PD-1). What is the normal function of PD-1?

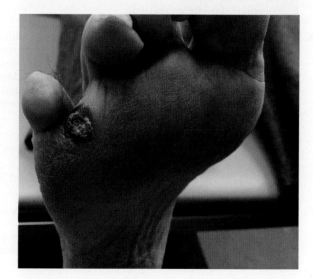

A. Membrane fusion
B. Cellular differentiation
C. Cellular growth and proliferation
D. Cell-cell adhesion
E. Inhibit activated T cells

A. Anti-MDA5
B. Anti-Scl-70
C. Anti-ECM-1
D. Anti-dsDNA
E. BPAG2

74. A patient comes to your office with these lesions on his hands as well as ulcers on his lower legs. He denies any muscle weakness but endorses worsening shortness of breath. Which autoantibody is most likely to be positive?

75. A 60-year-old man presents to your office with the pictured rash. Potassium hydroxide preparation shows yeast forms. What cell type within the epidermis is responsible for presenting the yeast antigens to lymphocytes?

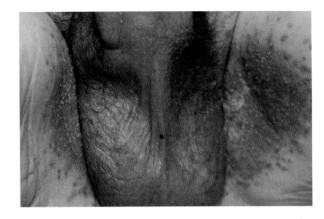

A. Melanocytes
B. Keratinocytes
C. Langerhans cell
D. Fibroblasts
E. Merkel cell

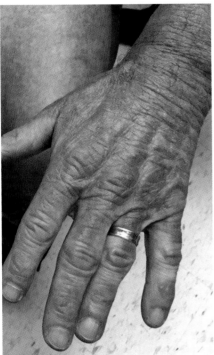

76. A 6-month-old infant presents with the lesions pictured. Which immunobullous disease targets the same antigen as the bacterial toxin produced in the lesions?

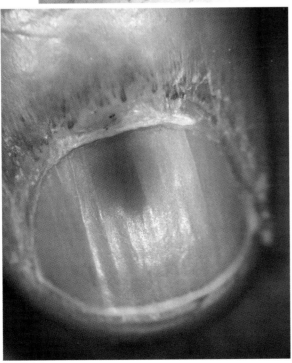

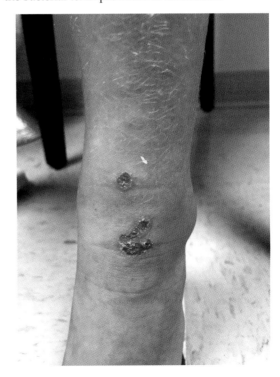

A. Pemphigus foliaceus
B. Epidermolysis bullosa
C. Bullous pemphigoid
D. Bullous lupus erythematosus
E. Linear IgA bullous dermatosis

77. A 25-year-old woman comes to the office with the rash shown. She just returned from a vacation in Hawaii. Laboratory analysis reveals an antinuclear antibody titer of 1:640. Biopsy demonstrates a subepidermal split with neutrophils. Which circulating autoantibody is most likely to be positive in this patient?

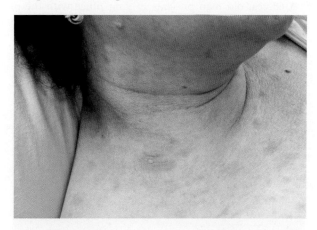

A. Desmoglein-3
B. Collagen VII
C. Collagen XVII
D. Desmoplakin
E. Desmocollin-1

78. A 65-year-old man was recently diagnosed with metastatic melanoma. Molecular analysis of the cancer is positive for *BRAF V600E* mutation and is treated with dabrafenib and trametinib. What type of protein is being targeted by trametinib?
A. G-protein coupled receptor
B. Growth factor receptor
C. Nuclear transcription factor
D. Intracellular kinase
E. Receptor tyrosine kinase

79. A 35-year-old woman with systemic lupus erythematosus comes to the office with new erythematous patches on her face. What molecular biology technique is used to detect antinuclear antibodies?
A. Mass spectroscopy
B. Enzyme-linked immunosorbent assay
C. Detection of specific proteins on sorted cells
D. Amplification of DNA
E. Nucleotide sequencing

80. A 75-year-old man comes to the office with a new lesion on his neck. A biopsy is performed and shows numerous small round blue cells with granular chromatin and nuclear molding. What immunotherapy is approved for patients with metastatic disease?

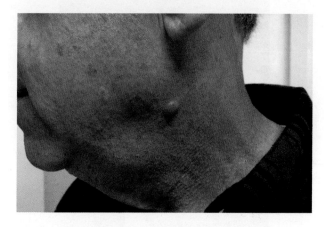

A. Anti–cytotoxic T-lymphocyte-associated protein-4
B. Recombinant interleukin-2
C. Talimogene laherparepvec
D. Anti–programmed cell death ligand 1
E. Anti–interleukin 17A

GENERAL DERMATOLOGY

1. C. Noninfectious granulomas
This patient has ataxia telangiectasia (AT), which is characterized by ataxia at a young age, oculocutaneous telangiectasias; immunodeficiency with sinopulmonary infections; increased sensitivity to ionizing radiation; and an increased risk of leukemia/lymphomas. It is caused by a mutation in the *ATM* gene, leading to a faulty response to DNA damage, particularly of double-stranded DNA breaks. Although patients with AT may develop gray hairs, diffuse graying of the hairs typically does not occur until adolescence if it occurs. Silvery hair is commonly seen is Chédiak-Higashi syndrome. Hyperimmunoglobulin E syndrome is commonly associated with early-onset eczematous dermatitis. Eczematous dermatitis has been reported in AT, but noninfectious granulomatous dermatitis is a more common clinical finding. Gingivitis/periodontitis is commonly seen in leukocyte adhesion deficiency.
Bolognia J, Schaffer J, Cerroni L, eds. *Dermatology.* [Philadelphia]: Elsevier, 2018 (ch. 60).

2. D. Quinacrine
Amiodarone may cause a slate-gray discoloration most commonly of sun-exposed skin, with the face being the most common site of discoloration. Chlorpromazine and diltiazem can also give slate-gray discoloration in sun-exposed skin. Quinacrine typically results in a yellow or yellow-brown pigmentation.
Bolognia J, Schaffer J, Cerroni L, eds. *Dermatology.* [Philadelphia]: Elsevier, 2018 (ch. 67).

3. D. t(17;22)
Dermatofibroma sarcoma protuberans (DFSP) is a locally aggressive sarcoma that is most commonly seen in young to middle-aged adults. The trunk, especially the shoulder and pelvic regions, is the most common location (50%–60%) of these tumors. DFSP begins as an indurated, usually skin-colored plaque that later develops into violaceous to red-brown nodules. The chromosomal abnormality seen in DFSP is a translocation between chromosome 17 and 22 that fuses the collagen type 1α1 (*COL 1A1*) gene with the platelet-derived growth factor (PDGF) β-chain gene (*PDGFB*). This translocation results in an overexpression of *PDGFB*, which stimulates the growth of mesenchymal cells. Imatinib targets the PDGF receptor (as well as other proteins with tyrosine kinase activity) and therefore can be used in patients with unresectable, recurrent, or metastatic DFSP. Mohs or wide local excision, however, is the preferred treatment for localized, primary tumors.

A translocation of (9;22) results in the chimeric *bcr-abl* gene seen in chronic myelogenous leukemia (CML); t(11;22) is found in Ewing's sarcoma.
Bolognia J, Schaffer J, Cerroni L, eds. *Dermatology.* [Philadelphia]: Elsevier, 2018 (ch. 116).

4. **A.** Simvastatin
Dermatomyositis is an autoimmune disease that in its classic form affects the skin and muscles. This picture demonstrates the "shawl sign," the photo-distributed poikiloderma involving the upper back that is characteristic of dermatomyositis. While the clinical and histopathologic findings in dermatomyositis can be difficult to distinguish from systemic lupus erythematosus, dermatomyositis is often intensely pruritic, which serves as a distinguishing feature. There is a high association with malignancy in adults presenting with dermatomyositis; however, drug-induced causes must also be considered. Medications known to induce dermatomyositis include hydroxyurea, lipid-lowering drugs (statins > gemfibrozil), TNF-α inhibitors, nonsteroidal antiinflammatory drugs (NSAIDs), cyclophosphamide, checkpoint inhibitors (e.g., ipilimumab), Bacillus Calmette–Guérin (BCG) vaccine, D-penicillamine, and single cases of alfuzosin (α-agonist for benign prostatic hyperplasia), articaine, etoposide, interferon-α-2b, ipecac (repeated exposures), omeprazole, phenytoin, sulfacetamide sodium ophthalmic drops, tegafur, terbinafine, and zoledronic acid.
Furosemide is a common culprit of drug-induced bullous pemphigoid. Thiazide diuretics (e.g., hydrochlorothiazide) can cause drug-induced lichenoid eruptions and drug-induced subacute cutaneous lupus erythematosus. Beta-blockers (e.g., metoprolol) are known to exacerbate psoriasis.
Bolognia J, Schaffer J, Cerroni L, eds. *Dermatology.* [Philadelphia]: Elsevier, 2018 (ch. 42).

5. **C.** Lung cancer
Immunoglobulin A (IgA) small vessel vasculitis in adults is sometimes referred to as adult Henoch-Schönlein purpura (HSP). While both typically present with palpable purpura on extensor extremities and/or buttocks, the clinical presentation and prognosis do have important differences. In adult IgA small vessel vasculitis, necrotic skin lesions are found in 60% of adults, while less than 5% of children with HSP have cutaneous necrosis. Adults with IgA vasculitis are also more likely than children to develop chronic renal insufficiency. IgA vasculitis is also often associated with malignancy (60%–90%), most commonly cancer of a solid organ. Lung cancer is the most common cancer associated with IgA vasculitis. In contrast, cutaneous small vessel vasculitis–associated malignancy is most often associated with hematologic malignancy.
Bolognia J, Schaffer J, Cerroni L, eds. *Dermatology.* [Philadelphia]: Elsevier, 2018 (ch. 24).

6. **A.** Intrapartum and postpartum hemorrhage
Intrahepatic cholestasis of pregnancy (ICP) is a genetically linked form of cholestasis that presents in the last trimester of pregnancy with significant pruritus without primary skin lesions. Elevated total serum bile acid levels are diagnostic, and treatment is with ursodeoxycholic acid. Reoccurrences in subsequent pregnancies are common (45%–70%). Associated fetal risks include prematurity, intrapartum fetal distress, and stillbirth. While overall maternal prognosis is good, approximately 10% develop jaundice, which can be associated with extrahepatic cholestasis and steatorrhea. This can lead to vitamin K deficiency, resulting in an increased risk of intra- and postpartum hemorrhage. The bile acids that cross the placenta are toxic and can lead to impaired fetal cardiomyocyte function but do not cause cardiac abnormalities

in the mother. There is no risk of permanent liver dysfunction to the mother. While ICP is associated with greater risks to the fetus, the mother is also at risk for complications as above.
Bolognia J, Schaffer J, Cerroni L, eds. *Dermatology.* [Philadelphia]: Elsevier, 2018 (ch. 27).

7. **D.** Squamous cell carcinoma
Erythema ab igne is a relatively common disorder caused by chronic exposure to local heat source. This patient had chronic abdominal pain due to his carcinoid and used a heating pad constantly to reduce his pain. This chronic heat exposure leads to reticulated erythema and later permanent reticulated hyperpigmentation, sometimes with secondary epidermal change such as atrophy or hyperkeratosis in later stages. Bullous lesions may develop as well. Increased risk of secondary cutaneous malignancies has been reported, namely squamous cell carcinoma and Merkel cell carcinoma. Rare reports of other malignancies, such as cutaneous marginal zone lymphoma, atypical cutaneous reactive angiomatosis, and poorly differentiated carcinoma, have been reported as well.
Bolognia J, Schaffer J, Cerroni L, eds. *Dermatology.* [Philadelphia]: Elsevier, 2018 (ch. 88).

8. **D.** Cutaneous collagenous vasculopathy
Cutaneous collagenous vasculopathy (CCV) is a benign condition of unknown etiology. It clinically can resemble generalized essential telangiectasia; however, the unique histologic findings can help distinguish them. Biopsy of CCV shows ectatic superficial blood vessels with hyalinization of the basement membranes of affected vessels. This material is PAS-positive and diastase-resistant. Biopsy of older lesions in patients with erythropoietic protoporphyria (EPP) also demonstrates Periodic acid-Schiff (PAS)-positive hyaline material around superficial blood vessels. Clinically, however, the photosensitive eruption of EPP is readily distinguishable from CCV. Hereditary hemorrhagic telangiectasia (HHT) presents with multiple telangiectasias most commonly on the face, tongue, lips, hands, and fingers. HHT may also have visceral involvement (e.g., gastrointestinal tract, lung, liver, CNS, etc.).
Bolognia J, Schaffer J, Cerroni L, eds. *Dermatology.* [Philadelphia]: Elsevier, 2018 (chs. 4 & 106).

9. **B.** Vemurafenib
Vemurafenib and other B-Raf (BRAF) inhibitors are associated with an increased production of squamous cell carcinomas (SCCs) and keratoacanthomas (KAs), the latter of which is depicted here. Up to 25% of patients receiving these therapies develop SCCs or KAs. They are more likely to develop in patients with photodamage and can begin within weeks of exposure to the medication. The addition of an mitogen-activated protein kinase kinase (MEK) inhibitor to a BRAF inhibitor significantly reduces the incidence of SCCs and KAs.
Trametinib is an MEK inhibitor. MEK inhibitors alone are not associated with an increased risk of SCCs and KAs. Some of the side effects seen with MEK inhibitors include rash, papulopustular eruptions, fatigue, peripheral edema, and diarrhea. Ipilimumab is a CTLA-4 inhibitor. Common side effects of CTLA-4 blockade include dermatitis, colitis, hepatitis, thyroiditis, hypophysitis, and vitiligo-like leukoderma. Nivolumab is a PD-1 inhibitor. Common side effects of PD-1 inhibitors are similar to those of CTLA-4 inhibitors, including dermatitis (in particular lichenoid, psoriasiform, and immunobullous), pneumonitis, nephritis, and colitis.
Bolognia J, Schaffer J, Cerroni L, eds. *Dermatology.* [Philadelphia]: Elsevier, 2018 (chs. 21 & 113).

10. A. Increased risk of recurrent *Neisseria meningitides* infections

Barraquer-Simons syndrome or acquired partial lipo-dystrophy (APL) is the second most common type of nonlocalized lipodystrophy. Onset is during childhood or prepuberty with a cephalocaudal pattern of subcutaneous fat loss. Women are affected more commonly than men, and nephritic syndrome is seen in one-fifth of patients. There is an association with autoimmune conditions such as lupus, dermatomyositis, hypothyroidism, celiac disease, and others. In addition, almost all those with APL have low levels of C3 and C3-nephritic factor. The low C3 level predisposes patients to recurrent *Neisseria meningitides* infections.

In congenital generalized lipodystrophy (Berardinelli-Seip syndrome) and acquired generalized lipodystrophy (Lawrence-Seip syndrome), liver disease is a significant cause of death. Generalized loss or absence of subcutaneous fat from birth is seen in congenital generalized lipodystrophy. Familial partial lipodystrophy (FPL) is associated with excess fat accumulation of the head and neck with characteristic acromegalic facies and double chin.

Bolognia J, Schaffer J, Cerroni L, eds. *Dermatology.* [Philadelphia]: Elsevier, 2018 (ch. 101).

11. D. HPV 16

The human papillomavirus is responsible for warts and papillomas, both benign and malignant. There are over 100 genotypes responsible for different manifestations of verrucae. High-risk HPV types are concerning due to their oncogenic potential. HPV 16 (D) and, less frequently, 18, 31, 33, and 45 have been detected in cervical and anal cancers. They have also been detected in a subset of some vaginal, vulvar, penile, oropharyngeal, and digital squamous cell carcinomas.

HPV 13 and 32 (A) are exclusively associated with focal epithelial hyperplasia, also called Heck disease. It clinically manifests as flat wartlike or condyloma-like lesions on the gingival, buccal, labial mucosa of children, especially from South America. HPV 2 and 7 (B) are associated with Butcher's warts, prevalent on the hands of meat and fish handlers. HPV 5 and 8 (C) are associated with squamous cell carcinomas in patients with epidermodysplasia verruciformis. HPV 6 and 11 (E) preferentially infect the anogenital mucosae and upper aerodigestive tract and are associated with condyloma acuminata (genital warts), Buschke-Löwenstein tumor, and recurrent oral papillomatosis.

Bolognia J, Schaffer J, Cerroni L, eds. *Dermatology.* [Philadelphia]: Elsevier, 2018 (ch. 79).

12. B. Foscarnet

Severe and chronic herpes simplex infection is often seen in immunocompromised patients (e.g., HIV, leukemia/lymphoma) or in patients following hematopoietic stem cell transplantation or solid organ transplantation on immunosuppressive therapy. The clinical manifestations may be atypical, including larger, chronic ulcers, which may be verrucous compared to the usual grouped vesicles and scalloped ulcerations seen in classical herpes simplex virus (HSV) infection. Acyclovir-resistant HSV infection is an emerging problem in immunocompromised patients that should be recognized. The treatment of choice for acyclovir-resistant HSV infection is foscarnet (B). Cidofovir has also shown promising results.

Azithromycin (A) is the treatment of choice for both chancroids and granuloma inguinale. Penicillin G (C) is the treatment of choice for syphilis. Famciclovir (D) is the prodrug form of penciclovir with increased oral bioavailability and is used to treat HSV infection in immunocompetent patients.

Bolognia J, Schaffer J, Cerroni L, eds. *Dermatology.* [Philadelphia]: Elsevier, 2018 (ch. 80).

13. A. Hospitalize and initiate intravenous acyclovir

Eczema herpeticum is a widespread HSV infection that typically affects infants and toddlers with atopic dermatitis. Adults with impaired skin barrier, such as Darier disease and Hailey-Hailey disease, are also at risk. It typically presents as acute onset of monomorphic punched-out erosions in areas of atopic dermatitis. Clinical features that may indicate a requirement for hospitalization and intravenous acyclovir treatment include male sex, age <1 year, fever, and systemic symptoms. Superficial wound culture, topical steroids, and oral antibiotics are used to treat atopic dermatitis with impetiginization. Bleach baths and mupirocin ointment are used for decolonization of staph aureus. Penciclovir cream is used in the treatment of herpes labialis.

Bolognia J, Schaffer J, Cerroni L, eds. *Dermatology.* [Philadelphia]: Elsevier, 2018 (ch. 80).

14. D. Type VII collagen

This patient has cicatricial pemphigoid or mucous membrane pemphigoid, which is a subepithelial blistering disorder that can lead to severe mucosal scarring. The oral mucosa and conjunctiva are the two most frequently affected mucous membranes. While there can be involvement of both mucosa and skin, this patient has only ocular findings (ocular mucous membrane pemphigoid), a variant associated with autoantibodies against alpha 6 beta 4 integrin. Antilaminin 332 and anti-BP180 antibodies are also associated with cicatricial pemphigoid. Autoantibodies against type VII collagen are seen in epidermolysis bullosa acquisita (EBA), not mucous membrane pemphigoid.

Bolognia J, Schaffer J, Cerroni L, eds. *Dermatology.* [Philadelphia]: Elsevier, 2018 (ch. 30).

15. D. Cytarabine

The patient developed neutrophilic eccrine hidradenitis (NEH), which is a toxic disorder of the sweat glands that is commonly associated with chemotherapeutic drugs. This eruption is thought to result from direct cytotoxic effects of chemotherapy on the eccrine glands. Commonly associated drugs include cytarabine, daunorubicin, bleomycin, and cyclophosphamide. Sorafenib is a tyrosine kinase inhibitor that is associated with hand-foot-skin reaction, among other dermatologic toxicities.

Bolognia J, Schaffer J, Cerroni L, eds. *Dermatology.* [Philadelphia]: Elsevier, 2018 (ch. 39).

16. D. Primary Epstein-Barr virus (EBV) infection

Large painful ulcers in prepubescent girls have been associated with primary EBV infection. These are non-sexually-acquired genital ulcerations and are also known as Lipschütz ulcers. They are more common in females and are occasionally associated with acute systemic illness, such as upper respiratory infection and gastroenteritis.

The most common cause of genital ulcers are due to herpes infection, typically HSV type 2, which manifests with grouped vesicles and scalloped ulcers. This is a sexually transmitted infection. Primary HIV infection typically presents as a mononucleosis-like illness approximately 1–6 weeks postexposure to HIV. It may present with a morbilliform exanthem, lymphadenopathy, and genital ulcers. Cytomegalovirus (CMV) has been found in genital ulcers in immunosuppressed patients. Behçet disease is a neutrophilic dermatosis that presents with recurrent oral and genital aphthous-like ulcers, as well as ocular involvement (uveitis, conjunctivitis, and retinal vasculitis). Patients may occasionally have cutaneous findings that

include facial/acral papulopustules, purpura, erythema nodosum-like lesions on the lower extremities, and a positive pathergy test.
Bolognia J, Schaffer J, Cerroni L, eds. *Dermatology*. [Philadelphia]: Elsevier, 2018 (ch. 2).

17. **B.** Spindle cells with slitlike spaces containing red blood cells
Kaposi sarcoma (KS) is a vascular neoplasm caused by Human Herpesvirus-8 (HHV-8) infection that typically manifests with blue-violaceous papules and nodules that favor the lower extremities. Four clinical variants include:
1. Classic: typically older men of Mediterranean and Ashkenazi Jewish descent; favors lower legs
2. African-endemic: typically young African males in endemic areas; may have lymph node involvement
3. Iatrogenic immunosuppression-associated: solid-organ transplant patients
4. AIDS-related epidemic: AIDS patients; typically widespread and may affect the oral mucosa

Histologically, nodular stage KS presents as a spindle cell proliferation with slitlike spaces containing red blood cells. The spindle cells may be plump but never as atypical and hyperchromatic as in angiosarcoma (choice C). All lesions KS will stain positive for HHV-8 or latency-associated nuclear antigen (LANA-1).
Leukocytoclastic vasculitis (LCV) is a small vessel vasculitis that demonstrates neutrophilic nuclear debris surrounding damaged blood vessels (choice A). Clinically, LCV presents as symmetric palpable purpura of the lower extremities and on pressure-dependent sites. Leukemia cutis (choice D) shows atypical and immature myeloid cells. They may dissect collagen fibers in a single-cell fashion, termed "Indian filing." There may be a clear unaffected area (Grenz zone) immediately under the epidermis.
Bolognia J, Schaffer J, Cerroni L, eds. *Dermatology*. [Philadelphia]: Elsevier, 2018 (ch. 80).

18. **C.** Recommend Zika diagnostic testing for the patient and his girlfriend
Zika virus infection is caused by a flavivirus, which also causes Dengue and Yellow fever. Only 20% of patients infected with Zika virus will become symptomatic, typically manifesting with fevers, arthralgias, headache, conjunctivitis, and a cephalocaudally spreading morbilliform exanthem. Large outbreaks have been reported in the Pacific Islands, Central and South America, Caribbean Islands, and Mexico. Zika has been linked to fetal microcephaly. The Center for Disease Control and Prevention currently recommends serum and urine real-time PCR (RT-PCR) and immunoglobulin M (IgM) serology diagnostic testing for all symptomatic patients with a possible exposure to Zika virus as well as asymptomatic pregnant patients with a possible exposure to Zika virus.
While supportive care including rest, hydration, and analgesics is recommended for Zika virus infection, appropriate diagnostic testing is paramount, especially for pregnant patients. Intravenous immunoglobulin is not an appropriate treatment option for Zika virus infection. Chikungunya virus infection (choice D) typically presents with high-grade fevers, severe arthralgias and headaches, retro-orbital pain, photophobia, and a morbilliform rash. While the manifestation may be similar to Zika virus infection, symptoms are typically much more severe.
Bolognia J, Schaffer J, Cerroni L, eds. *Dermatology*. [Philadelphia]: Elsevier, 2018 (ch. 81).

19. **D.** Calciphylaxis
Calciphylaxis presents as tender, indurated, deep subcutaneous plaques or nodules with a predilection for fat-bearing areas. Initial lesions typically manifest as ill-defined, painful erythema or retiform purpura and typically progress to ulceration. The lesions are usually rock hard and induration may extend beyond the boarder of the visible lesion. Classically, calciphylaxis occurs in patients with renal disease, although there is a subset of patients who do not have end-stage renal disease (i.e., nonuremic calciphylaxis). Other risk factors include obesity, diabetes, female gender, warfarin use, liver disease, hyperparathyroidism, and calcium and vitamin D supplementation. Infection with subsequent sepsis is the leading cause of death. Treatment includes early recognition, discontinuation of vitamin and calcium supplements, correction of calcium and phosphate metabolism, and increased frequency of dialysis (for those already on dialysis) with low calcium dialysate. Sodium thiosulfate, both intravenously and intralesionally, can also be used for treatment. Aggressive wound care is necessary, and hyperbaric oxygen has been successfully used. Other treatments reported to be effective include anticoagulation with low-molecular-weight heparin, vitamin K, and maggot therapy. Venous ulcers are most commonly found on the medial aspect of the lower leg with other signs of venous insufficiency, including varicosities, lipodermatosclerosis, and hemosiderin deposition. Arterial ulcers typically present as punched-out dry ulcerations, classically on the lateral malleoli. Surrounding skin may be atrophic and lack hair. Medium vessel vasculitis is on the differential diagnosis for calciphylaxis; however, tender lesions on fat-bearing sites in a patient with renal disease should prompt a high suspicion for calciphylaxis. Ecthyma is a bacterial infection usually caused by group A streptococcus that presents as punched-out ulceration with an eschar.
Bolognia J, Schaffer J, Cerroni L, eds. *Dermatology*. [Philadelphia]: Elsevier, 2018 (ch. 50).

20. **C.** Epidermolysis bullosa acquisita (EBA)
EBA is an acquired autoimmune mechanobullous disease characterized by antibodies against collagen type VII. The disease has various presentations but most commonly presents with noninflammatory bulla that heal with milia and scarring. Common locations include the dorsal hands, elbows, knees, dorsal feet, and toes. Less commonly, it can present with inflammatory bullous lesions similar to bullous pemphigoid. Mucous membranes may be involved and nail dystrophy may occur. Systemic lupus erythematosus, inflammatory bowel disease, and rheumatoid arthritis have been reported in association with EBA. Diagnosis is confirmed histologically and with immunohistological studies. Histologically, there is a subepidermal split with pauci-inflammatory infiltrate. Direct immunofluorescence shows linear immunoglobulin G (IgG) against the basement membrane, and IgG typically deposits on the dermal side of salt-split biopsies. Treatments include systemic steroids, immunosuppressants, dapsone, and IVIG.
Discoid lupus erythematosus can present with hypopigmented and hyperpigmented lesions that scar but are usually located on the head and neck. PCT is a mechanobullous eruption that heals with milia that usually presents on the dorsal hands in the setting of medications, alcoholism, and liver disease. Bullous pemphigoid is an inflammatory bullous disease that does not typically heal with scarring like in EBA. IgG typically deposits on the epidermal side of salt-split biopsies in its classical form. Dermatitis herpetiformis typically presents on extensor surfaces with pruritic vesicles and erosions. It is associated with gluten sensitivity, and patients should be screened for celiac disease.
Bolognia J, Schaffer J, Cerroni L, eds. *Dermatology*. [Philadelphia]: Elsevier, 2018 (ch. 32).

21. **D.** Glucose-6-phosphate dehydrogenase
Cyclosporine is used frequently in dermatology to treat psoriasis, drug hypersensitivity reactions, neutrophilic dermatosis, and other inflammatory conditions. A benefit of this treatment is its rapid onset of action. Side effects include nephrotoxicity, hyperkalemia, hypomagnesemia, hyperuricemia, hyperlipidemia, hypertension, paresthesia, hypertrichosis, and gingival hyperplasia. Prior to starting cyclosporine, blood pressure, lipid level, renal function, potassium, magnesium, and uric acid should be evaluated. Cyclosporine metabolism is not affected by glucose-6-phosphate dehydrogenase deficiency. This enzyme should be checked prior to initiation of certain medications, such as antimalarials and dapsone, as inherited deficiency of this enzyme may result in severe hemolysis with their use.
Bolognia J, Schaffer J, Cerroni L, eds. *Dermatology.* [Philadelphia]: Elsevier, 2018 (ch. 130).

22. **B.** Pancreatitis
The clinical picture is that of eruptive xanthomas, which present as dome-shaped red to yellow papules on the extensor surface of the arms, hands, and buttocks. They occur in the setting of primary or secondary hypertriglyceridemia. Obesity, diabetes, estrogen supplementation, and medications that can lead to hypertriglyceridemia are risk factors. Pancreatitis may be an associated complication of hypertriglyceridemia. Treatment consists of lowering the triglyceride level with oral lipid-lowering agents.
Dermatitis herpetiformis is the eruption associated with gluten enteropathy and typically presents with pruritic vesicles on the extremities, face, and scalp. Monoclonal gammopathy is not associated with eruptive xanthomas but rather with normolipemic plane xanthomas. Hypothyroidism can result in a secondary hyperlipidemia. Acute pancreatitis is more likely to be associated with eruptive xanthomas compared to hypothyroidism.
Bolognia J, Schaffer J, Cerroni L, eds. *Dermatology.* [Philadelphia]: Elsevier, 2018 (ch. 92).

23. **A.** Urine toxicology screen
The figure shows a purpuric patch on the ear, which is indicative of microvascular injury either due to vasculopathy and/or vasculitis. Retiform purpura on acral sites (i.e., ear, nose, distal extremities) may occur in various conditions such as levamisole toxicity (cocaine or heroin may be adulterated with levamisole), antiphospholipid syndrome, and type I cryoglobulinemia. Levamisole toxicity typically presents with retiform purpura with ulcerations and can favor acral sites. Pyoderma gangrenosum-like lesions may also occur. There may be systemic manifestations, including arthralgias, fevers, seizures, and glomerulonephritis. Additionally, leukopenia and neutropenia may occur as well as positive autoantibodies, including antineutrophil cytoplasmic antibody, antinuclear antibody, anti-double stranded DNA antibody, and lupus anticoagulant. Pathology typically shows both vasculitis and vasculopathy with intravascular thrombi and involvement of superficial and deep dermal vessels. Infective endocarditis can present with septic emboli, which may also favor distal acral sites and would be on the differential diagnosis. Type I cryoglobulinemia also presents with an occlusive vasculopathy favoring acral sites and is associated with a monoclonal gammopathy. Purpuric lesions on the ears may also be present with this entity.
Necrotizing infections can present with retiform purpura and may require a sterile tissue culture but are unlikely to be localized to the ear. Relapsing polychondritis is characterized by recurrent episodes of chondritis of the ear, nose, and tracheal cartilage. Antibodies to type II collagen may be found in this disease. The presentation here is consistent with purpura, not chondritis. X-ray is not indicated in the evaluation of acral retiform purpura.
Bolognia J, Schaffer J, Cerroni L, eds. *Dermatology.* [Philadelphia]: Elsevier, 2018 (ch. 23).

24. **D.** Phytophotodermatitis
The patient's leg was exposed to lime juice during sun exposure, resulting in phytophotodermatitis. This phototoxic reaction occurs with certain plants and citrus (limes, celery, rue, figs, lemon, parsley, parsnips, hogweed, bergamot orange). The furocoumarins are the most common culprit. Clinically, there is an initial erythema with or without bulla followed by postinflammatory hyperpigmentation, which may be streaky as demonstrated in the figure. Necrotizing fasciitis is a rapidly progressive infection that presents with dusky erythema, bullae, and tenderness out of proportion to examination, which may be a clinical clue as well as rapid progression and failure to respond to antibiotics. A brown recluse (Loxosceles) spider bite is a dermatonecrotic bite reaction that often manifests as erythema followed by purpura and ulceration. Shock, hemolysis, and disseminated intravascular coagulation may rarely occur.
Calciphylaxis (commonly associated with end-stage renal disease) presents as painful retiform purpura and tender plaques which may ulcerate, often in fat-bearing areas.
Bolognia J, Schaffer J, Cerroni L, eds. *Dermatology.* [Philadelphia]: Elsevier, 2018 (ch. 17).

25. **C.** Allergic contact dermatitis
There is erythema, vesicles, and crusting in the surrounding postoperative area. The patient had been applying neomycin/bacitracin/polymyxin to the wound and presented with this expanding rash and intense pruritus consistent with an allergic contact dermatitis. All postoperative eruptions should be evaluated for infection, which presents as erythema, pain, with or without fevers, and systemic symptoms. Antipseudomonal coverage (i.e., ciprofloxacin) should be considered. Chondritis is inflammation of the cartilage and may occur after ear surgery and can be managed with antiinflammatory drugs. It would not manifest with epidermal change as demonstrated in the figure. Tinea corporis can occur in the postoperative setting underneath an occlusive and moist bandage, and present with a sharper boarder, annular configuration with scale and/or pustules.
Bolognia J, Schaffer J, Cerroni L, eds. *Dermatology.* Philadelphia]: Elsevier, 2018 (ch. 14).

26. **B.** Corticosteroid-induced hypopigmentation
The patient has hypopigmentation secondary to intralesional injection of triamcinolone, with streaky hypopigmentation. With time the hypopigmentation often repigments. Vitiligo classically manifests with periorificial, acral, and genital depigmentation, with areas of follicular repigmentation. Hypopigmented mycosis fungoides typically presents as hypopigmented annular and polycyclic patches in photoprotected areas. Morphea would not present as streaky hypopigmentation but rather as sclerotic hyperpigmented plaques with an inflammatory halo in the acute stages. Lichen sclerosus presents with ivory white plaques, typically on the genital mucosa, but extragenital disease may occur as well.
Bolognia J, Schaffer J, Cerroni L, eds. *Dermatology.* [Philadelphia]: Elsevier, 2018 (ch. 125).

27. D. Renal cell carcinoma
The patient has familial cutaneous leiomyomatosis. This condition presents with multiple cutaneous leiomyomas, which typically manifest as tender erythematous papules/nodules. Patients have a predisposition to develop renal cell carcinoma and uterine leiomyomas. The genetic defect is in fumarate hydratase. It is important for patients to undergo surveillance for renal cell carcinoma.
Spontaneous pneumothoraces may occur in Birt-Hogg-Dube, which manifests with fibrofolliculomas, trichodiscomas, and acrochordons. Patients may also develop renal tumors. Mutation is in the gene coding for folliculin. Colorectal carcinoma may occur in Gardner syndrome due to mutations in the *APC* gene. Patients may also manifest with epidermoid cysts, pilomatricomas, lipomas, fibromas, and desmoid tumors. Gastrointestinal cancers may also develop in Peutz-Jeghers syndrome (hyperpigmented macules on mucosa surfaces), Cowden disease (trichilemmomas, cobblestoning of the oral mucosa, acral keratotic papules), and Muir-Torre syndrome (sebaceous neoplasms, multiple keratoacanthomas). Retinoblastoma and non–small cell lung carcinoma are not features of these syndromes.
Bolognia J, Schaffer J, Cerroni L, eds. *Dermatology.* [Philadelphia]: Elsevier, 2018 (ch. 53).

28. D. A & C
The kodachrome depicts macular amyloidosis, which manifests as rippled hyperpigmentation. It may be associated with notalgia paresthetica due to degenerative disc disease. In addition, multiple endocrine neoplasia type 2A (medullary carcinoma of the thyroid, pheochromocytomas, and hyperparathyroidism) has been associated with macular and lichen amyloidosis. A diagnosis of multiple endocrine neoplasia type 2A should be considered in young adults and children who present with extensive macular or lichen amyloid.
Confluent and reticulated papillomatosis presents as hyperpigmented macules, papules coalescing into patches/plaques with netlike configuration peripherally. It may be associated with insulin resistance, including diabetes mellitus and polycystic ovarian syndrome. Minocycline is the treatment of choice.
Bolognia J, Schaffer J, Cerroni L, eds. *Dermatology.* [Philadelphia]: Elsevier, 2018 (ch. 47).

29. A. Terbinafine
The patient has subacute cutaneous lupus erythematosus (SCLE), which is typically photosensitive and manifests with annular or papulosquamous plaques. It is important to consider drug-induced SCLE, which is associated with various common medications, including hydrochlorothiazide, terbinafine, calcium channel blockers, nonsteroidal antiinflammatory drugs (NSAIDs), griseofulvin, and antihistamines. Approximately 10%–15% of patients may develop systemic lupus. Titers for anti-SSA (Ro) may be elevated. The other medications are not typically associated with SCLE.
Penicillin commonly causes urticarial and exanthematous drug eruptions. Penicillamine may be associated with various reactions, including systemic lupus erythematosus, pemphigus vulgaris and foliaceus, pemphigoid, elastosis perforans serpiginosa, lichen planus, pseudoxanthoma elasticum-like eruption, and dermatomyositis-like reactions. Vemurafenib, the BRAF inhibitor, may be associated with various reactions, including maculopapular, keratosis pilaris-like, photosensitive, and erythema nodosum-like reactions. Prednisone may be associated with striae, dyspigmentation, and steroid-acne, which

typically manifests as monomorphic follicular papules and pustules.
Bolognia J, Schaffer J, Cerroni L, eds. *Dermatology.* [Philadelphia]: Elsevier, 2018 (ch. 41).

30. B. Serum immunofixation electrophoresis
The patient has scleromyxedema, a type of mucinosis characterized by a generalized symmetric eruption of waxy firm papules and induration and thickening of the skin. Infiltration of the hands with "donut sign" is classic, as illustrated in the kodachrome, and may be associated with decreased mobility. Involvement of the hands, forearms, face (leonine facies), neck, thighs, and upper trunk is typical. Patients should be screened for monoclonal gammopathy (paraproteinemia), which is associated with this condition, in particular IgG lambda. Noncutaneous manifestations may include myopathy, arthropathy, neuropathy, dysphagia, lung, and renal disease.
Elevated Anti-DNase B (for group A streptococcal infection) and hemoglobin A1C may be found in scleredema, which is marked by sclerodermoid infiltration of the upper back. Scleredema may also be associated with monoclonal gammopathy. Elevated ANA with systemic lupus erythematosus may be associated with a papulonodular mucinosis, which typically manifests on the trunk. ANA may also be elevated in scleroderma, which may manifest with nonpitting acral edema in the acute phase followed by sclerodactyly and digital ulcers or pits. Decreased oral aperture may occur with loss of wrinkles, salt and pepper vitiligo-like depigmentation, and sclerotic skin. Elevated ferritin levels are not associated with these mucinoses.
Bolognia J, Schaffer J, Cerroni L, eds. *Dermatology.* [Philadelphia]: Elsevier, 2018 (ch. 46).

31. A. Raynaud phenomenon
Raynaud phenomenon may uncommonly develop during intralesional bleomycin therapy, and patients should be asked if they have a history of existing Raynaud. Systemic bleomycin chemotherapy may be associated with alopecia, stomatitis, toxic erythema of chemotherapy, and hyperpigmentation (classically flagellate erythema and hyperpigmentation). Less frequently observed dermatologic complications include hyperkeratotic plaques on knees and elbows, nail changes, and scleroderma-like changes in the hands, which may result in digital gangrene. Lupus-like and dermatomyositis-like eruptions have not been associated with intralesional bleomycin.
Bolognia J, Schaffer J, Cerroni L, eds. *Dermatology.* [Philadelphia]: Elsevier, 2018 (ch. 21).

32. E. B & C
This kodachrome depicts *en coup de sabre*, a type of linear morphea that manifests on the forehead and scalp. Rarely, the sclerosis may progress to involve the meninges and even the brain, creating a potential focus for seizures. Hemifacial atrophy (Parry-Romberg syndrome) is a more severe variant. Linear morphea overlying a limb may impact joint mobility and in severe instances may involve the fascia, muscle, and tendons, resulting in limb shortening and contractures. Two-thirds of patients with linear morphea are under 18 years of age. In rapidly progressive inflammatory linear morphea, prompt and aggressive management with prednisone and methotrexate is recommended. Observation and doxycycline are options for patients without functional impairment.
Bolognia J, Schaffer J, Cerroni L, eds. *Dermatology.* [Philadelphia]: Elsevier, 2018 (ch. 44).

33. C. Bandlike lichenoid infiltrate and epidermal spongiosis with eosinophils

The figure depicts lichenoid dermatitis with features of hypertrophic lichen planus (note the Wickham striae overlying several plaques). Mucocutaneous lichenoid dermatitis is one of the most common reactions seen from anti-PD-1/PD-L1 immunotherapy (~15%–20% of patients). Patients present with pruritic lichenoid lesions and may have oral and anogenital mucosal involvement resembling erosive lichen planus. Other presentations include hypertrophic, generalized, palmar-plantar, and Grover-like presentations. Histopathology typically resembles that of lichen planus, with varying degrees of spongiosis and eosinophils. Other reactions seen from checkpoint inhibitors include maculopapular, eczematous, psoriasiform, granulomatous (sarcoid-like), and immunobullous reactions (typically resembling bullous pemphigoid).

Choice A describes bullous pemphigoid, choice B describes Grover disease, choice D describes psoriasis, and choice E describes sarcoidosis. All of these may occur during checkpoint inhibitor therapy but would not present with mucocutaneous papulosquamous lesions.

Bolognia J, Schaffer J, Cerroni L, eds. *Dermatology*. [Philadelphia]: Elsevier, 2018 (ch. 21).

34. C. The patient recently started sorafenib

Erythromelalgia manifests as erythema, tenderness, and burning of the extremities that is exacerbated by heat. The familial form of this condition is associated with mutations in the gene *SCN9A*, which encodes the voltage-gated sodium channel alpha subunit. Erythromelalgia can occur as a secondary phenomenon in myeloproliferative diseases, including thrombocytosis and polycythemia rubra vera. Both misoprostol and serotonin reuptake inhibitors have been used to treat this condition. Sorafenib has been associated with hand-foot-skin reaction, which manifests with erythema and focal hyperkeratotic plaques (may be callus-like) and erosions that can impact activities of daily living.

Bolognia J, Schaffer J, Cerroni L, eds. *Dermatology*. [Philadelphia]: Elsevier, 2018 (ch. 106).

35. C. Conjunctivitis

Dupilumab is an interleukin-4 (IL-4) receptor antagonist indicated for the treatment of adult patients with moderate-to-severe atopic dermatitis whose disease is not adequately controlled with topical prescription therapies or when those therapies are not advisable. The most common adverse reactions are injection-site reactions (~10%) and conjunctivitis (~10%). Less commonly blepharitis (<1%), oral herpes (4%), keratitis (<1%), eye pruritus (1%), and other herpes simplex virus infections (2%) may occur. It is important for dermatologists to be familiar with this efficacious agent, which is increasingly used in the management of patients with severe dermatitis.

Treister AD, Kraff-Cooper C, Lio PA. Risk factors for dupilumab-associated conjunctivitis in patients with atopic dermatitis. *JAMA Dermatol.* 2018;154(10):1208–1211.

36. B. Streptococcus

Cellulitis is an infection of the deep dermis and subcutaneous tissue that manifests as areas of erythema, swelling, warmth, and tenderness. Cellulitis in immunocompetent adults is most often caused by group A streptococci or staphylococcal aureus (more common in children). Lymphedema, alcoholism, diabetes mellitus, intravenous drug use, and peripheral vascular disease are all risk factors. Bullous and necrotizing forms of cellulitis (as depicted in kodachrome) are classically due to streptococcal infection. Immunosuppressed patients may have atypical organisms (including fungal and atypical mycobacterial).

Vibrio cellulitis typically develops from wounds acquired in or contaminated by seawater and manifests with erythematous, edematous, and painful lesions, typically with rapid evolution to hemorrhagic bullae. Pseudomonas (hot tub folliculitis, gram-negative toeweb, ecthyma gangrenosum) and Klebsiella (ecthyma gangrenosum, erysipelas-like, rhinoscleroma) are gram-negative bacterial organisms, which may be associated with various infections.

Bolognia J, Schaffer J, Cerroni L, eds. *Dermatology*. [Philadelphia]: Elsevier, 2018 (ch. 74).

37. B. Radiation

Post irradiation–induced morphea develops in approximately 1:500 individuals (particularly those treated for breast cancer) and classically involves the breast. Like morphea, the acute stage manifests with erythema and induration of the skin and may result in substantial sclerosis and deformity. The nipple is often spared.

Penicillamine may be associated with systemic lupus erythematosus, pemphigus vulgaris and foliaceus, pemphigoid, elastosis perforans serpiginosa, lichen planus, pseudoxanthoma elasticum-like eruption, and dermatomyositis-like reactions. Lymphedema may predispose patients to cellulitis, localized elephantiasis, lipodermatosclerosis, and rarely angiosarcoma.

PUVA may result in squamous cell carcinomas after typically 200 treatments and PUVA keratoses. Methotrexate is associated with various dermatologic toxicities, including photosensitivity, alopecia, other hair and nail changes, toxic erythema of chemotherapy, and ulceration of exiting psoriatic lesions.

Bolognia J, Schaffer J, Cerroni L, eds. *Dermatology*. [Philadelphia]: Elsevier, 2018 (ch. 44).

38. B. Hydroxyurea

Leg ulcerations have been reported in patients undergoing long-term hydroxyurea therapy for myeloproliferative diseases. The ulcers usually improve on discontinuation of the agent. Dermatomyositis-like reactions may occur as well.

Plaquenil and minocycline may result in mucocutaneous hyperpigmentation. Montelukast may result in Churg-Strauss-like reactions. Penicillamine may be associated with various immunobullous, connective tissue, and elastolytic disorders.

Bolognia J, Schaffer J, Cerroni L, eds. *Dermatology*. [Philadelphia]: Elsevier, 2018 (ch. 130).

39. E. Sweet syndrome

This kodachrome depicts Sweet syndrome, or acute febrile neutrophilic dermatosis, which typically manifests with erythematous and edematous plaques with a predisposition for the head, neck, upper torso, and upper extremities. Lesions may be strikingly edematous and appear pseudovesicular, as illustrated in the kodachrome. Bullous and extensive lesions are classically associated with malignancy (e.g., acute myeloid leukemia). Constitutional symptoms are frequently present, such as fevers and malaise. There are many associated conditions, including infections (especially URI due to streptococcus and gastrointestinal yersiniosis), malignancy (AML, gammopathy), inflammatory bowel disease, autoimmune disorders, drugs (such as Granulocyte-colony stimulating factor), and pregnancy.

The other listed conditions may present with vesicles and bullae. Bullous pemphigoid classically presents with urticarial plaques and tense bullae on an inflamed base. Acute

allergic contact dermatitis, such as to urushiol, may be vesicular but typically manifests with a geometric configuration in areas of contact with the allergen. Leukocytoclastic vasculitis typically presents with palpable purpura on the lower extremities, but hemorrhagic bullae may occur as well. Exaggerated arthropod reactions (e.g., in the setting of chronic lymphocytic leukemia) may vesiculate but would not present with as many widespread lesions.
Bolognia J, Schaffer J, Cerroni L, eds. *Dermatology*. [Philadelphia]: Elsevier, 2018 (ch. 26).

40. **C.** Excision with 2 cm margins and sentinel lymph node biopsy
Following histologic diagnosis of melanoma, the primary cutaneous lesion should be re-excised with an appropriate margin determined by the Breslow depth. Of note, while the following margins are recommended in surgically difficult anatomic sites such as the distal extremities, the mucous membranes, and lentigo maligna lesions on the face, an individualized surgical approach must be considered.
For melanoma in-situ, excision margins of 0.5 cm are recommended. For melanomas less than or equal to 1 mm, 1.0 cm margins are indicated. Lesions with Breslow depth 1.01–2 mm should be re-excised with 1.0–2.0 cm margins. Tumors greater than 2 mm in Breslow should be excised with 2.0 cm margins.
Numerous publications have identified the status of the sentinel lymph node as a strong prognostic factor for survival and recurrence. In addition, sentinel lymph node status may have implications for eligibility for adjuvant therapy. Recent clinical trial data demonstrated no clear survival benefit for patients with a tumor-involved sentinel node who underwent completion lymph node dissection compared with those who did not. Recent changes in the eighth edition of the American Joint Committee on Cancer (AJCC) include the definitions of T1a and T1b, which have been revised: T1a melanomas include those <0.8 mm without ulceration, while T1b melanomas include those 0.8–1 mm with or without ulceration and those <0.8 mm with ulceration. Mitotic rate is no longer a T1 category criterion but should be documented for all invasive primary melanomas. The joint ASCO-SSO guideline panel recommended sentinel lymph node biopsy (SLNB) for patients with primary melanomas >1.0 mm. Both the American Society of Clinical Oncology, Society of Surgical Oncology, and the National Comprehensive Cancer Network guidelines state that for patients with T1b (<0.8 mm with ulceration or 0.8–1.0 mm with or without ulceration) melanomas, SLNB may be considered and discussed with the patient.
Bolognia J, Schaffer J, Cerroni L, eds. *Dermatology*. [Philadelphia]: Elsevier, 2018 (ch. 113); and 8th edition of the AJCC guidelines. Gershenwald JE, Scolyer RA. Melanoma Staging: American Joint Committee on Cancer (AJCC) 8th Edition and Beyond. *Ann Surg Oncol*. 2018;25(8):2105–2110.

PEDIATRIC DERMATOLOGY

41. **B.** Pityriasis versicolor
Atopic dermatitis is a common inflammatory skin condition, and unlike in older children and adults where flexural involvement is predominant, infantile atopic dermatitis most often initially affects the cheeks and spares the central face (pictured in this image). Atopic dermatitis has a number of associated features, including keratosis pilaris, ichthyosis vulgaris, palmoplantar hyperlinearity, xerosis, Dennie-Morgan lines, periorbital darkening, and white dermatographism. Ocular complications include

allergic rhinoconjunctivitis, atopic and vernal keratoconjunctivitis, keratoconus, subcapsular cataracts, and very rarely retinal detachment. Pityriasis alba, not pityriasis versicolor, is more frequently found in children and adolescents with atopic dermatitis.
Bolognia J, Schaffer J, Cerroni L, eds. *Dermatology*. [Philadelphia]: Elsevier, 2018 (ch. 12).

42. **D.** Zinc oxide cream with frequent diaper changes
Irritant contact dermatitis in the diaper region is due to contact with urine and feces as well as occlusion, friction, and maceration. Irritant contact dermatitis causes erythema of the convex surfaces with relative sparing of the skin folds and is best treated with frequent diaper changes and barrier creams such as zinc oxide. Clotrimazole cream would be an appropriate treatment for candidiasis, which typically presents with satellite papules and pustules. Hydrocortisone ointment would be an appropriate treatment for psoriasis and may be an appropriate adjunctive treatment for irritant contact dermatitis. However, the best primary treatment for irritant contact dermatitis involves diaper changes immediately after urination or defecation along with thick ointments or pastes to improve the skin barrier. Triamcinolone ointment is a mid-potency halogenated topical steroid, which should be avoided in the diaper area for mild dermatoses such as this. Mupirocin ointment would be an appropriate treatment for impetigo or impetiginized dermatitis.
Bolognia J, Schaffer J, Cerroni L, eds. *Dermatology*. [Philadelphia]: Elsevier, 2018 (ch. 13).

43. **B.** Oral griseofulvin at 20 mg/kg/day
Tinea capitis, or dermatophyte infection of the scalp, is common in children and is due to members of the *Trichophyton* and *Microsporum* genera. In the United States, *T. tonsurans* is the most common cause, followed by *M. canis*. Patients most commonly present with alopecia with or without obvious scale; however, the clinical presentation may range from noninflammatory scaling with minimal alopecia to a severe pustular reaction with hair loss. Dermoscopy can reveal "comma," "corkscrew," and broken hairs, and many patients have posterior cervical lymphadenopathy. Treatment requires oral antifungals, such as griseofulvin (20–25 mg/kg/day) or terbinafine (125 mg/day if <25 kg, 187.5 mg if 25–35 kg, 250 mg if >35 kg), with griseofulvin preferred for treating disease caused by *M. canis*.
Treatment for trichotillomania includes habit reversal training/behavioral modification therapy, hypnosis, psychotherapy, and pharmacologic therapy. If pharmacologic treatment is planned, clomipramine is the recommended first-line medication. Doxycycline is used to treat a number of alopecias, including central centrifugal cicatricial alopecia, acne keloidalis, dissecting cellulitis of the scalp, and folliculitis decalvans. Intralesional triamcinolone is frequently used to treat localized alopecia areata. Topical clindamycin is a treatment option for folliculitis decalvans.
Bolognia J, Schaffer J, Cerroni L, eds. *Dermatology*. [Philadelphia]: Elsevier, 2018 (chs. 69 and 77).

44. **E.** Superficial fungal infection
Cutaneous candidiasis is a superficial fungal infection that commonly involves the diaper area in infants. Infants present with beefy red plaques with satellite papules and pustules, and treatment typically consists of topical nystatin or an azole antifungal. Diaper candidiasis may be a complication of systemic antibiotics or steroids and may also develop in the setting of underlying seborrheic dermatitis, psoriasis, irritant contact dermatitis, or acrodermatitis enteropathica. Mutation of the *SLC39A4* gene is responsible for inherited zinc deficiency in acrodermatitis enteropathica. Overabundance of

IL-17, along with dysregulation of additional cytokines, is a pathogenic factor in psoriasis. IL-17 plays a role in host defense against candida, and therefore psoriasis medications that inhibit IL-17 have been associated with candidal infections. Exposure to proteases and lipases in stool is a pathogenic factor in irritant contact diaper dermatitis. Langerhans cell histiocytosis is caused by a clonal proliferation of Langerhans cells, which are antigen-presenting cells.
Bolognia J, Schaffer J, Cerroni L, eds. *Dermatology*. [Philadelphia]: Elsevier, 2018 (ch. 77).

45. B. Ibuprofen
This patient has urticaria pigmentosa, a form of cutaneous mastocytosis. Nonsteroidal antiinflammatory drugs are among the list of medications that may stimulate mast cells (B). This list also includes aspirin, narcotics, anticholinergics, dextromethorphan, some systemic anesthetics, and iodine-based radiographic dyes. The other choices are not associated with mast cell degranulation (A, C, D, E).
Bolognia J, Schaffer J, Cerroni L, eds. *Dermatology*. [Philadelphia]: Elsevier, 2018 (ch. 118).

46. B. Vitamin A
After a 10- to 14-day incubation period, measles presents with a prodrome of fever accompanied by cough, coryza, and conjunctivitis (the "3 Cs"). Koplik spots appear on the buccal mucosa during the prodrome period, after which a morbilliform exanthem begins on the forehead and spreads in a cephalocaudal manner classically. There is no antiviral therapy available for measles; however, the World Health Organization recommends that children with severe measles, such as those who are hospitalized, be treated with vitamin A, as low serum vitamin A levels are associated with increased morbidity and mortality. Unvaccinated individuals who have been exposed to measles may benefit from administration of the MMR vaccine within 3 days of exposure or with intramuscular or intravenous immunoglobulin within 6 days of exposure, but that does not apply to the patient in this vignette.
Bolognia J, Schaffer J, Cerroni L, eds. *Dermatology*. [Philadelphia]: Elsevier, 2018 (ch. 81).

47. C. Nonaccidental injury
Thermal burns due to dunking in scalding water occur most frequently in infants and toddlers. Lesions are typically symmetric on the hands, feet, or diaper area. Those on the buttocks may be associated with abuse during the process of toilet training.
Staphylococcal scalded skin syndrome causes flaccid blisters and desquamation that is accentuated on flexural surfaces, classically with perioral radial fissures and crusts. Acrodermatitis enteropathica causes sharply demarcated periorificial and acral scaly red eczematous and vesiculobullous plaques that may become eroded. Stevens-Johnson syndrome is characterized by dusky, ill-defined macules with central epidermal necrolysis as well as mucosal involvement. Diaper irritant contact dermatitis can cause erythema or, when severe, bullae and erosions over the convexities of the buttocks. However, such erosions are generally accompanied by well-circumscribed papules or nodules and are multiple, small, punched-out erosions that have been termed Jacquet erosive dermatitis.
Bolognia J, Schaffer J, Cerroni L, eds. *Dermatology*. [Philadelphia]: Elsevier, 2018 (ch. 90).

48. A. Blistering and erosions
Epidermolytic ichthyosis, previously known as bullous congenital ichthyosiform erythroderma, is a disorder of cornification due to a mutation in keratin 1 or 10 that presents at birth with erythroderma, blistering, and erosions.

While hyperkeratosis may be present, it more frequently develops later in infancy. Patients later develop hyperkeratosis with a cobblestone pattern over extensors and ridged or "corrugated cardboard" pattern that is most prominent over the flexures. Patients have variable erythroderma, palmoplantar involvement, and blistering.
Patients with Harlequin ichthyosis are born with thick yellow-brown plates of scale separated by bright red fissures. There may be an eclabium or ectropion. Patients with Netherton syndrome present at birth or shortly thereafter with erythroderma and generalized fine white scaling. Patients with neutral lipid storage disease with ichthyosis may also present at birth with generalized fine white scaling and variable erythema. Collodion membrane at birth is a common presenting feature in patients with lamellar ichthyosis, congenital ichthyosiform erythroderma, and self-improving collodion ichthyosis. A collodion membrane may also be present in trichothiodystrophy and is rarely present in Sjögren-Larsson syndrome and infantile Gaucher disease.
Bolognia J, Schaffer J, Cerroni L, eds. *Dermatology*. [Philadelphia]: Elsevier, 2018 (ch. 57).

49. E. Lymphangioma circumscriptum
The clinical image depicts clusters of papulovesicles with clear and blood-tinged fluid on the tongue of a young child, consistent with a lymphangioma circumscriptum. These lesions represent superficial lymphatic malformations that generally present during infancy and can affect any area of skin or mucosa. Oral lesions are common.
Oral candidiasis on the tongue presents as thrush with adherent white plaques that can be scraped off. HSV infection presents as grouped vesicles on an erythematous base, and may favor the hard palate of the oral mucosa in otherwise healthy individuals. Herpangina is most often caused by a Coxsackie virus infection, which more commonly involves the posterior oropharynx with pronounced erythema and small papulovesicles. Infantile hemangiomas are solid lesions that present as vascular papules, plaques, or nodules.
Bolognia J, Schaffer J, Cerroni L, eds. *Dermatology*. [Philadelphia]: Elsevier, 2018 (ch. 104).

50. C. Peripheral neuropathy
The clinical image depicts pinpoint vascular papules in a bandlike distribution on the lower abdomen around the umbilicus, characteristic of angiokeratoma corporis diffusum, a finding seen in patients with Fabry disease. Fabry disease is an X-linked recessive lysosomal storage disease due to deficiency of alpha-galactosidase, leading to lipid accumulation in multiple organs. Additional manifestations include peripheral neuropathy, cardiac abnormalities, cerebrovascular accidents, and renal failure. Treatment involves enzyme replacement therapy.
Arteriovenous malformations are seen in hereditary hemorrhagic telangiectasia. Truncal ataxia is a feature of ataxia telangiectasia, a primary immunodeficiency that also presents with telangiectasia on the conjunctivae, face, and ears. There is an association with the development of lymphoma and leukemia. Patients with liver failure often present with multiple spider angiomas. Petechiae can be seen in patients with hematologic malignancy.
Bolognia J, Schaffer J, Cerroni L, eds. *Dermatology*. [Philadelphia]: Elsevier, 2018 (ch. 65).

DERMATOPATHOLOGY

51. C. Granular parakeratosis
The figure illustrates a prominent stratum corneum with parakeratosis, hyperkeratosis, and retention of keratohyaline

granules. The underlying epidermis shows mild acanthosis. These findings are diagnostic of granular parakeratosis, which is a disorder of keratinization that affects intertriginous areas.

Both acanthosis nigricans and confluent and reticulated papillomatosis demonstrate acanthosis, hyperkeratosis, and hypergranulosis and cannot be differentiated from each other on histology alone. However, neither of these two entities show retained keratohyaline granules within the stratum corneum. Ichthyosis vulgaris shows loss of granular layer, which appears to be intact in the image shown.

52. **B.** Cowden syndrome

Sclerotic fibroma (also known as storiform collagenoma) is a well-demarcated nodule within the dermis composed of storiform, hyalinized collagen bundles with clefts ("plywood" appearance). Sclerotic fibromas may be seen in Cowden syndrome, in addition to other cutaneous manifestations that include trichilemmomas, oral fibromas, and punctate palmoplantar keratoses.

Erythema elevatum diutinum demonstrates sclerosis with neutrophils, and early lesions show vasculitis and may be associated with a monoclonal gammopathy. Leiomyoma is composed of fascicles of spindle cells with eosinophilic cytoplasm and blunt-ended nuclei, while neurofibromas contain bland spindle cells with tapered nuclei within a pale-pink stroma. Multiple leiomyomas may occur in Reed syndrome also known as hereditary leiomyomatosis and renal cell cancer syndrome. Diffuse neurofibromas are found in neurofibromatosis.

Bolognia J, Schaffer J, Cerroni L, eds. *Dermatology.* [Philadelphia]: Elsevier, 2018 (ch. 63).

53. **B.** Discoid lupus erythematosus

The figure illustrates interface dermatitis, with superficial and deep perivascular and periadnexal lymphocytic infiltrate, follicular plugging, and interstitial mucin. Taken together, these findings are most compatible with the diagnosis of discoid lupus erythematosus. Dermatomyositis also presents with interface change, however the density of inflammation is much less than that seen in lupus. Lichen sclerosus shows homogenization of the superficial dermis; follicular plugging and a bandlike lymphocytic infiltrate are also typical features. Flegel disease (hyperkeratosis lenticularis perstans) demonstrates epidermal atrophy and interface change with overlying hyperkeratosis and parakeratosis.

Bolognia J, Schaffer J, Cerroni L, eds. *Dermatology.* [Philadelphia]: Elsevier, 2018 (ch. 41).

54. **B.** Acquired digital fibrokeratoma

Acquired digital fibrokeratoma is a pedunculated lesion on acral skin that shows vertical streaking of collagen bundles within the dermis. The onset is often in adulthood. Accessory digit presents in childhood and demonstrates all normal components of acral skin, including nerve bundles and tactile corpuscles. Verruca vulgaris shows hypergranulosis with coarse keratohyaline granules, which are not seen here. Histopathological features of punctate palmoplantar keratoderma include hyperkeratosis overlying areas of epithelial depression.

Bolognia J, Schaffer J, Cerroni L, eds. *Dermatology.* [Philadelphia]: Elsevier, 2018 (ch. 116).

55. **D.** Xanthogranuloma

The photomicrograph illustrates the characteristic features of xanthogranuloma—multiple Touton-like giant cells (with an eosinophilic center surrounded by a wreathlike arrangement of nuclei and foamy cytoplasm at the periphery) admixed with foamy histiocytes and a mixed infiltrate containing eosinophils.

Necrobiotic xanthogranuloma demonstrates areas of necrobiosis surrounded by bizarre giant cells and cholesterol clefts. Reticulohistiocytoma is composed of giant cells with eosinophilic, finely granular, ground glass cytoplasm. Giant cell tumors of tendon sheath often have osteoclast-like giant cells, foamy histiocytes, and hemosiderin deposition.

Bolognia J, Schaffer J, Cerroni L, eds. *Dermatology.* [Philadelphia]: Elsevier, 2018 (ch. 91).

56. **D.** Tuberous sclerosis

The figure demonstrates a dome-shaped lesion with increased blood vessels within the dermis with surrounding fibrous tissue and stellate fibroblasts. The findings are characteristic of an angiofibroma. Multiple facial angiofibromas or "adenoma sebaceum" are associated with tuberous sclerosis.

Neurofibromas would be seen in type I neurofibromatosis, multiple leiomyomas would be seen in Reed syndrome, and telangiectasias (without surrounding sclerosis) would be seen in hereditary hemorrhagic telangiectasia.

Bolognia J, Schaffer J, Cerroni L, eds. *Dermatology.* [Philadelphia]: Elsevier, 2018 (ch. 61).

57. **B.** Metastatic signet ring cell carcinoma

Within the dermis, there is a proliferation of signet ring cells with intracellular mucin that displaces the nucleus to one side. Signet ring cell carcinomas most commonly arise in the gastrointestinal tract and may metastasize to skin. A xanthoma is composed of foamy cells without intracellular mucin, while lepromatous leprosy shows a proliferation of histiocytes with clear cytoplasm distended with large groups of leprosy bacilli. Cutaneous silicone deposition is seen as multiple empty vacuoles of varying sizes within histiocytes and giant cells where the silicone is lost during processing.

58. **C.** *NEMO*

The photomicrograph illustrates aggregates of dyskeratotic cells along with eosinophilic spongiosis. These findings in an infant are indicative of incontinentia pigmenti, which may be present in the following stages: vesicular (eosinophilic spongiosis with dyskeratosis), verrucous (hyperkeratosis, papillomatosis, and dyskeratosis), linear hyperpigmentation (pigment incontinence), and linear hypopigmentation (epidermal atrophy with loss of adnexal structures). Mutations in nuclear factor-kappa B (NF-κB) essential modulator (*NEMO*) have been implicated in the development of incontinentia pigmenti. *NEMO* is involved in inhibiting tumor necrosis factor (TNF)-induced apoptosis. *ATP2A2* is mutated in Darier's disease. *KRT1* mutation is found in epidermolytic hyperkeratosis. *TGM1* mutation is found in lamellar ichthyosis.

Bolognia J, Schaffer J, Cerroni L, eds. *Dermatology.* [Philadelphia]: Elsevier, 2018 (ch. 62).

59. **C.** Epidermolytic ichthyosis

The clinical image shows an epidermal nevus. Histologic features include: epidermal hyperplasia, hyperkeratosis, and acanthosis. Other features, including epidermolytic hyperkeratosis (as pictured here), can be seen. The cardinal histologic feature of epidermolytic hyperkeratosis is the granular and vacuolar degeneration of the upper layers of the epidermis shown here. The granular layer may be described as looking "chewed up" in epidermolytic hyperkeratosis.

Epidermal nevi are caused by somatic mosaicism. When the biopsy of a solitary epidermal nevus shows epidermolytic hyperkeratosis, the epidermal nevus could be caused by mosaic keratin 1 or 10 (*KRT1* or *KRT10*) mutation. Given the mosaic nature of the disorder, there is also risk for gonadal *KRT1* or *KRT10* mosaicism and risk for passing down epidermolytic ichthyosis. Epidermolytic ichthyosis (formerly bullous congenital ichthyosiform erythroderma) is typically an autosomal dominant disorder caused by *KRT1* or *KRT10* mutations. Patients typically present at birth with erythroderma, bullae, and denuded skin, which evolves into verrucous hyperkeratotic plaques with flexural involvement, and palmoplantar keratoderma. Genetic counseling would be recommended in this patient when he is of reproductive age.

Epidermal nevus syndrome classically refers to nonepidermolytic verrucous epidermal nevi with widespread mosaicism. Solitary epidermal nevi are somatically acquired lesions and so cannot be inherited.

Bolognia J, Schaffer J, Cerroni L, eds. *Dermatology*. [Philadelphia]: Elsevier, 2018 (ch. 57).

60. A. Emperipolesis—Rosai-Dorfman

Skin lesions in Rosai-Dorfman consist of yellow-brown papules or nodules. Rarely pustules, annular granuloma annulare-like lesions, and macular erythema have also been reported. Other typical findings of Rosai-Dorfman include massive cervical lymphadenopathy, other sites of lymphadenopathy, leukocytosis, anemia, and a polyclonal hypergammaglobulinemia. Emperipolesis is thought to represent a cell, usually a lymphocyte (lymphocytes pictured here) or neutrophil, passing through another cell (typically histiocytes) without phagocytosis (so the cell will appear normal with an intact cell membrane, as pictured here).

Cutaneous findings in hemophagocytic lymphohistiocytosis (HLH) are variable, and hemophagocytosis is rarely seen in the skin but often present in the bone marrow. Hemophagocytosis, if it were present in the biopsy, would be characterized by uptake and degradation of erythrocytes (greater than other cell types) by histiocytes. Thus the cells/cell membrane also would not appear intact as in emperipolesis. HLH presents with fever, splenomegaly, cytopenia, hypertriglyceridemia, and hyperferritinemia. The diagnosis requires histopathologic evidence of hemophagocytosis.

The photomicrograph does not represent parasitized macrophages as would be seen in leishmaniasis. Multinucleate giant cells are not a primary feature of the photomicrograph. Xanthoma disseminatum presents with yellow-red papules and nodules affecting flexures.

Bolognia J, Schaffer J, Cerroni L, eds. *Dermatology*. [Philadelphia]: Elsevier, 2018 (ch. 91).

PROCEDURAL DERMATOLOGY

61. A. Air embolism

Air embolism is an uncommon complication of dermatologic surgery, with reports occurring from Mohs micrographic surgery (MMS) and foam sclerotherapy. Two reports of air emboli from MMS have been described, both involving excision of large scalp tumors with calvarial invasion, and both patients were treated in the upright position. Seated positions contribute to lower hydrostatic pressures in venous structures above the heart and can allow for air to enter the venous circulation. A paradoxical embolism may occur from a right-to-left shunt, such as due to a patent foramen ovale. Dermatologic surgery on the scalp is typically very safe, as the venous drainage is external and venous structures highly collapsible. However, the venous structure of the bony skull drain internally.

The other answer choices have not been described as a direct complication of MMS of the scalp.

Bolognia J, Schaffer J, Cerroni L, eds. *Dermatology*. [Philadelphia]: Elsevier, 2018 (ch. 150).

62. B. Sonidegib

Vismodegib and sonidegib are FDA-approved treatments for locally advanced (not amenable to curative surgical or radiation treatment) or metastatic basal cell carcinoma. These oral medications inhibit signaling via the smoothened receptor, which is abnormally activated by mutations in the hedgehog signaling pathway in nearly all basal cell carcinomas. These medications have been shown to have an overall response rate of 30%–60% in clinical trials of locally advanced or metastatic basal cell carcinoma.

Ipilimumab is an anti-CTLA-4 monoclonal antibody approved as immunotherapy for melanoma. Erlotinib is a small molecule inhibitor of the epidermal growth factor receptor (EGFR) tyrosine kinase approved as treatment for non–small cell lung cancer. Interferon alpha is an immunomodulatory agent that has been used off-label for treatment of various types of skin cancer; there is limited data on efficacy. 5-Fluorouracil is a nucleoside analog chemotherapeutic used as topical therapy for actinic keratoses and superficial basal cell carcinoma.

Bolognia J, Schaffer J, Cerroni L, eds. *Dermatology*. [Philadelphia]: Elsevier, 2018 (chs. 107 and 108).

63. C. Polidocanol

Polidocanol can cause a disulfiram-like reaction, as described in the question. Hypertonic saline and sodium tetradecyl sulfate risks include pain, cramping, necrosis of the skin, and hyperpigmentation. Glycerin may also cause pain and cramping but has a low risk of hyperpigmentation. Sodium morrhuate has the highest risk of anaphylaxis.

Bolognia J, Schaffer J, Cerroni L, eds. *Dermatology*. [Philadelphia]: Elsevier, 2018 (ch. 155).

64. A. Polymethylmethacrylate

Polymethylmethacrylate (PMMA) is FDA-approved for deep wrinkles and folds and acne scarring. The PMMA microspheres are suspended in a water-based carrier gel. Fibroblasts encapsulate the microsphere and are stimulated to ultimately lead to collagen production. Calcium hydroxylapatite and poly-L-lactic acid are considered semipermanent fillers. Hyaluronic acid and bioengineered human collagen transfer are temporary fillers.

Bolognia J, Schaffer J, Cerroni L, eds. *Dermatology*. [Philadelphia]: Elsevier, 2018 (ch. 158).

65. D. 26%–45%

Infiltrative, morpheaform, and micronodular subtypes of basal cell carcinoma (BCC) have an increased risk of subclinical extension (microscopic extension beyond grossly visible tumor margins) and local recurrence. BCCs on the central face (including the nose) also have an increased risk of subclinical extension and local recurrence. Definitive excisional surgery with thorough pathologic evaluation of surgical margins (such as with Mohs micrographic surgery) is recommended for treatment of infiltrative and central facial BCCs. Retrospective data has confirmed that infiltrative BCCs treated with ED+C alone have a 27% rate of local recurrence, and infiltrative BCCs on the nose have a 43% rate of local recurrence. This is significantly greater than recurrence rates of less than 5% reported with Mohs micrographic surgery.

Bolognia J, Schaffer J, Cerroni L, eds. *Dermatology*. [Philadelphia]: Elsevier, 2018 (ch. 150).

66. C. Expected progression without treatment, greater than 10% rate of local recurrence with complete excision

This presentation is diagnostic of dermatofibrosarcoma protuberans (DFSP), which has aggressive local behavior but low potential for metastasis. Conservative excision of DFSP is associated with local recurrence rates of 30%–60%, while wide local excision (>2 cm margins) is associated with local recurrence rates of 10%–15%. Mohs micrographic surgery has been reported to have a less than 5% rate of local recurrence. Distant metastasis is rare for DFSP, with an overall rate of less than 5%. DFSP with fibrosarcomatous pathologic features appears to have a significantly increased rate of metastasis.
Bolognia J, Schaffer J, Cerroni L, eds. *Dermatology.* [Philadelphia]: Elsevier, 2018 (ch. 116).

67. **A.** Linear repair with long axis of ellipse oriented vertically
This orientation of linear repair will place the primary tension vector in a horizontal direction, parallel to the lower lid margin, and prevent any downward or inferior tension on the lower lid.
Linear repair with the long axis of the ellipse oriented horizontally would place the primary tension vector in a vertical direction, perpendicular to the lower lid margin. This would cause direct downward tension on the lower lid margin and promote ectropion. Healing by second intention (granulation) may generate unpredictable contractile forces on the thin skin of the lower eyelid and could contribute to lower lid ectropion. Wedge repair of the lower eyelid is not indicated for this lesion that does not affect the lid margin. Flap repair with superior advancement of the mid-cheek would place the primary tension vector in a vertical direction, perpendicular to the lower lid margin. This would cause direct downward tension on the lower lid margin and promote ectropion. Advancement/rotation flap repair with medial and inferior rotation of the lateral cheek and temple (not one of the options here) may be considered, as exemplified by the Mustarde flap.
Bolognia J, Schaffer J, Cerroni L, eds. *Dermatology.* [Philadelphia]: Elsevier, 2018 (chs. 142, 144, and 147).

68. **C.** Primary nodular basal cell carcinoma arising within prior radiation treatment field on the neck, 0.5 cm diameter
Appropriate use criteria (AUC) for Mohs surgery have been published by the American Academy of Dermatology, American College of Mohs Surgery, and American Society for Dermatologic Surgery. Any BCC or SCC arising within a prior radiation field at any anatomic location has an increased risk of subclinical extension and local recurrence and is noted as appropriate for Mohs surgery in the AUC.
Primary nodular BCC on the female breast (not on nipple or areola) of less than 2 cm in diameter is a low-risk lesion that is listed as either inappropriate (diameter less than 1 cm) or uncertain (diameter 1.1–2 cm). Primary superficial basal cell carcinoma of the forehead less than 0.5 cm diameter is listed as uncertain for Mohs surgery and is amenable to other forms of treatment. Actinic keratosis with focus of SCC in situ is not appropriate for Mohs surgery at any anatomic location. Primary SCC without aggressive features on a low-risk anatomic location such as the shoulder with diameter less than or equal to 1 cm is listed as inappropriate for Mohs surgery.
Ad Hoc Task Force, Connolly SM, Baker DR, Coldiron BM, et al. AAD/ACMS/ASDSA/ASMS 2012 appropriate use criteria for Mohs micrographic surgery: a report of the American Academy of Dermatology, American College of Mohs Surgery, American Society for Dermatologic Surgery Association, and the American Society for Mohs Surgery. *J Am Acad Dermatol.* 2012;67(4):531–550.

69. **E.** Retina
The Q-switched alexandrite laser has a wavelength of 755 nm with melanin being the target chromophore. Lasers or light sources that target melanin or hemoglobin can lead to retinal damage given that the retina is highly pigmented. Pulsed dye laser (595 nm) and Ruby (694 nm) lasers also have risk of retinal damage. Lasers that have water as a chromophore, including the CO2 (10600 nm) and Erb:yag (2940 nm), can cause corneal damage. The excimer laser (308 nm) poses risk to the cornea and lens.
Bolognia J, Schaffer J, Cerroni L, eds. *Dermatology.* [Philadelphia]: Elsevier, 2018 (chs. 136 and 137).

70. **B.** Croton oil
The efficacy of a Baker-Gordon peel is most strongly related to Croton oil, which is extracted from the seed of the Croton tiglium plant. It promotes penetration of the phenol component of the peel. Septisol helps with more homogenous peeling. Water acts as a vehicle for the phenol. Mineral oil is not found in Baker-Gordon peels.
Bolognia J, Schaffer J, Cerroni L, eds. *Dermatology.* [Philadelphia]: Elsevier, 2018 (ch. 154).

BASIC SCIENCE

71. **C.** Janus kinase
Ruxolitinib is a Janus kinase (JAK) inhibitor that has recently been used for the treatment of alopecia areata and vitiligo. In addition, there are ongoing studies for its use in graft-versus-host disease. Other JAK inhibitors such as tofacitinib have been increasingly used in dermatology over the past several years in a variety of conditions, including psoriasis, vitiligo, atopic dermatitis, and alopecia areata. Topical formulations are under investigation as well. Topical mTOR inhibitors such as sirolimus can be used to treat angiofibromas in tuberous sclerosus (A); topical calcineurin inhibitors including tacrolimus and pimecrolimus are used to treat dermatitis in facial and flexural sites; topical imiquimod targets toll-like receptor 7 and is approved for the treatment of warts, actinic keratoses, superficial basal cell carcinomas, and squamous cell carcinoma in-situ, with off-label use in lentigo maligna, particularly after excision with positive margins (D). Targeted cancer drugs that inhibit NF-kB signaling are being investigated.
Bolognia J, Schaffer J, Cerroni L, eds. *Dermatology.* [Philadelphia]: Elsevier, 2018 (chs. 69 and 128).

72. **D.** Herpes simplex virus type I
Talimogene laherparepvec (T-VEC) is the first oncolytic virus approved by the FDA in 2015. It is a modified herpes simplex virus type I (HSV)–expressing granulocyte macrophage colony-stimulating factor (GM-CSF), which stimulates antitumor immunity. It is important to note that although T-VEC reduces tumor burden, it has not been shown to reduce mortality in long-term follow-up studies. Its use in combination with immune checkpoint inhibitors has shown promising results in phase 1 and 2 studies.
Bolognia J, Schaffer J, Cerroni L, eds. *Dermatology.* [Philadelphia]: Elsevier, 2018 (ch. 113).

73. **E.** Inhibit activated T cells
Nivolumab and pembrolizumab are monoclonal antibodies against programmed death 1 receptor (PD-1) that are FDA-approved for the treatment of melanoma, as well as a variety of other malignancies. PD-1 normally functions to inhibit antigen stimulated T cells and thus acts as an

"immune checkpoint." When PD-1 is blocked by either nivolumab or pembrolizumab, immune responses against tumors are enhanced. This type of immunotherapy is often likened to "taking the brakes off the immune system." Adhesion molecules between keratinocytes such as desmosomes are comprised of cadherins, including desmogleins (D). Desmogleins are targeted by auto-antibodies in pemphigus.

Extracellular growth factor receptors, such as epidermal growth factor receptor (EGFR), promote tumor growth and are targeted for cancer treatment (e.g., cetuximab) (C). Downstream signaling events of growth receptors result in activation of MAP kinase pathway (i.e., RAS, RAF), which stimulate cell growth and proliferation. Intracellular vesicular membrane fusion proteins, such as synaptobrevin, syntaxin, and SNAP-25, are involved in the fusion of synpatic vesicles with cell membrane, resulting in the release of acetylcholine into the neuronal synapse (A). These proteins are blocked by multiple subtypes of botulinum toxin.

Bolognia J, Schaffer J, Cerroni L, eds. *Dermatology.* [Philadelphia]: Elsevier, 2018 (chs. 113 and 128).

74. **A.** Anti-MDA5

The clinical photo shows Gottron papules of the dorsal hand and dilated nailfold capillary loops in dermatomyositis. The autoantibody anti–melanoma differentiation-associated gene 5 (MDA-5) is a marker of amyopathic dermatomyositis associated with rapidly progressive interstitial lung disease. In addition, this subset of dermatomyositis patients is more likely to develop vasculopathy-associated ulcers.

Anti–extracellular matrix protein 1 (ECM-1) is positive in 80% of patients with lichen sclerosus. Patients with systemic sclerosus are often positive for anti-Scl-70 antibodies. Collagen XVII, also known as bullous pemphigoid antigen 2 (BPAG2) or BP180, is targeted in bullous pemphigoid and linear IgA bullous dermatosis.

Bolognia J, Schaffer J, Cerroni L, eds. *Dermatology.* [Philadelphia]: Elsevier, 2018 (chs. 40 and 42).

75. **C.** Langerhans cell

Langerhans cells are professional antigen presenting cells that reside within the epidermis. These cells function as epidermal dendritic cells which uptake, process, and then present antigens to lymphocytes to induce adaptive immune response, including the activation of CD4 T-cells. The clinical photo shows cutaneous candidiasis and Langerhans cells have been demonstrated to present Candida antigens.

Bolognia J, Schaffer J, Cerroni L, eds. *Dermatology.* [Philadelphia]: Elsevier, 2018 (chs. 4 and 77).

76. **A.** Pemphigus foliaceus

Desmoglein-1 is targeted by exfoliative toxin A produced by *Staphylococcus aureus* in bullous impetigo (local) and in staphylococcal scalded skin syndrome (systemic). In pemphigus foliaceus, autoantibodies also target desmoglein 1. Epidermolysis bullosa is an inherited genodermatosis with mutations in *keratin 5, keratin 14, laminin 5,* and *collagen VII* as well as other structural proteins critical for skin integrity. Collagen VII may also be targeted in bullous lupus erythematosus. Bullous pemphigoid and linear IgA bullous dermatosis are autoimmune blistering diseases caused by autoantibodies against *collagen XVII* (*BP180* or *BPAG2*). Chronic bullous disease of childhood is another name for linear IgA bullous dermatosis when it occurs in children.

Bolognia J, Schaffer J, Cerroni L, eds. *Dermatology.* [Philadelphia]: Elsevier, 2018 (chs. 29 and 34).

77. **B.** Collagen VII

This patient has bullous systemic lupus erythematosus (SLE), which is a rare manifestation of acute cutaneous lupus characterized by bullous lesions, elevated antinuclear antibody, and biopsy, demonstrating a subepidermal split with a neutrophil rich infiltrate. Circulating autoantibodies against collagen VII are thought to be responsible for the bullous presentation. Desmocollin-1 is targeted by autoantibodies in subcorneal pustular dermatosis or IgA pemphigus. Bullous pemphigoid antigen 2 (BPAG2) is the same as collagen XVII and BP180, which is targeted in bullous pemphigoid. Patients with bullous pemphigoid are typically elderly and have spongiosis or subepidermal split with eosinophils on biopsy and typically do not have positive ANA. Desmoplakin is targeted by autoantibodies in paraneoplastic pemphigus.

Bolognia J, Schaffer J, Cerroni L, eds. *Dermatology.* [Philadelphia]: Elsevier, 2018 (chs. 40 and 41).

78. **D.** Intracellular kinase

BRAF is a member of the MAP kinase signaling pathway and functions as an intracellular signal transduction kinase that helps stimulate cell division, differentiation, and secretion. Melanoma often has activating mutations in *BRAF* (e.g., V600E) that contribute to melanoma growth. The V600E mutation in BRAF can be inhibited by the small molecule inhibitors dabrafenib or vemurafenib. Trametinib is a small molecule inhibitor of MEK, another MAP kinase family member.

Bolognia J, Schaffer J, Cerroni L, eds. *Dermatology.* [Philadelphia]: Elsevier, 2018 (chs. 113 and 128).

79. **B.** Enzyme-linked immunosorbent assay

Enzyme-linked immunosorbent assay (ELISA) is used to detect specific immunoglobulins such as circulating antinuclear antibodies (ANA), including anti-dsDNA in systemic lupus erythematosus. A modified ELISA technique is used to detect specific proteins in tissue (immunohistochemistry). Mass spectroscopy separates ions based on mass-to-charge ratios. Polymerase chain reaction (PCR) amplifies specific segments of DNA that is used to help identify malignant T-cell receptor clones in cutaneous T-cell lymphoma (CTCL). Flow cytometry is a biotechnology that separates cells through a narrow, rapidly flowing stream of liquid and then employs lasers to detect fluorescent antibodies bound to the cells. Sequencing of DNA nucleotides is used for immunophenotyping of malignant T-cell clones in CTCL.

Bolognia J, Schaffer J, Cerroni L, eds. *Dermatology.* [Philadelphia]: Elsevier, 2018 (chs. 3 and 40).

80. **D.** Anti–programmed cell death ligand 1

Merkel cell carcinoma (MCC) is a rare, neuroendocrine tumor of the skin with an aggressive clinical behavior. Risk factors include both ultraviolet radiation and infection with Merkel cell polyomavirus. Anti–programmed cell death ligand 1 (anti-PD-L1; avelumab) therapy was approved by the FDA in 2017 for metastatic Merkel cell carcinoma. Avelumab blocks the interaction between PD-L1 expressed on tumor cells and myeloid cells and its receptor, programmed cell death 1 (PD-1) on T cells, which normally inhibits T-cell function. Therefore, blocking PD-L1 results in enhanced T-cell activity against cancers, including MCC. Currently for cutaneous tumors, PD-1 inhibitors are approved for metastatic melanoma (nivolumab, pembrolizumab) and advanced cutaneous squamous cell carcinoma (cemiplimab), and PD-L1 inhibitor (avelumab) is approved for metastatic MCC.

Bolognia J, Schaffer J, Cerroni L, eds. *Dermatology.* [Philadelphia]: Elsevier, 2018 (chs. 115 and 128).

GENERAL DERMATOLOGY

1. An otherwise healthy 60-year-old woman presents with new ulcers 3 weeks after surgery for removal of a benign tumor. What is the next best step?

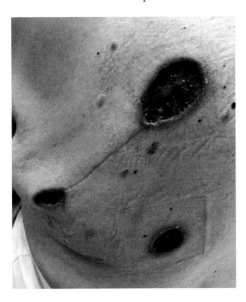

A. Surgical debridement
B. Hospitalize for intravenous vancomycin
C. Biopsy for H&E and tissue culture
D. Prednisone (if negative cultures)
E. C & D

2. A 55-year-old African American woman presents to the emergency department with facial and oral swelling as well as episodic abdominal pain. Upon further history, the patient states that her primary doctor prescribed a new antihypertensive 2 weeks ago. What is the pathogenesis of the patient's symptoms?
A. Low C4 levels
B. Low bradykinin levels
C. Elevated bradykinin levels
D. C1 esterase inhibitor deficiency
E. Increased C1 esterase inhibitor

3. A 6-year-old child presents with well-demarcated erythematous, large, scaly plaques on his bilateral elbows, knees, forearms, shins, back, and scalp. What is the most common HLA association with this patient's skin findings?
A. Human Leukocyte Antigen-B27
B. HLA-Cw6
C. HLA-B13
D. HLA-B17
E. HLA-DR3

4. A 55-year-old man with a history of HIV on antiretroviral therapy presents with a 2-month history of nonhealing, enlarging tender lesions on his legs. He has endured a persistent cough for the past month. He visited his brother in Ohio several weeks ago. He denies fevers and chills, as well as travel outside of the United States. He was previously treated with oral doxycycline and clindamycin without improvement. A sterile biopsy was performed and smear of the cultured organism showed the following morphology. What is the most likely culprit?

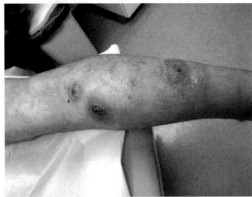

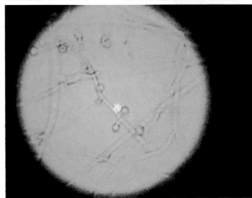

A. Blastomyces dermatitidis
B. Mycobacterium kansasii
C. Histoplasma capsulatum
D. Trichophyton rubrum
E. Secondary cutaneous B cell lymphoma

5. Which of the following is NOT a feature of Graham-Little-Piccardi-Lassueur syndrome?
A. Scarring alopecia of the scalp
B. Nonscarring loss of the pubic and axillary hairs
C. Scarring loss of pubic and axillary hairs
D. Disseminated follicular papules
E. Cutaneous or mucosal lichen planus

6. The patient has had the following pruritic eruption for many years. He has tested negative for HIV and hepatitis, and laboratory evaluation was negative for anemia, renal dysfunction, or liver dysfunction. The patient was treated for scabies on multiple occasions. His itching is unbearable and remains refractory to antihistamines, topical steroids, gabapentin, and light therapy. The most appropriate next step is:

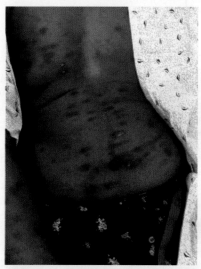

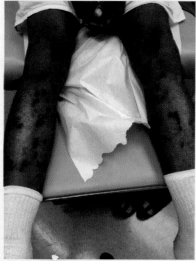

A. Psychiatric evaluation
B. Biopsy for histology and direct immunofluorescence
C. Biopsy for histology
D. No further workup; initiate high-dose oral prednisone taper
E. CT scan of the chest, abdomen, and pelvis

7. A 23-year-old female seeks consultation for evaluation and management of acne. She has seen over 10 other providers in the past year and expresses unhappiness with the provided treatment regimens. On examination, she has no cysts, inflammatory papules, or comedones. There are few pitted scars on her cheeks. There is no postinflammatory hyperpigmentation. Her chest and back are completely clear. She is tearful in the room over the severity of her acne and demands to be placed on isotretinoin. She states her acne makes her feel inferior, and she does not want to be seen in public. The next best step is:
A. Urine pregnancy test in anticipation of isotretinoin initiation
B. Reassure her that her acne is not noticeable
C. Recommend hyaluronic acid fillers for her acne scars
D. Assess for suicidality

8. An 18-year-old college student in the Northeast presented with tender nodules on the bilateral lower extremities. She has no other symptoms including cough, diarrhea, sore throat, fevers, or arthralgias. She has never traveled outside of the Northeast. Her only medication is an oral contraceptive pill. The patient has had two negative purified protein derivative (PPD) tests 1 month ago for her volunteer job at the hospital emergency room. Appropriate next steps may include (choose 4):

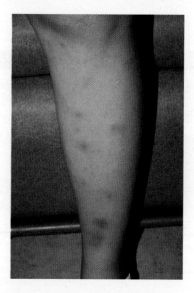

A. Skin biopsy
B. Skin biopsy and request PCR for mycobacteria
C. Treatment with itraconazole
D. Discontinuation of oral contraceptives
E. Pregnancy test
F. Amylase and lipase
G. Chest x-ray
H. Colonoscopy
I. Recommend compression stockings

9. The patient has been on hydroxychloroquine for 6 months without improvement. Which of the following has been associated with failure of antimalarials?

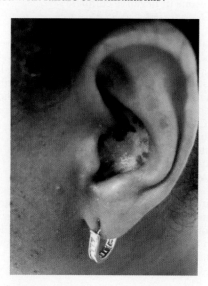

A. Uveitis
B. Smoking
C. Positive antinuclear antibody (ANA)
D. UV exposure

10. Which marker would be positive?

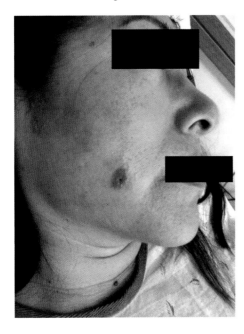

A. ACE
B. P63
C. BCL-6
D. Desmin
E. Cd34+

11. A patient with bullous pemphigoid on azathioprine for the past 5 years presents with high-spiking fevers and chills. He has a history of gout and was started on full-dose allopurinol by an outside physician. Which of the following would you expect on laboratory evaluation?
A. Eosinophilia
B. Neutropenia
C. High thiopurine S-methyltransferase (TPMT) activity
D. Creatine phosphokinase (CPK)
E. International normalized ratio (INR)

12. What is the diagnosis?

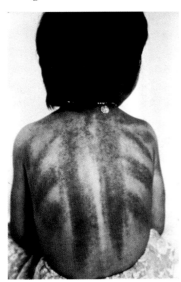

A. Abuse
B. Gardner-Diamond syndrome
C. Coining
D. Pigmented purpuric dermatosis

13. What condition is shown on dermoscopy?

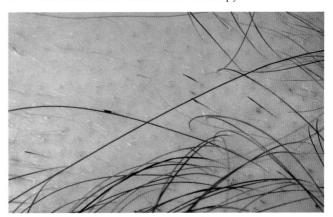

A. Tinea capitis
B. Lichen planopilaris
C. Discoid lupus
D. Alopecia areata

14. What is the diagnosis based on the dermoscopic figure?

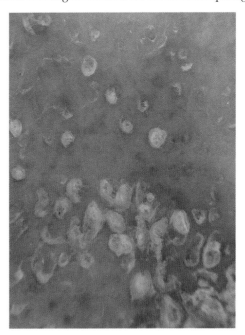

A. Lichen planopilaris
B. Discoid lupus erythematosus
C. Folliculitis decalvans
D. Androgenic alopecia
E. Alopecia areata

15. The patient is referred for a gradual onset of dark lesions on the bilateral lower extremities. What part of the patient's medical history is most relevant to the diagnosis?

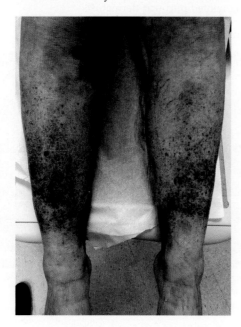

A. History of varicose veins on the lower extremities
B. History of prolonged minocycline use
C. History of motor vehicle accident
D. History of bladder surgery

16. Diagnosis:

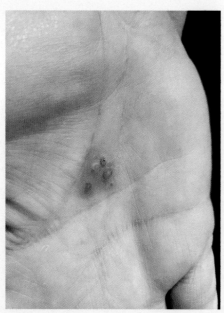

Photo courtesy Barry Ginsburg, Birmingham, AL.

A. Coxsackie
B. Varicella zoster virus
C. Erythema multiforme
D. Orf
E. Allergic contact dermatitis

17. The patient presents with the following eruption, and biopsy is obtained. Once the likely diagnosis is confirmed, what is the next step in evaluation?

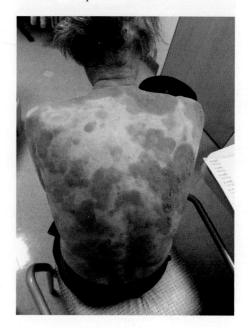

A. Repeat biopsy to confirm diagnosis
B. ANA, SSA (Rho), SSB (La) titers
C. Desmoglein 1, desmoglein 3 titers
D. Flow cytometry, T-cell PCR
E. Direct immunofluorescence

18. What is the best diagnosis?

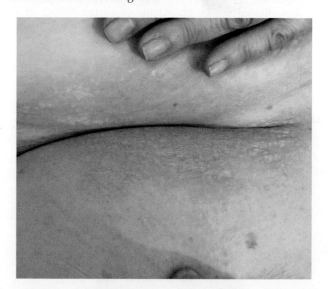

A. Lichen sclerosus
B. Lichen planus
C. Lichen striatus
D. Lichen amyloid
E. Lichen aureus

19. A 65-year-old man presents with decreased mobility of the wrists and elbows as well as stiffening of his skin. He has a history of acute myelogenous leukemia and underwent allogeneic stem cell transplantation 6 months previously.

His current posttransplant regimen includes sirolimus and tacrolimus. A complete blood count notes peripheral eosinophilia of 15%. Which two classes of medications have shown promise in the management of this condition?

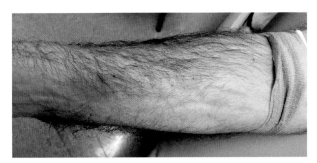

A. cytotoxic T-lymphocyte-associated protein 4 (CTLA-4) and Programmed cell death protein 1 (PD-1) inhibitors
B. Janus kinase (JAK) and Bruton tyrosine kinase inhibitors
C. BRAF and MEK inhibitors
D. Interleukin (IL)-17 and IL-12/23 inhibitors
E. IL-4 inhibitors and Immunoglobulin E (IgE) inhibitors

20. What is the best diagnosis?

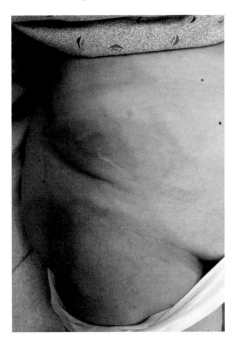

A. Cutaneous T-cell lymphoma
B. Annular elastolytic giant cell granuloma
C. Annular lichen planus
D. Inflammatory morphea
E. Granuloma annulare

21. The patient was referred to Mohs surgery for squamous cell carcinoma. On evaluation by the Mohs surgeon, the patient is noted to have multiple keratotic plaques on the extremities. A review of histopathology is most likely to reveal which diagnosis?

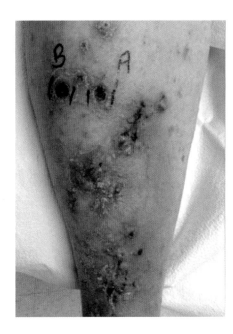

A. Squamous cell carcinoma
B. Pemphigus vulgaris
C. Hypertrophic lichen planus
D. Psoriasis
E. Subacute cutaneous lupus erythematosus

22. A pregnant 35-year-old woman presents with the following eruption. She reports chills and notes that the rash developed shortly after tapering prednisone. Which four management options below are most acceptable?

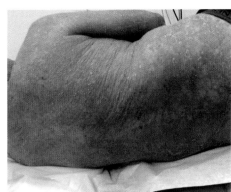

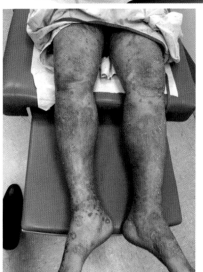

A. Hospitalize
B. Treat as outpatient
C. Topical steroids, sauna suit, open-wet dressings
D. Check complete blood count, comprehensive metabolic panel, calcium
E. Begin acitretin
F. Begin methotrexate
G. Begin adalimumab

23. Which nail finding is NOT associated with this eruption?

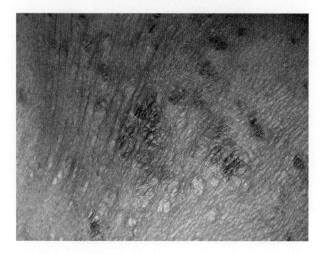

A. Ventral pterygium
B. Trachyonychia
C. Red lunulae
D. Onycholysis

24. What autoantibody is most strongly associated with this condition?

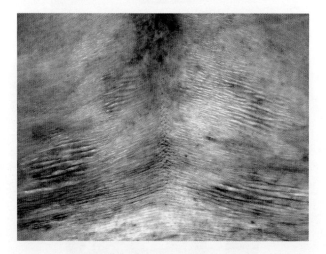

A. DNA topoisomerase I
B. Extracellular Matrix Protein 1 (ECM-1)
C. Nuclear matrix protein (NXP-2)
D. Antinuclear

25. An abnormality in which lab result is most commonly associated with the image shown?

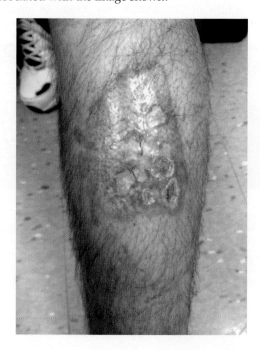

A. Lipase
B. Liver enzymes
C. Calcium
D. Glucose

26. A 57-year-old female has a long-standing history of psoriasis well controlled with 10 mg of methotrexate weekly along with daily folic acid. She develops burning pain with urination and goes to urgent care for treatment. She subsequently develops extreme fatigue, easy bruising, and epistaxis. Which medication is likely given?
A. Cephalexin
B. Sulfamethoxazole/trimethoprim
C. Ciprofloxacin
D. Azithromycin

27. Which medication most likely caused the pictured reaction?

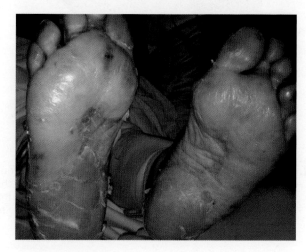

A. Hydroxyurea
B. Allopurinol
C. Bleomycin
D. Capecitabine

28. This nail finding is associated with what disorder?

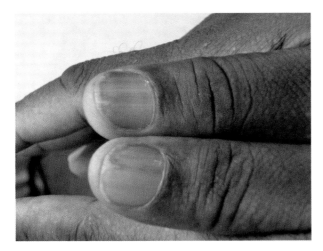

- **A.** Lichen planus
- **B.** Onychopapilloma
- **C.** Keratosis follicularis (Darier disease)
- **D.** Psoriasis

29. Immunohistochemical staining of this lesion would most likely be positive for all of the following EXCEPT:

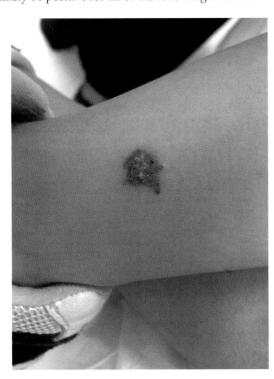

- **A.** Thrombospondin
- **B.** Podoplanin
- **C.** LYVE-1
- **D.** Prox1

30. Treatment for this condition includes (choose all that apply):

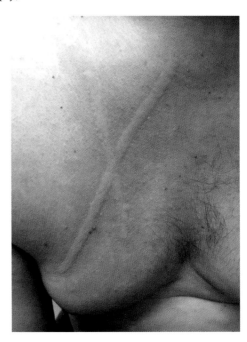

- **A.** Ibuprofen
- **B.** Doxepin
- **C.** Fexofenadine
- **D.** Dupilumab

31. Diagnosis:

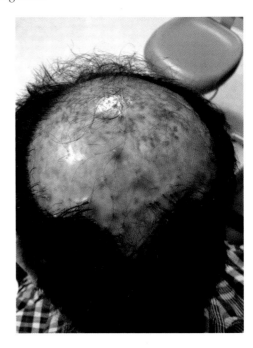

- **A.** Folliculitis decalvans
- **B.** Discoid lupus
- **C.** Lipedematous scalp
- **D.** Acne conglobata

32. A 25-year-old female presents with this asymptomatic eruption. A workup for which of the following should be considered?

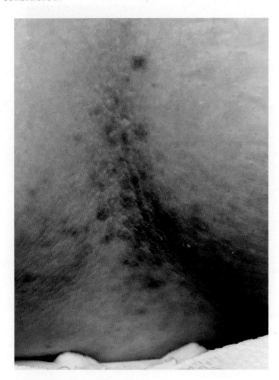

A. Medullary thyroid cancer
B. Lymphoma
C. Diabetes Mellitus
D. Monoclonal gammopathy

33. Other findings may include:

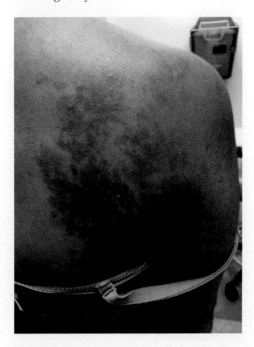

A. Smooth muscle hamartoma
B. Resolution with atrophy and fibrofatty changes
C. Diabetes mellitus
D. Propionibacterium acnes

34. Which of the following is the best next step?

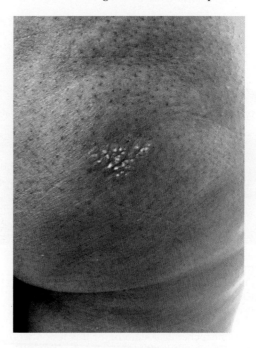

A. Bacterial culture
B. KOH
C. Direct fluorescent antibody
D. Biopsy

35. A patient presented with the pictured concern. What is the likely cause?

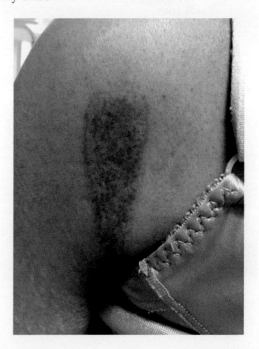

A. UV radiation
B. Chronic rubbing
C. An object
D. Spray perfume

36. The diagnosis is:

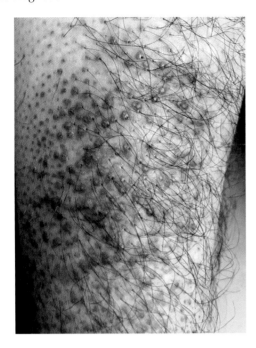

- **A.** Hypertrophic lichen planus
- **B.** Lichen amyloidosis
- **C.** Prurigo nodularis
- **D.** Papular mucinosis

37. A 63-year-old man presents with the pictured findings, as well as diffuse prurigo nodules with intractable pruritus. Complete blood count and lipid panel are normal. What other lab test is most likely to be elevated?

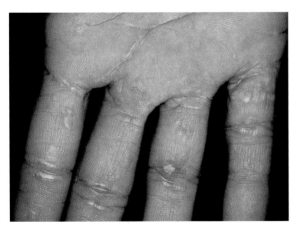

With permission from James WD, Berger TG, et al. Andrews' Diseases of the Skin, 2016, Elsevier, 45–61.e2 (fig. 4-3).

- **A.** BP180
- **B.** Bilirubin
- **C.** c-reactive protein
- **D.** Angiotensin-converting enzyme

38. A 16-year-old woman presents as shown. All of these disorders can be associated EXCEPT:

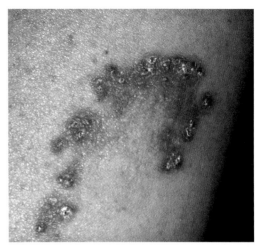

With permission from James WD, Abnormalities of dermal fibrous and elastic tissue, in *Andrews' Diseases of the Skin*, 25, Copyright © 2016, Elsevier, 500–508.e1.

- **A.** Rothmund-Thomson syndrome
- **B.** Pseudoxanthoma elasticum
- **C.** Netherton syndrome
- **D.** Down syndrome
- **E.** Marfan syndrome

39. A 28-year-old man with history of severe atopic dermatitis returns to your office after failing topical corticosteroids and phototherapy with narrow band UVB. You place him on a monoclonal antibody that blocks IL-4 receptor signaling. What is the most common side effect of this drug?
- **A.** Serum sickness–like reaction
- **B.** Lupus-like syndrome
- **C.** Hepatitis B reactivation
- **D.** Conjunctivitis

40. A 15-year-old boy has the following recalcitrant plaques as shown. He has had these plaques wax and wane since he was an infant. He also has a history of sterile osteolytic bone lesions on x-rays of his hands. The patient has failed therapy with topical corticosteroids, phototherapy, TNF-alpha inhibitors, and immunosuppressive agents, including cyclosporine. Which treatment should be started?

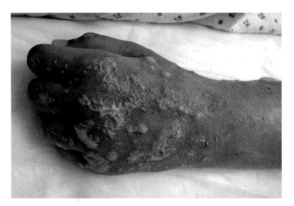

- **A.** Anakinra
- **B.** Dupilumab
- **C.** Dapsone
- **D.** Apremilast

PEDIATRIC DERMATOLOGY

41. A 2-year-old boy is brought to your clinic for evaluation of pink scaly patches and plaques and poor hair growth. He is small for his age and his mother notes a history of several food allergies. Based on your suspicion, a bedside test is performed. What is the most likely diagnosis?

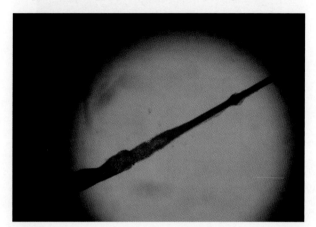

With permission from Yu-Pei Lo, Desale Snehal, Chao-Jen Shih, and Po-Yuan Wu, in Erythroderma and bamboo hair at birth: A case of Netherton syndrome and literature review, *Dermatologica Sinica*, 2018, 36(3):159–160.

    A. Atopic dermatitis
    B. Menkes kinky hair syndrome
    C. Bazex-Dupre-Christol syndrome
    D. Netherton syndrome
    E. Trichothiodystrophy

42. You are asked to evaluate a young boy with loose, distensible skin. Examination is shown. What is the most likely associated feature?

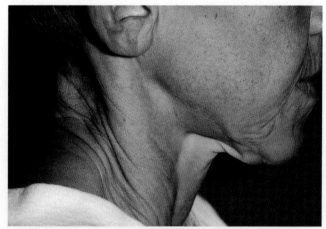

With permission from Paller AS, Mancini AJ (eds), Hereditary disorders of the dermis, in *Hurwitz Clinical Pediatric Dermatology*, 5th edition, 2016, Elsevier, 119–135 (fig. 6-8).

    A. Angioid streaks
    B. Pulmonary emphysema
    C. Gastrointestinal hemorrhage
    D. Ectopia lentis
    E. Blue sclerae

43. A 9-year-old boy is brought to the emergency department for evaluation of a rash on his upper and lower extremities that has fluctuated over the past 10 days. The week prior to rash onset, the patient experienced fevers and myalgias. What is the most likely diagnosis?

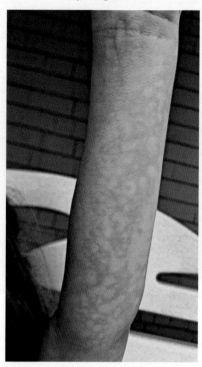

Courtesy Oleg Akilov, MD, PhD, Pittsburgh, PA.

    A. Erythema infectiosum
    B. Mononucleosis
    C. Rubeola
    D. Exanthem subitum
    E. Rubella

44. A child presents for evaluation of facial scarring. Examination is shown. Which of the following is the most likely associated clinical finding?

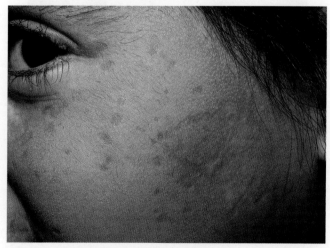

With permission from Paller AS, Mancini AJ (eds), Hereditary disorders of the dermis, in *Hurwitz Clinical Pediatric Dermatology*, 5th edition, 2016, Elsevier, 119–135 (fig. 6-20).

A. Hepatosplenomegaly
B. Developmental delay
C. Hoarseness
D. Alopecia
E. Lymphadenopathy

45. A 17-year-old girl is referred for evaluation of skin findings. Her ocular exam is shown. Which of the following findings are most likely to be present on the remainder of her cutaneous exam?

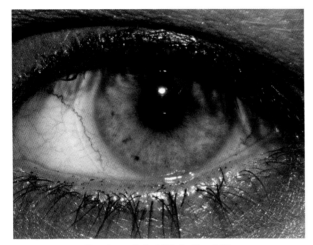

Courtesy Julie V Schaffer, MD.

A. White-yellow papules along the lateral neck
B. Multiple red facial papules
C. Hypopigmented macules and patches
D. Triangular lunulae
E. Axillary freckling

46. A young girl is brought to your office for evaluation of photosensitivity and facial erythema. She is small for her age and has a history of recurrent infections. Based on your suspicions, the patient undergoes chromosomal instability testing, which reveals a characteristic pattern of breakage and rearrangement. Which of the following is the best diagnosis?
A. Rothmund-Thomson syndrome
B. Xeroderma pigmentosum
C. Cockayne syndrome
D. Bloom syndrome
E. Trichothiodystrophy with photosensitivity

47. You are called to the neonatal Intensive Care Unit (NICU) to evaluate a newborn girl with the pictured cutaneous examination. The pregnancy was complicated by premature delivery. Her parents are very concerned about her diagnosis and prognosis. Which of the following is the most likely diagnosis?

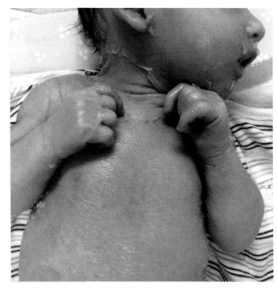

With permission from James WD, Elston DM, McMahon P, Genodermatoses and congenital anomalies, in *Andrews' Diseases of the Skin Clinical Atlas*, 2018, Elsevier, 379–404 (fig. 27.59).

A. Epidermolytic ichthyosis
B. Autosomal recessive congenital ichthyosis
C. Neutral lipid storage disease
D. Sjögren-Larsson syndrome

48. A young girl is sent to your office for evaluation of skin findings. Cutaneous examination is notable for widespread linear atrophic papules with telangiectasia and soft yellow-red nodules on the legs. Femoral x-ray reveals characteristic osteopathia striata. Which of the following genes is mutated in this disorder?
A. *ECM1*
B. *PORCN*
C. *LEMD3*
D. *NEMO*
E. *FBN1*

49. You are asked to evaluate an infant with the pictured cutaneous examination. A skin biopsy from an adult with this condition is most likely to show which of the following findings?

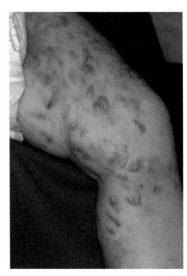

With permission from Paller AS, Mancini AJ (eds), Disorders of pigmentation, in *Hurwitz Clinical Pediatric Dermatology*, 5th edition, 2016, Elsevier, 245–278 (fig. 11-28).

A. Epidermal atrophy, loss of melanin in the basal layer, and absence of pilosebaceous units
B. Papillomatosis, hyperkeratosis, and acanthosis
C. Intraepidermal vesicles with eosinophils and necrotic keratinocytes
D. Marked pigment incontinence with dermal melanophages
E. Large epitheloid endothelial cells with dense infiltrate of lymphocytes and eosinophils

50. A 5-year-old boy with a history of mild atopic dermatitis presents with this eruption involving the face. His mom also notes that his eczema is flaring. He had a low-grade fever 2 days ago and some mild diarrhea but otherwise is acting normally. What is the most appropriate course of treatment?

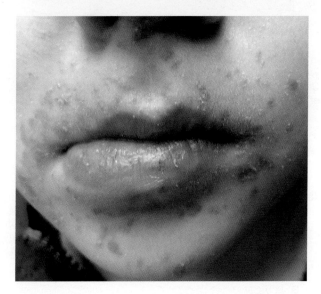

A. Reassurance
B. Cefadroxil
C. Acyclovir
D. Mupirocin ointment
E. Prednisolone

DERMATOPATHOLOGY

51. A 5-year-old boy presents with a 1-year history of a growing lesion on the face. On exam, an 8-mm, firm, bluish papule is noted on the left cheek. Exam also revealed several epidermal inclusion cysts. Family history is positive for colon cancer at a young age. Biopsy is performed as illustrated. Genetic testing should be considered for which of the following conditions:

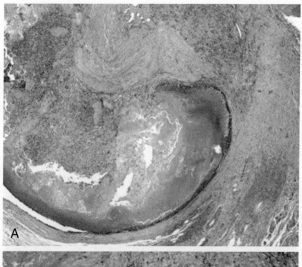

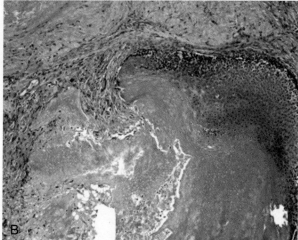

With permission from Hernandez-Nunez, et al. *Actas Dermosifiliographicas*, 2014, volume 105, issue 7, 699–705 (fig. 4, p. 703).

A. Turner syndrome
B. Cowden syndrome
C. Peutz-Jeghers syndrome
D. Gardner syndrome
E. Myotonic dystrophy

52. A 50-year-old man presents with multiple flesh-colored, translucent-appearing papules around the eyes and eyelids. A biopsy shows the following image. Further questioning reveals that the patient has a similarly affected family member who has a documented *WNT10A* mutation. Examination of the hands and feet in this patient would be expected to show:

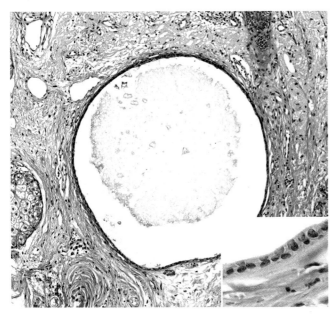

With permission from Bolognia J, et al., in *Dermatology*, 4th ed., 2018, Elsevier, 1925 (ch. 110, fig. 110.18).

A. Brachydactyly
B. Pseudoainhum
C. Palmoplantar keratoderma
D. Anonychia
E. Palmar pits

53. A biopsy is performed and shows the pictured histologic pattern. What is the diagnosis?

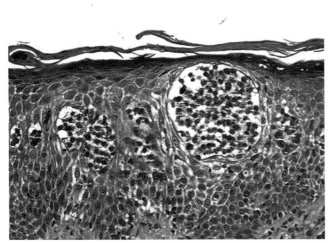

With permission from Agero, et al., *J Am Acad Dermatol*, 2007, volume 57, issue 3, 439 (fig. 2C).

A. Cutaneous T-cell lymphoma
B. Acute allergic contact dermatitis
C. Tinea corporis
D. Subcorneal pustular dermatosis (Sneddon-Wilkinson disease)
E. Dyshidrotic eczema

54. A 10-year-old boy presents with dozens of hypopigmented macules and minimally elevated papules on the trunk, and a few scattered on the face and upper extremities. Biopsy of the lesion is illustrated in the figure. The correct diagnosis is:

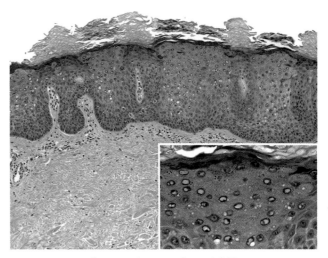

Courtesy Lorenzo Cerroni, MD.

A. Multiple tumors of follicular infundibulum
B. Idiopathic guttate hypomelanosis
C. Epidermodysplasia verruciformis
D. Pityriasis lichenoides chronica
E. Hypopigmented mycosis fungoides

55. A 50-year-old previously healthy woman presents with red-brown papules around the eyes. A detailed physical exam reveals a few, similarly appearing lesions on the scalp and one on her neck. A biopsy of a lesion on the scalp is illustrated in the figure. Chart review reveals that she has also recently been complaining of fevers and was recently diagnosed with diabetes insipidus by her primary care provider. CT scans showed adrenal and central nervous system lesions. Mutational testing of lesional skin was sent and revealed *BRAFV600E* mutation. The correct diagnosis is:

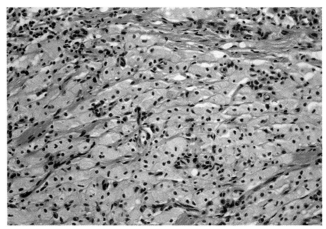

With permission from Caputo et al., *J Am Acad Dermatol*, 2007, volume 57, issue 6, 1031–45 (fig. 8, p. 1040).

A. Metastatic melanoma with balloon cell change
B. Metastatic renal cell carcinoma
C. Erdheim-Chester disease
D. Langerhans cell histiocytosis (Hand-Schüller-Christian disease)
E. Xanthelasma with unrelated systemic disorder

56. A 25-year-old female presents with a subcutaneous nodule on her index finger. It is light pink, 0.5 cm in size, and is otherwise asymptomatic. A biopsy is performed and is shown in the figure. The most appropriate diagnosis in this setting would be:

With permission from Frey, et al., *J Am Acad Dermatol*, 2009, volume, 60, issue 2, 331–9 (fig. 3, p. 333).

A. Mucinous carcinoma
B. Aggressive digital papillary adenocarcinoma
C. Hidradenoma papilliferum
D. Digital syringoma
E. Desmoplastic trichoepithelioma

57. What is the best diagnosis?

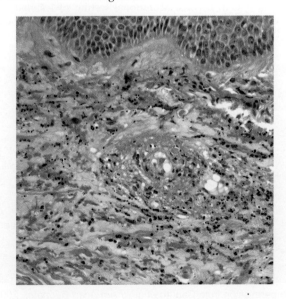

A. Urticaria
B. Sweet syndrome
C. Leukocytoclastic vasculitis
D. Intravascular lymphoma

58. A 45-year-old woman with a history of systemic lupus erythematosus presents with a 6-month history of mildly tender, subcutaneous nodules on the legs with slight overlying erythema. A deep biopsy is performed and shows the pattern in the figure. The next correct step in diagnosis and/or treatment would be as follows:

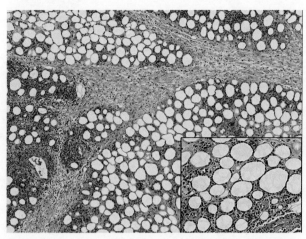

With permission from Sluzevich, et al., *J Am Acad Dermatol*, 2012, volume 67, issue 5 (fig. 2, p. e224).

A. Check dsDNA titers.
B. Increase hydroxychloroquine dose from 2.5 mg/kg to 5 mg/kg.
C. Keep hydroxychloroquine dose at 2.5 mg/kg and start prednisone 0.5 mg/kg.
D. Check peripheral blood flow cytometry and T cell receptor (TCR) gene rearrangement clonality by V-beta.
E. Recommend patient stops taking oral contraceptive pills.

59. A patient presents with a 4.0 cm thin pink plaque on the hand. A biopsy is performed and shown in the figure. The most appropriate diagnosis would be:

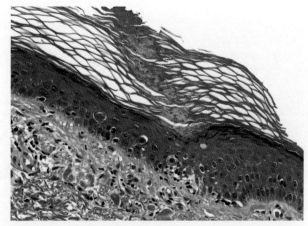

With permission from Bolognia J, et al., *Dermatology*, 4th ed., Elsevier, 1904 (ch. 109, fig. 109.9).

A. Porokeratosis
B. Tinea corporis
C. Lichen planus like keratosis
D. Bowen disease
E. Seborrheic keratosis

60. A 65-year-old man with a history of actinic keratosis, basal cell carcinoma, and cutaneous squamous cell carcinoma presents with a 1-cm, tender, crusted nodule on the left antihelix. A biopsy is performed and the entire lesion is removed (see figure). The next correct step in management is:

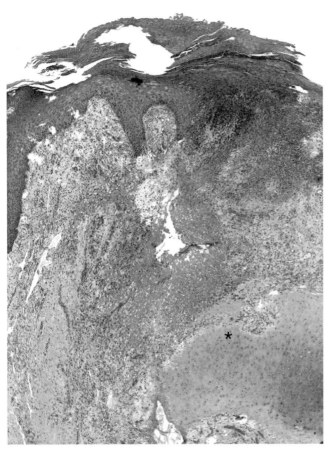

Courtesy Lorenzo Cerroni, MD.

A. Refer for Mohs.
B. Refer for excision with sentinel lymph node biopsy.
C. Refer for excision with sentinel lymph node biopsy and adjuvant radiation.
D. Reassure the patient.

PROCEDURAL DERMATOLOGY

61. A 42-year-old man presents with clinical findings shown. He has a history of two pathologically atypical nevi on the trunk (both with moderate atypia). He has a family history of surgically excised cutaneous melanoma in his mother at 68 years of age. What is the appropriate diagnostic workup to evaluate risk of future malignancy?

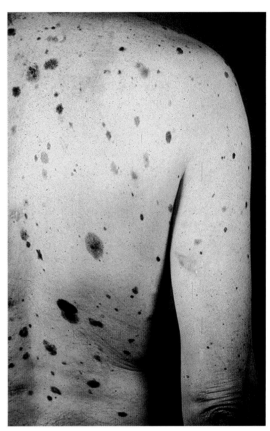

Courtesy of New York University Ronald O Perelman Department of Dermatology.

A. Biopsy of several clinically atypical nevi
B. Genetic testing for *MC1R* mutation
C. Genetic testing for *CDKN2A* mutation
D. Genetic testing for *BRAF* mutation
E. Computed tomography scan to screen for pancreatic cancer

62. What is the maximum dose of lidocaine for tumescent liposuction?
A. 25 mg/kg
B. 85 mg/kg
C. 55 mg/kg
D. 35 mg/kg
E. 65 mg/kg

63. A patient presents with ringing in her ears after having a chemical peel. What type of chemical peel was performed?
A. Glycolic acid peel
B. Trichloroacetic (TCA) 20% peel
C. Trichloroacetic (TCA) 50% peel
D. Baker-Gordon peel
E. Salicylic acid peel

64. An African American woman presents to inquire about laser hair removal of her axillae. What is the safest laser to use for this patient?
A. Diode
B. Alexandrite
C. Nd:YAG
D. IPL
E. Ruby

65. A patient presents complaining that too much of her upper gums show when she smiles. She inquires about treatment options. Which muscle would you inject with botulinum toxin to remedy the patient's complaint?

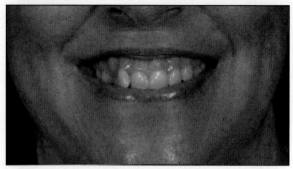

With permission from Maher IA, Flynn TC, Treatment of the midface with botulinum toxin, in Carruthers A, Carruthers J (eds), *Botulinum Toxin: Procedures in Cosmetic Dermatology Series*, 2018, Elsevier, 133–138 (fig. 20.3 A).

A. Nasalis
B. Levator labii superioris alaeque nasi
C. Orbicularis oris
D. Zygomatis major
E. Depressor anguli oris

66. Which of the following sclerosing agents is associated with the highest risk of anaphylaxis?
A. Polidocanol
B. Sodium tetradecyl sulfate
C. Glycerin
D. Sodium morrhuate
E. Ethanolamine oleate

67. For primary cutaneous melanoma, which of the following factors has the greatest impact on prognosis? Choose the best two answers.
A. Breslow depth
B. Sentinel lymph node biopsy
C. Gender
D. Ulceration of primary tumor
E. >1 mitosis per high-powered field

68. A 72-year-old immunocompetent man presents with two separate biopsy-confirmed squamous cell carcinomas (SCCs) and several additional gritty papules on the scalp. After definitive surgical treatment of the two SCCs, which of the following interventions has been shown to decrease the risk of subsequent skin cancer?

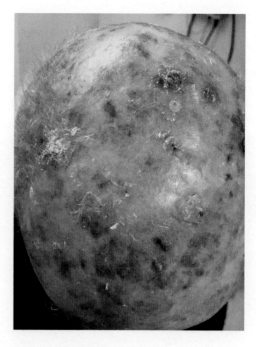

A. Rigorous sun protection
B. Topical fluorouracil
C. Photodynamic therapy
D. Oral niacinamide
E. All of the above

69. During excisional surgery and reconstruction of a large basal cell carcinoma on the scalp, a 150-lb patient is given 42 ml of 1% lidocaine with epinephrine. What is the expected result?
A. Excellent anesthesia
B. Sinus tachycardia
C. Ventricular tachycardia
D. Perioral paresthesia
E. Muscular rigidity

70. During Mohs surgery for SCC on the scalp, the following intraoperative histology is observed. Which of the following is true?

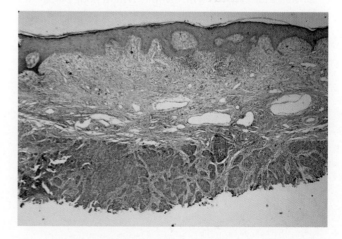

A. Tumor is noted at the superficial surgical margin. Additional staged excision is required.
B. Tumor is noted at the deep surgical margin. Additional staged excision is required.

C. Tumor is noted on the slide but is not involving the surgical margin. No additional excision is required.

D. Tumor is noted on the slide and is too extensive for additional excision. Additional workup is required in preparation for adjuvant treatment.

E. Benign changes of inflammation and fibrosis are noted on the slide. No additional excision is required.

BASIC SCIENCE

71. A patient with a history of chronic sun exposure presents with the lesion shown. Which cancer-associated gene is most commonly mutated?

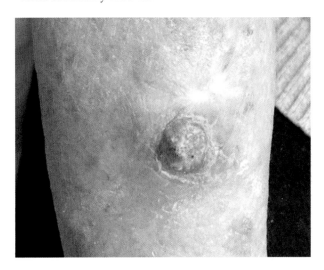

A. *BRAF*
B. *GNAQ*
C. *TP53*
D. *PTCH1*
E. *c-KIT*

72. A 10-year-old boy with recent bone marrow transplant presents with the lesions below. What other dermatologic condition is caused by a distinct but related virus?

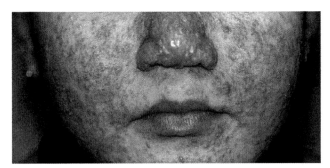

Courtesy Len Sperling, MD.

A. Squamous cell carcinoma
B. Merkel cell carcinoma
C. Burkitt lymphoma
D. Lipschütz ulcer
E. Rosai-Dorfman disease

73. A 68-year-old man developed the painful rash pictured. At what anatomic site does viral latency occur?

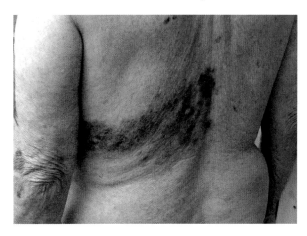

A. Cutaneous nerve fibers
B. Dorsal root ganglion
C. Pacinian corpuscle
D. Keratinocyte
E. Schwann cells

74. A 35-year-old man with metastatic melanoma was treated with targeted cancer therapy and presented with the reaction depicted. What is the function of the protein targeted by this drug?

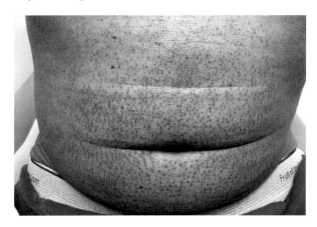

A. PDGF inhibition
B. mTOR inhibition
C. Checkpoint inhibition
D. Phosphorylation

75. A patient with Gorlin syndrome has several advanced basal cell carcinomas and is placed on vismodegib. What is the mechanism of vismodegib?

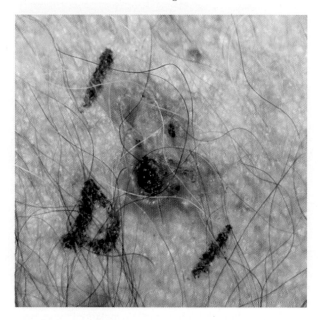

   A. Activates *Patched*
   B. Inhibit *Sonic Hedgehog* binding
   C. Inhibits *Smoothened*
   D. Activates *GL1*
   E. Inhibits *Patched*

76. An 80-year-old man with multiple keratinocyte carcinomas presents with the lesion shown. Six months after removal of the lesion, he develops lymphadenopathy, and CT scan shows metastatic disease. What is the next appropriate therapy?

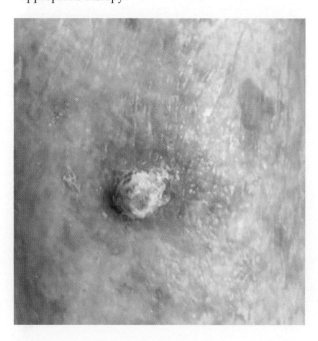

   A. Anti-cytotoxic T-lymphocyte-associated protein-4
   B. Recombinant interleukin-2
   C. Talimogene laherparepvec
   D. Anti-programmed cell death 1
   E. Anti-interleukin 17A

77. A patient presents with worsening rash (shown in the image) and joint stiffness. Which potential therapy increases risk of cutaneous candidiasis?

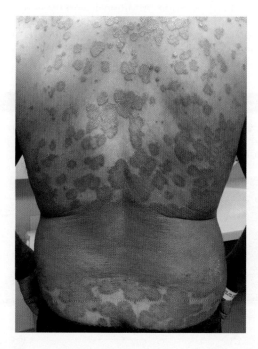

   A. Anti-tumor necrosis factor alpha
   B. Anti-interleukin 4a receptor
   C. Mycophenolate mofetil
   D. Anti-programmed cell death 1
   E. Anti-interleukin 17A

78. This patient presents with a worsening pruritic rash, as depicted. Two weeks after starting a new medication for this rash, he complains of eye irritation and redness. Which targeted therapy did he start?

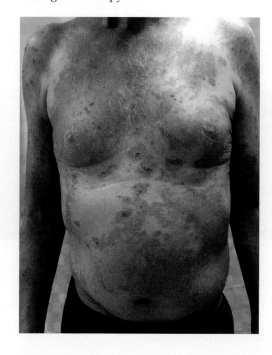

A. Anti-tumor necrosis factor alpha
B. Anti-interleukin 4 receptor alpha
C. Anti-interleukin 13
D. Anti-programmed cell death 1
E. Anti-interleukin 17A

79. A 50-year-old man complains of chronic blistering rash for the past two decades. His ANA is negative. Which circulating autoantibody is associated with this disease?

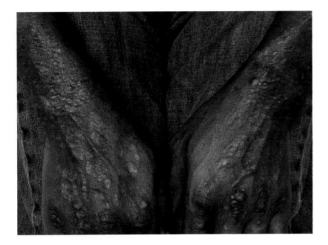

A. Desmoglein-3
B. Collagen VII
C. Collagen XVII
D. Desmoplakin
E. Desmocollin-1

80. A 45-year-old man presents with worsening rash (as shown) despite phototherapy, topical steroids, and methotrexate. He is interested in starting a "biologic" for his disease. What is a unique feature of "biologic" drugs?

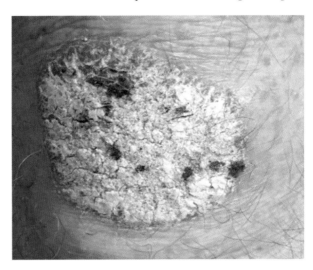

A. Chemically synthesized in a laboratory
B. Binds to receptors on cells
C. Injected intradermally
D. Produced by living organisms or cells
E. Have more side effects

GENERAL DERMATOLOGY

1. E. C & D

It is important for clinicians to recognize postoperative pathergic pyoderma gangrenosum, a neutrophilic dermatosis that classically manifests with ulcerations with a violaceous and undermined rim. Pathergy is a prominent feature, and surgical debridement may worsen the lesions and in some instances may result in severe complications, including death. In general, these ulcers should be biopsied for hematoxylin & eosin and tissue culture to rule out other entities (e.g., medium vessel vasculitis, ecthyma). Granulomatosis with polyangiitis and levamisole toxicity can present with pyoderma gangrenosum-like lesions and are important entities to consider in the differential diagnosis. Treatment of choice is prednisone, while anti-tumor necrosis factor agents have been used as well. Intravenous vancomycin is not indicated if there is no evidence of infection.
Bolognia J, Schaffer J, Cerroni L, eds. *Dermatology*. [Philadelphia]: Elsevier, 2018 (ch. 26).

2. C. Elevated bradykinin levels

The patient's primary care physician most likely prescribed an angiotensin-converting enzyme inhibitor such as lisinopril. Drug-induced angioedema may occur in 0.2% of new users. There is a higher risk in black patients, and most cases occur within the first month of use. ACE inhibitors block kinase II, which leads to elevated bradykinin levels. Another common cause of drug-induced angioedema are nonsteroidal antiinflammatory drugs. Low C4 levels are seen in hereditary angioedemas and acquired angioedema due to B-cell lymphoproliferative disorders, plasma cell dyscrasias, or autoimmune connective tissue diseases. C1 esterase inhibitor deficiency is found in hereditary angioedema type I. Normal or increased levels of C1 esterase inhibitor is seen in type II hereditary angioedema.
Bolognia J, Schaffer J, Cerroni L, eds. *Dermatology*. [Philadelphia]: Elsevier, 2018 (ch. 19).

3. B. HLA-Cw6

HLA-Cw6 has the strongest association with psoriasis. It is found in approximately 90% of cases of early-onset psoriasis and 50% of cases of late-onset psoriasis. It is associated with 10–15 times increased risk for psoriasis. HLA-B27 is associated with sacroiliitis, psoriatic arthritis, and pustular psoriasis. HLA-B13 and HLA-B17 are associated with guttate and erythrodermic psoriasis. HLA-DR3 is associated with palmoplantar pustulosis.
Bolognia J, Schaffer J, Cerroni L, eds. *Dermatology*. [Philadelphia]: Elsevier, 2018 (ch. 8).

4. A. Blastomyces dermatitidis

B. dermatitidis is a dimorphic fungus typically found in soil and moist, decaying wood endemic to eastern North America, the Great Lakes, Ohio River, and Mississippi River basins. It is classically described as a broad-based budding yeast when cultured at body temperature. In nature and culture, however, the filamentous moldlike structures produce short conidiophores with individual conidia at the apex resembling lollipops (seen in the figure). Pulmonary infection is the most common manifestation of disease, while cutaneous blastomycosis is most often due to secondary lymphohematogenous dissemination. Cutaneous lesions are commonly papulopustular but may develop into well-demarcated verrucous plaques. Central ulceration can also occur. Itraconazole and amphotericin B, in severe cases, are the treatments of choice.

Mycobacterium kansasii (B) is an atypical mycobacterial infection. Pulmonary involvement mimicking tuberculosis is most common. Cutaneous lesions may display sporotrichoid spread and are often seen in immunocompromised patients. *M. kansasii* is a slow-growing intracellular mycobacteria and often difficult to culture. Acid-fast stain may reveal broad rods of bacilli.

Histoplasma capsulatum (C) is the causative agent of histoplasmosis. Similar to blastomycosis, pulmonary infection in the most common manifestation of disease and hematogenous spread can lead to internal organ and skin involvement, especially in patients with HIV. While *H. capsulatum* is classically an intracellular yeast at body temperature, in culture the mold produces tuberculate macroconidia and smooth-walled spherical microconidia. Clinically, cutaneous lesions are nonspecific but tend to be molluscoid/umbilicated in immunocompromised hosts. Oral lesions may develop as well. Treatment is the same as for blastomycosis.

Trichophyton rubrum (D) is the most common cause of tinea corporis, a superficial mycosis.

Bolognia J, Schaffer J, Cerroni L, eds. *Dermatology*. [Philadelphia]: Elsevier, 2018 (ch. 77).

5. C. Scarring loss of pubic and axillary hairs
Graham-Little-Piccardi-Lassueur syndrome is a variant of lichen planopilaris, which is characterized by cutaneous or mucosal lichen planus, scarring alopecia of the scalp, and nonscarring alopecia of the pubic and axillary hair with disseminated spinous/follicular papules.

Frontal fibrosis alopecia is another variant of lichen planopilaris characterized by scarring hair loss of the frontal scalp, which slowly progresses. Eyebrow loss may also occur.

Bolognia J, Schaffer J, Cerroni L, eds. *Dermatology*. [Philadelphia]: Elsevier, 2018 (ch. 11).

6. B. Biopsy for histology and direct immunofluorescence
Prurigo nodularis (PN) results from chronic scratching or picking of the skin and may occur in patients with primary cutaneous disease such as atopic dermatitis or as a manifestation of a systemic disorder that may result in itching (i.e., lymphoma, liver or renal disease). The differential diagnosis includes perforating disorders, pemphigoid nodularis (variant of bullous pemphigoid with prurigo nodularis-like lesions), hypertrophic lichen planus, scabetic nodules, or persistent bite reactions. In order to confirm histology and exclude other diagnoses, including pemphigoid nodularis, a biopsy for histology and direct immunofluorescence should be performed. Biopsy for histology alone is another acceptable first step, but the diagnosis of pemphigoid nodularis should be considered, especially in refractory cases. In addition, dermatitis herpetiformis should be considered for pruritic lesions on extensor surfaces, and DIF again is helpful in ruling this out.

Workup for PN should include testing for infections such as HIV, hepatitis, and parasites, and systemic disease including anemia, thyroid, renal, or kidney dysfunction. Although PN and pruritus may be associated with

malignancies (i.e., lymphoma), flow cytometry, chest x-ray, and CT scan would not be the best next step without first confirming the clinical diagnosis and ruling out other primary cutaneous dermatoses. Psychiatric diseases such as obsessive-compulsive disorder and anxiety may be associated with PN; however, workup to exclude a primary cutaneous dermatosis or systemic disease is necessary.

Treatment for PN includes super-potent topical steroids, intralesional steroids, antihistamines, phototherapy, and other antipruritic agents including antidepressants (SSRIs), neuropathic agents (e.g., gabapentin, pregabalin, nortriptyline), and thalidomide. Oral prednisone may be used in the short term for symptomatic relief or while transitioning to steroid-sparing immunosuppressive medications (i.e., cyclosporine).

Bolognia J, Schaffer J, Cerroni L, eds. *Dermatology*. [Philadelphia]: Elsevier, 2018 (ch. 6).

7. D. Assess for suicidality
The patient has signs of body dysmorphic disorder (BDD), including fixation on a mild flaw in appearance. She also expresses signs of depression. It is important for dermatologists to recognize BDD and not perform unnecessary cosmetic treatments (choice C). Additionally, the patient should not dictate treatment if it is not medically necessary (choice A). It is important to not only address such patient's concerns but to ensure that there is no associated suicidal ideation if depressive signs are apparent. The link between BDD and suicidality should be noted, and patients should be screened and referred to psychiatry if deemed medically necessary.

Bolognia J, Schaffer J, Cerroni L, eds. *Dermatology*. [Philadelphia]: Elsevier, 2018 (ch. 7).

8. A. Skin biopsy
   D. Discontinuation of oral contraceptives
   E. Pregnancy test
   I. Recommend compression stockings
Erythema nodosum is a septal panniculitis, which presents as painful nodules on the lower legs (anterior > posterior) but can also be seen on thighs, buttocks, and, less commonly, upper extremities. Common associations include infections (streptococcal, viral upper respiratory infection, bacterial gastroenteritis, coccidioidomycosis), medications (Oral Contraceptive Pills, tumor necrosis factor-alpha inhibitors, BRAF-inhibitors), and systemic disease such as sarcoidosis, inflammatory bowel disease (Crohn's > ulcerative colitis), or Behçet's disease. Pregnancy may also be associated with erythema nodosum. One-third to one-half of cases are idiopathic. Workup for erythema nodosum should include a thorough review of symptoms for recent infections and full medication history. In this vignette, the patient has no other systemic symptoms and has not traveled or lived in an area endemic to coccidioidomycosis. Obtaining a skin biopsy is reasonable to confirm the diagnosis and rule out other entities in the differential, including other panniculitides or a neutrophilic dermatosis. The diagnosis can be made clinically in patients who have a classic presentation. In addition, a pregnancy test should be performed given the association of erythema nodosum with pregnancy. A trial off OCPs (or other medication triggers) is advised to see if there is improvement. Compression and rest/elevation should be recommended for all patients. Other treatment options include NSAIDs, saturated solution of potassium iodide (SSKI), colchicine, and other immunosuppressant medications.

Unlike other panniculitides (i.e., pancreatic panniculitis, erythema induratum, or infectious panniculitis), there is usually no drainage or breakdown of the lesions. Erythema

induratum (EI) or nodular vasculitis presents on the posterior lower legs and may have associated ulceration. Biopsy would reveal a lobular panniculitis or mixed panniculitis. Classically EI is associated with tuberculosis but also may be idiopathic or triggered by other infections. PCR for mycobacterium may be performed with initial biopsy if there is suspicion for EI. In this case, empiric treatment with itraconazole is not indicated, since this patient has not travelled to an area endemic for coccidioidomycosis. Amylase and lipase are part of the workup for pancreatic panniculitis. Chest x-ray and colonoscopy may be performed in the workup of EN if there were signs and symptoms of sarcoidosis or inflammatory bowel disease, respectively. Synovitis, diarrhea, abnormal chest x-ray, preceding infectious symptoms, elevated anti-streptolysin O and/or anti-DNase B titers, or positive purified protein derivative (PPD) are all features associated with a systemic cause of EN; none of which are present in this vignette, making these unnecessary.
Bolognia J, Schaffer J, Cerroni L, eds. *Dermatology*. [Philadelphia]: Elsevier, 2018 (ch. 100).

9. B. Smoking
The patient has discoid lupus erythematosus with a scarred hyper- and hypopigmented plaque in the conchal bowl, a fairly classic presentation. Antimalarials such as hydroxychloroquine, in addition to UV protection, are first-line treatment. Cigarette smoking in patients with lupus is associated with decreased efficacy of antimalarials. Systemic lupus erythematosus may develop in 10%–20% of patients with discoid lupus erythematosus. Uveitis may occur in systemic lupus erythematosus but does not predict antimalarial failure. A percentage of DLE patients may have a positive antinuclear antibody (ANA) (~5%–15%), and this has no association with antimalarial failure. UV radiation plays a role in the pathogenesis of DLE.
Side effects of antimalarial therapy include retinopathy, cytopenias, hemolysis in patients with G6PD deficiency, and gastrointestinal upset, including diarrhea or nausea. Blue-gray or black pigmentation may occur on the shins, nailbed, face, or palate. Morbilliform or urticarial drug hypersensitivity reactions may occur more commonly in patients with dermatomyositis. Lichenoid drug reactions are also a cutaneous side effect. Quinacrine is associated with yellow discoloration. Quinacrine can be added to hydroxychloroquine (HCQ); however, chloroquine should not be added to HCQ due to increased risk of retinopathy and ocular toxicity. HCQ has lower risk of retinopathy than chloroquine does, and risk of toxicity is dependent on daily dosage. All patients on antimalarials should undergo screening with an ophthalmologist given risk of retinopathy. The American Academy of Ophthalmology guidelines (revised 2016) recommends a maximum dose of 5.0 mg/kg real weight for HCQ and 2.3 mg/kg for chloroquine. A baseline fundus exam should rule out preexisting disease within the first year of treatment followed by yearly screening after 5 years for low-risk patients. Patients with higher risk of retinopathy (greater than 5.0 mg/kg of HCQ, duration of use greater than 5 years, renal disease, concurrent use of tamoxifen, macular disease) may require more frequent monitoring.
Bolognia J, Schaffer J, Cerroni L, eds. *Dermatology*. [Philadelphia]: Elsevier, 2018 (ch. 41 and 130).

10. C. BCL-6
The patient has a violaceous papulonodule on the face, depicting follicle center B-cell lymphoma. Clinical features include solitary or grouped papules, plaques, or nodules with predilection for the head and neck in elderly patients. There may be extracutaneous disease in 5%–10% of patients. Prognosis is excellent, with 95% 5-year survival. Treatment options include intralesional steroids, radiation, and, in severe disease, rituximab. Follicular center B-cell lymphoma is BCL-2 negative and BCL-6 positive. It is important to note that if BCL-2 is positive in follicular cells, this favors a systemic lymphoma with secondary cutaneous involvement. The differential diagnosis includes acneiform or epidermal inclusion cysts, pseudolymphoma, arthropod bite reaction, nonmelanoma skin cancer including Merkel cell carcinoma, cutaneous metastasis, and other cutaneous lymphomas.
Marginal zone B-cell lymphoma typically presents as papules, nodules, or plaques on the trunk and upper extremities in younger patients. Extracutaneous disease is rare. BCL-2 is typically positive, and condition is indolent with excellent survival rate of 99% at 5 years.
Serum ACE levels may be elevated in 60% of sarcoidosis patients. P63 may be positive in spindle cell squamous cell carcinomas. Dermatofibrosarcoma protuberans, a locally aggressive fibrous skin tumor, is CD34+. It is most commonly found on the trunk (shoulder or chest area) as a red-brown firm plaque or nodule that slowly grows.
Bolognia J, Schaffer J, Cerroni L, eds. *Dermatology*. [Philadelphia]: Elsevier, 2018 (ch. 119).

11. B. Neutropenia
Azathioprine is an antiinflammatory and immunosuppressive agent used to treat a host of dermatologic diseases including immunobullous disorders. It is processed through three different pathways: two of these result in inactive metabolites (xanthine oxidase and thiopurine methyl transferase [TPMT]), and the third pathway (through hypoxanthine-guanine phosphoribosyl transferase [HGPRT]) results in an active metabolite. If either of the first two pathways become inactivated, then more active metabolite becomes available, which may result in cytopenias or excessive immunosuppression. Allopurinol is a xanthine oxidase inhibitor, thus when given in combination with azathioprine, a pancytopenia may result.
TPMT activity should be evaluated prior to initiating azathioprine, as those with low levels may be at increased risk of cytopenias. Eosinophilia may occur in azathioprine hypersensitivity syndrome, a clinical syndrome that usually begins within the first month of therapy and manifests as fever, morbilliform eruption, hepatotoxicity, and respiratory and gastrointestinal distress. Permanent discontinuation is required should this develop.
Azathioprine may decrease the effectiveness of warfarin, thus monitoring of the INR is necessary for patients on this combination. Captopril may also increase risk of leukopenia. Other side effects of azathioprine include the development of nonmelanoma skin cancers with long-term use, lymphoma, and pancreatitis or hepatitis. Elevated creatine phosphokinase (CPK) may occur with drug reaction with eosinophilia and systemic symptoms (DRESS) or with rhabdomyolysis, which are not relevant to the clinical scenario of the vignette.

12. C. Coining
There are numerous dermatoses that can result from cultural practices. Linear ecchymosis occurs from rubbing the skin with a coin, which may be used as a remedy for fevers, cough, and headaches. The pattern usually

resembles a pine tree. Coining must be distinguished from child abuse. Gardner diamond syndrome (autoerythrocyte sensitization syndrome or psychogenic purpura) presents as the spontaneous development of ecchymosis on the trunk and extremities in middle-aged females. There is an association with emotional trauma and psychiatric disease. The ecchymosis are not linear or geometric as with coining. Pigmented purpuric dermatoses typically manifest as brown-yellow patches or plaques and with varying morphology (lichen aureus, eczematous, lichenoid).

Other cultural practices include cupping and moxibustion. Cupping occurs through local suction/vacuum application to the skin and results in round purpuric patches that may heal with hyperpigmentation. Moxibustion is when moxa (dried plant materials) is burned onto the skin and may result in vesicles and bulla as well as second- or third-degree burns.

13. D. Alopecia areata

This image shows exclamation point hairs, which are found in alopecia areata, especially at the border of lesions. The hairs are tapered (distal end is broader than the proximal ends). Tinea capitis often has broken short hairs, which may appear like commas. Lichen planopilaris is a scarring alopecia that presents with perifollicular erythema and scale. Trichoscopy would show discrete white dots due to loss of melanin and perifollicular fibrosis. Follicular red dots are present in discoid lupus erythematosus on trichoscopy.
Bolognia J, Schaffer J, Cerroni L, eds. *Dermatology*. [Philadelphia]: Elsevier, 2018 (ch. 69).

14. B. Discoid lupus erythematosus

Absence of follicular openings, keratin plugs, and red dots are features of DLE on dermoscopy. Lichen planopilaris (LPP) also has absence of follicular openings and white patches but lacks the red dots seen in DLE. Other features of LPP include perifollicular erythema and blue-gray dots. Peripilar casts may also be present. Androgenic alopecia usually has brown hallows around the follicular ostia and hairs of varying diameters. Black dots, exclamation point hairs, and yellow dots are present in alopecia areata. In folliculitis decalvans, tufted hairs and perifollicular pustules are present.
Bolognia J, Schaffer J, Cerroni L, eds. *Dermatology*. [Philadelphia]: Elsevier, 2018 (ch. 69).

15. B. History of prolonged minocycline use

The kodachrome demonstrates hyperpigmentation secondary to minocycline. There are three types that can occur: blue-black discoloration in sites of inflammation and scars; blue-gray hyperpigmentation within normal skin, typically the shin (as seen in the figure); and diffuse muddy-brown pigmentation most prominent in sun-exposed sites. The discoloration may also involve nails, teeth, and mucosae (eyes, oral). The differential includes antimalarial hyperpigmentation (i.e., to hydroxychloroquine), which may manifest as gray to blue-black pigmentation with a predilection for pretibial skin, as well as other sites including the face, hard palate, sclerae, and subungual skin. Unlike hydroxychloroquine, quinacrine may result in yellowish-brown diffuse discoloration.

Varicose veins, a sign of venous hypertension, may result in venous stasis purpura (often golden-brown, petechial). A motor vehicle accident may result in silica granuloma (tattooing of silicon dioxide from dirt/asphalt), which are often geometric and appear at the site of injury. Prior bladder surgery may result in lymphedema and changes of lymphedema, which may include lipodermatosclerosis and elephantiasis nostras verrucosa at severe stages.
Bolognia J, Schaffer J, Cerroni L, eds. *Dermatology*. [Philadelphia]: Elsevier, 2018 (ch. 67).

16. B. Varicella zoster virus

The kodachrome depicts group vesicles on an inflamed base, some of which are starting to crust. Herpes viral infections, including herpes simplex and herpes zoster, may present on the palm and should be considered in the differential diagnosis of vesicular palmar lesions. Coxsackie is another viral infection that also presents on acral skin but with small, discrete vesicles and papules (often white-gray), which are usually oval-shaped and follow the dermatoglyphics. Erythema multiforme presents with targetoid or atypical targetoid lesions on acral skin with central necrosis. Associated mucosal lesions (ocular, genital, and mouth) may also occur. Orf is a self-limited parapox viral infection, which is contracted from animals, especially sheep and goats. The presentation is a firm vesiculobullous or pustular lesion. Acute allergic contact dermatitis may also present with inflamed vesicles but often with a geometric configuration. The grouped vesicles in the kodachrome is typical of a herpes virus infection.
Bolognia J, Schaffer J, Cerroni L, eds. *Dermatology*. [Philadelphia]: Elsevier, 2018 (ch. 80).

17. D. Flow cytometry, T-cell PCR

The patient has cutaneous T-cell lymphoma with polycyclic, annular papulosquamous lesions that are generalized >10% body surface area (stage 1B). In general, lesions of mycosis fungoides have a predilection for sun-protected sites. Evaluation for systemic involvement is indicated with flow cytometry and T-cell PCR, as well as thorough physical examination, including lymph node examination.

Repeat biopsies may be indicated in presentations of cutaneous T-cell lymphoma whereby prior biopsies are nondiagnostic. In fact, many patients have prior biopsies demonstrating eczematous or psoriasiform dermatitis. Repeated biopsies and close surveillance are indicated in these patients. ANA, SSA, and SSB titers may be obtained in subacute cutaneous lupus erythematosus. These papulosquamous or annular lesions often favor photoexposed and seborrheic sites. Desmoglein titers are obtained in pemphigus vulgaris (dsg 3) or foliaceous (dsg1). Direct immunofluorescence is obtained to evaluate for immunobullous disorders.
Bolognia J, Schaffer J, Cerroni L, eds. *Dermatology*. [Philadelphia]: Elsevier, 2018 (ch. 120).

18 A. Lichen sclerosus

This kodachrome depicts extragenital lichen sclerosus (LS). LS is a chronic inflammatory disease with predilection for anogenital sites. Pruritus is common, and advanced disease may result in scarring and loss of normal architecture of the vulva in women and phimosis in men. Lesions are generally ivory-white and atrophic, and follicular plugging may be present in nonglabrous skin. Active lesions may show purpura and hemorrhage, while bullous lesions are less common. Extragenital presentations typically favor the submammary skin, shoulders, neck, and wrists. Surveillance of genital lesions is indicated given the risk of squamous cell carcinoma development. Treatment is with high-potency topical steroids and topical calcineurin inhibitors. Circumcision may be required in cases of refractory phimosis in men with LS (aka balanitis xerotica obliterans).

The other lichen conditions manifest differently. Lichen planus presents with violaceous flat-topped papules to hypertrophic papules/plaques and may involve the oral or anogenital mucosae. Lichen striatus typically manifests with a linear configuration of lichenoid papules. Lichen amyloidosis presents with pruritic, hyperkeratotic red-brown papules. Lichen aureus, a type of pigmented purpuric dermatosis, typically presents as golden-brown petechial patches or plaques that favor the lower extremities.

Bolognia J, Schaffer J, Cerroni L, eds. *Dermatology*. [Philadelphia]: Elsevier, 2018 (ch. 73).

19. **B.** Janus kinase (JAK) and Bruton tyrosine kinase inhibitors
The vignette and kodachrome depict the diagnosis of eosinophilic fasciitis (EF)-like presentation of chronic graft-versus-host disease (GVHD) post–stem cell transplantation. Patients with EF typically present with a rippled appearance and irregular nodular texture to the skin due to involvement of subcutaneous tissues, and decreased joint mobility may occur. In the earlier, more edematous phase, the presence of hypereosinophilia is a clue to diagnosis. Standard of care includes immunosuppression in the management of GVHD, and prednisone and methotrexate have been classically used. More recently, use of the JAK inhibitor ruxolitinib (selective for JAK 1, 2) has gained traction in the management of chronic GVHD off-label and is currently under investigation. Ibrutinib, a Bruton tyrosine kinase inhibitor, has been recently approved in the treatment of GVHD following failure of one or more lines of systemic therapy. Other presentations of chronic GVHD include lichenoid, morpheaform, sclerodermoid, dyspigmentation, icthyosiform, and eczematous forms.
CTLA-4 and PD-1 blockers are immune checkpoint inhibitors approved for the use of multiple cancers, most notably melanoma, lung, and genitourinary cancers. BRAF and MEK inhibitors are targeted chemotherapeutic agents used in the treatment of BRAF V600E mutant melanomas. IL-17 inhibitors are used in psoriasis (i.e., ixekizumab, secukinumab), as well as IL-12/23 inhibitors (ustekinumab), while guselkumab is a selective IL-23 blocker. Dupilimumab is an IL-4 and IL-13 biologic inhibitor approved for atopic dermatitis, and omalizumab is a monoclonal antibody directed against IgE approved for chronic urticaria and severe allergic asthma. It has been used off-label in patients with bullous pemphigoid and elevated IgE titers with varying degrees of success.

Bolognia J, Schaffer J, Cerroni L, eds. *Dermatology*. [Philadelphia]: Elsevier, 2018 (ch. 52).

20. **D.** Inflammatory morphea
Plaque-type morphea is the most frequent variant of morphea and is characterized by the insidious onset of a slightly elevated erythematous or violaceous plaque that expands centrifugally. The central portion of the progressing lesion may become hyperpigmented and sclerotic. The kodachrome highlights the classic lilac border of inflammatory morphea.
Annular elastolytic giant cell granuloma typically manifests on photoexposed sites as annular patches with a classic hypopigmented center. Annular lichen planus classically occurs on the genitals. Cutaneous T-cell lymphoma may present with papulosquamous patches and plaques, which are polycyclic or reniform in photoprotected sites. Granuloma annulare classically manifests with annular dermal papules and plaques. The hyperpigmented, sclerotic center would not be present.

Bolognia J, Schaffer J, Cerroni L, eds. *Dermatology*. [Philadelphia]: Elsevier, 2018 (ch. 44).

21. **C.** Hypertrophic lichen planus
This kodachrome illustrates hypertrophic lichen planus. It is important for dermatologists to recognize lesions that may mimic squamous cell carcinoma (SCC) both clinically and histologically (due to pseudoepitheliomatous hyperplasia)—including hypertrophic lichen planus and hypertrophic discoid lupus. Lesions of hypertrophic lichen planus typically manifest on the extremities, and clues for the diagnosis include multiple lesions and lichenoid inflammation on histopathology. More conservative approaches including topical and intralesional steroids, methotrexate or 5-fluorouracil, as well as acitretin should be considered.
Pemphigus vulgaris, psoriasis, and subacute cutaneous lupus erythematosus do not typically present with pseudoepitheliomatous hyperplasia mimicking SCC. While pemphigus vegetans may have epidermal hyperplasia, acantholysis and eosinophilic abscesses are distinguishing features.

Bolognia J, Schaffer J, Cerroni L, eds. *Dermatology*. [Philadelphia]: Elsevier, 2018 (ch. 11).

22. **A.** Hospitalize
C. Topical steroids, sauna suit, open-wet dressings
D. Check CBC, CMP, calcium
G. Begin adalimumab
The vignette and figures depict a case of generalized pustular psoriasis, which may occur in the setting of rapid tapering of systemic steroids and pregnancy (impetigo herpetiformis). Patients with acute erythroderma and generalized pustular psoriasis often require hospitalization for close monitoring. In particular, patients may be at risk for thermal dysregulation and dehydration/electrolyte imbalance. The patient in the vignette is pregnant, which should prompt close surveillance and hospitalization. Skin-directed therapy with topical steroids and sauna suit/open-wet dressings is helpful and can lead to rapid improvement and symptomatic control. Laboratory evaluation is indicated as well, and in particular checking for hypocalcemia, which may be a trigger of generalized pustular psoriasis in pregnancy. Acitretin is absolutely contraindicated in pregnant women and is generally avoided in women of childbearing age. It is a severe teratogen, with studies showing increased risk of spontaneous abortion or congenital malformation. Additionally, women should avoid pregnancy for at least 2 years after taking acitretin. Methotrexate is absolutely contraindicated and is used in medical abortions. Women should wait at least 1 month after discontinuation of methotrexate prior to conceiving, and men should wait at least 3 months. Adalimumab and other TNF inhibitors were formerly considered pregnancy category B. While many patients elect to hold treatment with biologic agents in the setting of pregnancy, overall studies suggest that they do not cause fetal harm. It is therefore reasonable to treat with adalimumab or etanercept in cases of severe pustular generalized psoriasis during pregnancy.

Bolognia J, Schaffer J, Cerroni L, eds. *Dermatology*. [Philadelphia]: Elsevier, 2018 (ch. 8).

23. **A.** Ventral pterygium
Nail abnormalities are seen in approximately 10% of patients with lichen planus. Nail thinning, longitudinal ridging and fissuring, and dorsal pterygium are common in nail lichen planus. Dorsal pterygium is a result of adhesion of the proximal nail fold to the nail bed due to matrix

destruction and disappearance of the nail plate. Nail bed lichen planus can result in onycholysis, nail thickening, and yellow discoloration. Trachyonychia, also known as twenty-nail dystrophy, refers to nail plate roughness due primarily to excessive longitudinal ridging. The inflammatory condition most commonly associated with trachyonychia is alopecia areata; however, it can also be associated with lichen planus, eczema, and psoriasis. Red lunulae are seen in approximately 30% of patients with nail lichen planus. Ventral pterygium is seen in autoimmune connective tissue disorders, especially systemic sclerosis.

Bolognia J, Schaffer J, Cerroni L, eds. *Dermatology*. [Philadelphia]: Elsevier, 2018 (ch. 71).

24. B. ECM-1

IgG autoantibodies against extracellular matrix protein 1 (ECM-1) are seen in approximately 80% of patients with lichen sclerosus. Females with lichen sclerosus have a higher incidence of autoimmune diseases and positive antinuclear antibody (ANA); however, ANA is not specific to lichen sclerosus and can be seen in a variety of autoimmune conditions. DNA topoisomerase I (formerly Scl-70) autoantibodies are seen in scleroderma. Nuclear matrix protein (NXP-2) autoantibodies are associated with 1%–15% of adults and 20%–25% of juveniles with dermatomyositis.

Bolognia J, Schaffer J, Cerroni L, eds. *Dermatology*. [Philadelphia]: Elsevier, 2018 (chs. 40 & 44).

25. D. Glucose

Necrobiosis lipoidica diabeticorum (NLD) is a granulomatous condition of unknown cause. Key clinical features include atrophic red-brown to yellow plaques with a translucent center with telangiectasia usually found on the lower legs. Ulcerations may occur. The differential includes granuloma annulare, lipodermatosclerosis, granulomatous infections, and sarcoid. NLD is associated with diabetes mellitus. As many as 15% to 65% of patients with NLD have diabetes mellitus; however, only 0.3% of patients with diabetes mellitus have NLD. While it is not proven that poor glycemic control will lead to the development of NLD, diabetic patients with NLD have higher rates of diabetes-associated complications such as peripheral neuropathy, retinopathy, and joint immobility.

There is no association with abnormalities of lipase, liver enzymes, or calcium with NLD. Of note, a retrospective review found thyroid dysfunction in 13% of patients with NLD.

Bolognia J, Schaffer J, Cerroni L, eds. *Dermatology*. [Philadelphia]: Elsevier, 2018 (ch. 93).

26. B. Sulfamethoxazole/trimethoprim

When taken along with methotrexate, trimethoprim, dapsone, and other sulfonamides inhibit the folate metabolic pathway. This inhibition leads to a markedly increased risk of pancytopenia. Sulfamethoxazole/trimethoprim is a commonly prescribed antibiotic for urinary tract infections, but great care should be taken to avoid its use in patients on methotrexate due to this potentially life-threatening interaction.

Additional drugs that elevate methotrexate blood levels include NSAIDs, salicylates, chloramphenicol, phenothiazines, phenytoin, and tetracyclines. Dipyridamole and probenecid increase intracellular accumulation of methotrexate. Systemic retinoids and alcohol should also be avoided in patients taking methotrexate due to synergistic liver damage.

Bolognia J, Schaffer J, Cerroni L, eds. *Dermatology*. [Philadelphia]: Elsevier, 2018 (ch. 130).

27. D. Capecitabine

Toxic erythema of chemotherapy (TEC) is an all-encompassing term to describe the toxic cutaneous side effects of some chemotherapies that results in symmetric erythematous to dusky patches with associated edema, erosions, desquamation, and/or purpura, with a predilection for acral and intertriginous zones. Additional terms may be used to describe the reaction depending on the location. Here the reaction favors an acral site; therefore "palmoplantar erythrodysesthesia" and "hand-foot syndrome" are sometimes used.

Of the listed medications, capecitabine is most likely responsible. TEC may be seen following administration of a variety of agents, including cytarabine, anthracyclines, 5-fluorouracil and its prodrugs (e.g., capecitabine), taxanes, methotrexate, busulfan, and cisplatin.

Hydroxyurea cutaneous adverse events include a dermatomyositis-like eruption on the dorsal hands, diffuse cutaneous and mucosal hyperpigmentation, and lower leg ulcers (classically on the lateral malleolus). Allopurinol may cause an exanthematous drug eruption, DRESS, or Stevens–Johnson syndrome / toxic epidermal necrolysis. Bleomycin may cause flagellate hyperpigmentation and digital ulcers.

Bolognia J, Schaffer J, Cerroni L, eds. *Dermatology*. [Philadelphia]: Elsevier, 2018 (ch. 21).

28. C. Keratosis follicularis (Darier disease)

Nail findings associated with Darier disease (keratosis follicularis) include multiple red and white longitudinal streaks with wedge-shaped "V-nicking" and fissuring at the distal margin of the nail plate. The key to the diagnosis is the presence of multiple bands. A single red longitudinal band with distal subungual hyperkeratosis can be seen in both benign tumors (e.g., onychopapilloma, glomus), Bowen's disease or amelanotic melanoma. Nail changes found in psoriasis include inflammatory onycholysis, subungual hyperkeratosis, oil spots, and nail plate pits.

Bolognia J, Schaffer J, Cerroni L, eds. *Dermatology*. [Philadelphia]: Elsevier, 2018 (ch. 71).

29. A. Thrombospondin

Microcystic lymphatic malformation ("lymphangioma circumscriptum") is the most common type of lymphatic malformation. They are ill-defined aggregates of abnormal lymphatic channels. Histopathology of microcystic lymphatic malformations demonstrates enlarged, distorted lymphatic channels with smooth muscle cells in their walls and a very thin endothelium. The lymphatic endothelium can be identified by immunohistochemical staining for podoplanin, LYVE-1, Prox1, and VEGFR-3. Thrombospondin (TSP-1 and TSP-2) are endogenous inhibitors of skin angiogenesis and are expressed in normal human skin. TSP-1 is expressed by dermal cells and epidermal keratinocytes and is deposited at the basement membrane zone.

Bolognia J, Schaffer J, Cerroni L, eds. *Dermatology*. [Philadelphia]: Elsevier, 2018 (ch. 102 & 104).

30. B. Doxepin
C. Fexofenadine

Symptomatic dermographism is the most common of the physical urticarias. Patients are often young adults and complain of pruritus. The course is typically unpredictable but can improve over time. Mucosal involvement does not occur, but vulvar swelling has been reported during

intercourse. Associations may include pregnancy, thyroid disease, and atopic dermatitis. Treatment is with antihistamines such as fexofenadine or doxepin. Ibuprofen can trigger urticaria and is not used in the treatment of dermatographism. Dupilumab is approved in the treatment of atopic dermatitis and asthma.
Bolognia J, Schaffer J, Cerroni L, eds. *Dermatology*. [Philadelphia]: Elsevier, 2018 (ch. 18).

31. A. Folliculitis decalvans
The kodachrome displays scarring alopecia with highly inflammatory papules and pustules indicative of folliculitis decalvans. Staph aureus is often cultured from the pustules. Treatment with oral or topical antibiotics is usually necessary, including tetracycline or a combination of rifampin and clindamycin. Discoid lupus of the scalp is also a scarring alopecia that may have classic features of DLE, including dyschromia, erythema, and plugged follicles, whereas papules and pustules are not a typical feature. Lipedematous scalp or lipedematous alopecia is characterized by a boggy scalp in association with alopecia and is usually found in females. Acne conglobata is part of the follicular occlusion tetrad that includes hidradenitis suppurativa, dissecting cellulitis, and pilonidal cyst.
Bolognia J, Schaffer J, Cerroni L, eds. *Dermatology*. [Philadelphia]: Elsevier, 2018 (ch. 69).

32. C. Diabetes mellitus
Confluent and reticulated papillomatosis (CARP) presents as reticulated keratotic papules and plaques that usually manifest on the chest, back, or abdomen. It usually occurs during puberty and can be associated with obesity, menstrual irregularities, diabetes mellitus, and pituitary and thyroid disorders. Lesions are asymptomatic or rarely, mildly pruritic. Treatment is difficult but oral minocycline is most effective. Lichen amyloid may be found in the multiple endocrine neoplasia 2a syndrome, which also has medullary thyroid cancer, pheochromocytoma, and parathyroid abnormalities as part of the syndrome. Lymphomas may present with persistent pruritus, dermal hypersensitivity reactions, erythema annular centrifugum, cutaneous involvement, and other paraneoplastic disorders; however, CARP is not a harbinger of lymphoma. Monoclonal gammopathies are associated with a myriad of dermatologic diseases, including diffuse normolipemic plane xanthomas, neutrophilic dermatoses, scleromyxedema, necrobiotic xanthogranuloma, and erythema elevatum diutinum, among others.
Bolognia J, Schaffer J, Cerroni L, eds. *Dermatology*. [Philadelphia]: Elsevier, 2018 (ch. 109).

33. A. Smooth muscle hamartoma
Becker's nevus is a unilateral, hyperpigmented, and often hypertrichotic patch or slightly elevated plaque. The hyperpigmentation has irregular borders. It often presents in adolescent men and on the shoulder, as well as upper lateral trunk. Hyperpigmentation may arise during the first decade, but lesions most often appear during adolescence. Hyperpigmentation usually precedes the hypertrichosis. Thickening found in Becker's nevus may be associated with an underlying smooth muscle hamartoma. Lesions are difficult to treat but laser surgery may be useful.
Infantile hemangiomas may leave atrophy and fibrofatty changes upon involution. Diabetes mellitus can be associated with CARP or acanthosis nigricans. *P. acnes* has been implicated in the pathogenesis of acne and progressive macular hypomelanosis, which presents as ill-defined hypopigmented macules on the trunk.

Bolognia J, Schaffer J, Cerroni L, eds. *Dermatology*. [Philadelphia]: Elsevier, 2018 (ch. 112).

34. C. Direct fluorescent antibody
This kodachrome depicts group vesicles on a red base on the buttocks, a common presentation of herpes simplex virus (HSV). Direct fluorescent antibody assay is frequently performed as an initial diagnostic test in HSV due to greater sensitivity than other tests and the ability to distinguish between HSV and varicella zoster virus, as well as the ability to give rapid results. Alternatively, PCR for HSV may be obtained when available. Viral culture usually takes 2–5 days. Bacterial culture would be considered if there is concern for a bacterial folliculitis. KOH would be considered for candida/tinea. Biopsy would be unnecessary in this classic presentation of HSV.
Bolognia J, Schaffer J, Cerroni L, eds. *Dermatology*. [Philadelphia]: Elsevier, 2018 (ch. 80).

35. C. An object
This lesion was obtained from an accidental thermal burn from an iron. The triangular shape is the most important clue to indicate an outside job. Lichenoid eruptions or phytophotodermatitis may be induced by UV radiation and result in hyperpigmentation (often streaky when due to phytophotodermatitis) but not in this triangular geometric configuration. Chronic rubbing results in lichen simplex chronicus, which presents as hyperpigmented lichenified plaques. Spray perfume could result in berloque dermatitis, which presents as hyperpigmented macules and patches on the neck and chest. This entity is less common in recent years as bergapten (5-methoxypsoralens) is restricted in cosmetic products.
Bolognia J, Schaffer J, Cerroni L, eds. *Dermatology*. [Philadelphia]: Elsevier, 2018 (ch. 88).

36. B. Lichen amyloidosis
The kodachrome depicts lichen amyloidosis, the most common form of primary cutaneous amyloidosis. It usually presents on extensor surfaces as coalescing pruritic, discrete, firm, and often scaly papules. Hypertrophic lichen planus and prurigo nodularis may also present on the extensor extremities, but the lesions are often thicker and may be violaceous with white scales in the case of lichen planus. Waxy papules (as opposed to scaly papules) best characterize papular mucinosis (also known as lichen myxedematosus). Lichen amyloidosis can be found in Multiple endocrine neoplasia, type 2A (MEN 2A) autoimmune connective tissue disorders, and primary biliary cirrhosis. There are also familial forms of lichen amyloidosis.
Bolognia J, Schaffer J, Cerroni L, eds. *Dermatology*. [Philadelphia]: Elsevier, 2018 (ch. 47).

37. B. Bilirubin
The patient has evidence of plane xanthomas of the palmar crease, x*anthoma striatum palmare*, which is seen in dysbetalipoproteinemia (type III hyperlipoproteinemias). Palmar plane xanthomas may also occur in secondary forms of hyperlipidemia, including primary biliary cirrhosis (PBC), which this vignette depicts (note the diffuse itching and prurigo nodules, which are also a presenting cutaneous manifestation of PBC). Plane xanthomas may also be found in normolipemic patients that have underlying monoclonal gammopathy, most commonly IgG. Other lymphoproliferative disorders are also associated, including B-cell lymphoma and Castleman disease. BP180 (BPAG2) would be elevated in bullous pemphigoid, which does not present with xanthomas. Elevated CRP is

a nonspecific marker of inflammation. ACE levels may be elevated in sarcoidosis.
Bolognia J, Schaffer J, Cerroni L, eds. *Dermatology.* [Philadelphia]: Elsevier, 2018 (ch. 92).

38. C. Netherton syndrome
Elastosis perforans serpiginosa is a rare perforating dermatosis consisting of papules arranged in a serpiginous pattern commonly found on the neck, face, and arms. About 40% of cases are associated with genetic diseases, including Rothmund-Thomson syndrome, Ehlers-Danlos syndrome, osteogenesis imperfecta, Down syndrome, pseudoxanthoma elasticum, and acrogeria. Netherton syndrome is an ichthyosis that presents with erythroderma, hair anomalies (trichorrhexis invaginata), and food allergies. Ichthyosis linearis circumflexa (ILC) is the characteristic cutaneous finding in Netherton syndrome. ILC presents as serpiginous plaques with double-edged scale.
Bolognia J, Schaffer J, Cerroni L, eds. *Dermatology.* [Philadelphia]: Elsevier, 2018 (ch. 96).

39. D. Conjunctivitis
The patient has been placed on dupilumab, an IL-4 receptor antagonist. The most common side effects are injection-site reaction and conjunctivitis. Dupilumab has not been associated with hepatitis B reactivation, lupus-like syndromes, or serum sickness–like reactions.
Bolognia J, Schaffer J, Cerroni L, eds. *Dermatology.* [Philadelphia]: Elsevier, 2018 (ch. 128).

40. A. Anakinra
The patient has DIRA—deficiency of IL-1 receptor antagonist. This is an autosomal recessive disorder that presents typically early in life with erythematous plaques studded with pustules that looks similar to pustular psoriasis. Osteolytic bone lesions may also occur. The recalcitrant nature of his pustular psoriasiform eruption suggests a potential genetic basis of his disease, namely deficiency of IL1RN. Anakinra (IL-1 receptor antagonist) has been shown to be an effective therapy for this condition.
Bolognia J, Schaffer J, Cerroni L, eds. *Dermatology.* [Philadelphia]: Elsevier, 2018 (ch. 45 and 130).

PEDIATRIC DERMATOLOGY

41. D. Netherton syndrome
The trichogram depicted here shows trichorrhexis invaginata, also referred to as "bamboo hair," which is characteristically seen in patients with Netherton syndrome. Failure to thrive and food allergies, which the vignette also describes, are additional features of this syndrome, which is due to mutations in *SPINK5* (*serine protease inhibitor LEKTI*).
Menkes kinky hair syndrome and Bazex-Dupre-Christol present with sparse or absent hair that shows flattened, twisted hairs referred to as pili torti with light microscopy. Trichorrhexis nodosa is a feature of trichothiodystrophy. Atopic dermatitis is not associated with increased hair shaft fragility.
Bolognia J, Schaffer J, Cerroni L, eds. *Dermatology.* [Philadelphia]: Elsevier, 2018 (ch. 57).

42. B. Pulmonary emphysema
The clinical image and vignette suggest a diagnosis of inherited cutis laxa, which manifests in birth to early childhood with severe skin and internal organ involvement.

Key clinical features include an aged facial appearance with loose, sagging skin. Lung involvement presenting as emphysema is common and can be fatal.
Angioid streaks and GI hemorrhage are prominent features of pseudoxanthoma elasticum, which presents with yellowish papules in flexural areas. Ectopia lentis is a manifestation of Marfan syndrome, and blue sclerae is seen in Ehlers-Danlos syndrome.
Bolognia J, Schaffer J, Cerroni L, eds. *Dermatology.* [Philadelphia]: Elsevier, 2018 (ch. 97).

43. A. Erythema infectiosum
The clinical image and vignette support a diagnosis of erythema infectiosum, which is caused by parvovirus B19 infection. The infection begins with a prodrome of fever, headache, and malaise, and the exanthem typically presents 1–2 weeks later. Prominent erythema of the cheeks is the classic presentation, but a development of a lacy, reticulated maculopapular eruption over the extremities is also characteristic (as seen in the figure). Arthritis is another accompanying feature, particularly in adult women. Infection of the fetus may result in anemia, fetal hydrops, or death.
Mononucleosis presents in young adults with fever, pharyngitis, and lymphadenopathy. A nonspecific exanthem may occur, and a morbilliform eruption may develop after unnecessary treatment with amoxicillin. Rubeola or measles typically presents with cough, coryza, and conjunctivitis (three C's). Rubella can resemble measles, though typically milder, with an eruption that spreads in a cephalocaudal fashion. Exanthem subitum (also called roseola or "sixth" disease) presents with several days of high fevers followed by the appearance of a generalized eruption.
Bolognia J, Schaffer J, Cerroni L, eds. *Dermatology.* [Philadelphia]: Elsevier, 2018 (ch. 81).

44. C. Hoarseness
The image depicts a child with ice-pick scarring on the face and waxy, beaded papules along the eyelid margin, suggesting a diagnosis of lipoid proteinosis. This is an autosomal recessive deposition disorder caused by mutations in the extracellular matrix protein 1 (*ECM1*) gene. Hyaline-like deposition occurs in multiple organs, namely the skin, oral mucosa, laryngeal mucosa, and brain. Hoarseness or weak cry is often the first sign and begins in infancy. Other cutaneous signs include skin-colored papulonodules or verrucous changes of the elbows, firm tongue with papules, and waxy yellowish plaques on the back. Respiratory infections are common and can lead to early death.
Hepatosplenomegaly, developmental delay, alopecia, and lymphadenopathy are not classical features associated with lipoid proteinosis.
Bolognia J, Schaffer J, Cerroni L, eds. *Dermatology.* [Philadelphia]: Elsevier, 2018 (ch. 48).

45. E. Axillary freckling
This question requires the recognition of Lisch nodules, an ocular finding characteristically seen in patients with neurofibromatosis. Axillary freckling, also referred to as Crowe sign, is a diagnostic cutaneous feature of this syndrome. Facial red papules (adenoma sebaceum) and hypopigmented macules and patches (ash-leaf and confetti macules) are features of tuberous sclerosus. These patients can develop retinal phakomas, which require ophthalmoscopy and retinoscopy to be seen. White-yellow papules along the neck are seen in patients with pseudoxanthoma elasticum. These patients can develop angioid streaks that also require

ophthalmoscopy to be seen. Finally, triangular lunulae are seen in patients with nail-patella syndrome. These patients may have a lester iris, seen as hyperpigmentation of the pupillary margin of the iris.
Bolognia J, Schaffer J, Cerroni L, eds. *Dermatology*. [Philadelphia]: Elsevier, 2018 (ch. 61).

46. D. Bloom syndrome
The vignette is suggestive of a DNA repair disorder associated with photosensitivity, of which there are many. However, chromosomal instability and increased rates of sister chromatid exchange are characteristic of Bloom syndrome. Additional features include growth impairment, photosensitivity, and malar erythema, as described previously. Patients often have a narrow face and high-pitched voice. Decreased IgA and IgM predispose patients to recurrent infections. There may be increased frequency of leukemia, lymphoma, and GI adenocarcinoma.
Rothmund-Thomson syndrome results from mutations in a DNA helicase that functions in DNA replication and repair of UV damage. Poikiloderma is a characteristic feature. Xeroderma pigmentosum and trichothiodystrophy with photosensitivity result from mutations in the nucleotide excision repair pathway. Cockayne syndrome results from defective transcription-coupled nucleotide excision repair.
Bolognia J, Schaffer J, Cerroni L, eds. *Dermatology*. [Philadelphia]: Elsevier, 2018 (ch. 87).

47. B. Autosomal recessive congenital ichthyosis
The clinical image depicts a newborn baby with a collodion membranea shiny, transparent covering formed from thickened stratum corneum. This finding may be the initial manifestation of several different disorders, but the most common among them are autosomal recessive congenital ichthyoses (lamellar ichthyosis and nonbullous congenital ichthyosiform erythroderma). Infants with self-healing collodion baby syndrome by definition are born with a collodion membrane, but this condition is very rare. Neutral lipid storage disease and Sjögren-Larsson syndrome can present with collodion membranes but rarely do so. Epidermolytic ichthyosis does not present with a collodion membrane and manifests with erythroderma, denuded skin, and erosions at birth, followed by hyperkeratosis that predominates later on.
Bolognia J, Schaffer J, Cerroni L, eds. *Dermatology*. [Philadelphia]: Elsevier, 2018 (ch. 57).

48. B. *PORCN*
The vignette describes clinical and radiographic features of focal dermal hypoplasia, or Goltz syndrome, which is an X-linked dominant disorder caused by mutations in the porcupine (*PORCN*) gene. The disorder is typically lethal in males, thus is predominately seen in females. Ectrodactyly (lobster claw deformity) and dental anomalies are common.
ECM1 is mutated in lipoid proteinosis. *LEMD3* is mutated in Buschke-Ollendorf syndrome, in which the characteristic bone findings are osteopoikilosis. *NEMO* is mutated in incontinentia pigmenti. *FBN1* is mutated in Marfan syndrome.
Bolognia J, Schaffer J, Cerroni L, eds. *Dermatology*. [Philadelphia]: Elsevier, 2018 (ch. 55).

49. A. Epidermal atrophy, loss of melanin in the basal layer, and absence of pilosebaceous units
The clinical image depicts blaschkoid vesicular lesions characteristic of incontinentia pigmenti. The spectrum of clinical findings encompasses four distinct stages of disease, though not all patients manifest all stages of the disease. The first is the vesicular stage, characterized histologically by intraepidermal vesicles with eosinophils and necrotic keratinocytes with onset at or around birth. The second stage is the verrucous stage, characterized histologically by papillomatosis, hyperkeratosis, and acanthosis. This stage generally resolves spontaneously within the first 2 years of life. The third stage is the hyperpigmented stage, characterized histologically by marked pigment incontinence with dermal melanophages and can persist through adolescence. The fourth stage, which manifests as atrophic, hypopigmented thin streaks favoring the calves, is characterized histologically by epidermal atrophy, loss of melanin in the basal layer, and absence of pilosebaceous units. Choice E describes the histologic features of angiolymphoid hyperplasia with eosinophilia.
Bolognia J, Schaffer J, Cerroni L, eds. *Dermatology*. [Philadelphia]: Elsevier, 2018 (ch. 34).

50. A. Reassurance
This patient has hand-foot-mouth disease (HFMD) caused by coxsackievirus. Coxsackievirus A6 has been associated with an atypical cutaneous presentation, often with marked perioral involvement and accentuation in areas of atopic dermatitis—so-called "eczema coxsackium"—in addition to typical areas affected by HFMD. This condition is self-limited with an excellent prognosis. Cefadroxil or mupirocin would be appropriate choices for bullous impetigo, which often affects the perioral skin but shows honey-colored crusting and collarettes of scale (B, D); acyclovir is the treatment of choice for eczema herpeticum, which is on the differential diagnosis but presents with more monomorphic, punched out erosions (C); and prednisolone is not indicated for this self-limited viral illness (E).
Bolognia J, Schaffer J, Cerroni L, eds. *Dermatology*. [Philadelphia]: Elsevier, 2018 (ch. 81).

DERMATOPATHOLOGY

51. D. Gardner syndrome
The biopsy shows a pilomatricoma (PMX): a wall of basaloid cells that transition abruptly to cornified cells with only scant nuclear remnants termed ghost (or shadow) cells. PMXs usually present as firm, flesh-colored, or bluish nodules on hair-bearing surfaces, most commonly the head and upper trunk, and usually arise during childhood or adolescence. Multiple PMXs are sometimes associated with myotonic dystrophy, Turner syndrome, and Gardner syndrome. Here, the presence of a PMX and epidermal inclusion cysts in a young patient with a family history of colon cancer specifically raise the possibility of Gardner syndrome. Other findings of Gardner syndrome include polyposis, colon cancer, and the presence of osteomas, epidermoid cysts, desmoid tumors, cutaneous fibromas, and ocular findings of CHRPE (congenital hypertrophy retinal pigment epithelium).
Multiple PMXs can also be found in myotonic dystrophy and Turner syndrome, but a family history of colon cancer would not be expected. Cowden syndrome is associated with GI, breast, and thyroid cancer and is caused by Phosphatase and tensin homolog (*PTEN*) gene mutations. Cowden syndrome would be expected to present with multiple facial papules (often trichilemmomas), perioral lentigines, cobblestoning of the oral mucosa, acral keratotic papules, and lipomas. Sclerotic fibromas are a histopathologically characteristic lesion in Cowden syndrome.

Peutz-Jeghers syndrome (*STK11* mutation) is associated with an increased risk of breast, ovarian, pancreatic, and multiple other cancer types (including GI) and typically presents with cutaneous findings of melanotic macules on mucosal surfaces and not PMX.
Bolognia J, Schaffer J, Cerroni L, eds. *Dermatology*. [Philadelphia]: Elsevier, 2018 (ch. 53).

52. C. Palmoplantar keratoderma
The biopsy shows an eccrine hidrocystoma. Eccrine hidrocystomas are histologically composed of a cystic space lined by two layers of cuboidal epithelium and often contain the histologic equivalent of clear fluid (as pictured here). Apocrine hidrocystomas (not pictured here) are another variant that can be multiloculated and show decapitation secretion by lining epithelial cells. The patient has Schopf-Schulz-Passarge syndrome (SSPS), which falls under the umbrella of odonto-onycho-dermal dysplasia (is also sometimes called PPK with cystic eyelids). These diseases result from *WNT10A* mutations. Clinical features of SSPS include diffuse palmoplantar keratoderma, facial telangiectasias or reticulate erythema, hypodontia, nail dystrophy, and hypotrichosis in addition to development of multiple hidrocystomas of the eyelids (as in this patient). Patients with SSPS can also develop poromas and tumors of the follicular infundibulum.
Brachydactyly is not a typical feature of SSPS. Pseudoainhum, or constricting keratotic bands of the digits, is not seen in SSPS but can be seen in a variety of other genodermatoses, including Vohwinkel syndrome, Mal de Meleda, and others (Bolognia et al, ed. 4, Table 58.3). Anonychia (absence of nails) is not a typical feature of SSP. Palmar pits are seen in a variety of genodermatoses, including Gorlin syndrome, Cowden syndrome, and Darier disease, but not in SSPS.
Bolognia J, Schaffer J, Cerroni L, eds. *Dermatology*. [Philadelphia]: Elsevier, 2018 (ch. 55 and 58).

53. A. Cutaneous T-cell lymphoma
Pictured in the above photomicrograph are Pautrier microabscesses, which are intraepidermal clusters of atypical lymphocytes found in cutaneous T-cell lymphoma (CTCL). Despite having "abscess" in the name, the cells clustered in the epidermis here are not neutrophils. Other typical histologic features of CTCL include: lymphocytes lining up along the DEJ (simulating vacuolar interface dermatitis); large, dark lymphocytes with irregular nuclei and perinuclear halos; and absence of marked spongiosis in the surrounding epidermis. Note the lack of spongiosis in the above photomicrograph.
Allergic contact dermatitis and dyshidrotic eczema should have more spongiosis and fewer intraepidermal lymphocytes; acral skin would favor dyshidrotic dermatitis, and the presence of eosinophils would favor allergic contact dermatitis. While it is always good to consider tinea, one might expect to see round hyphae in the stratum corneum if this were the diagnosis. In dermatophyte infections, subcorneal collections of neutrophils (not atypical lymphocytes) are often noted. Sneddon Wilkinson would also be predicted to have subcorneal pustules (neutrophils), which are not seen here.
Bolognia J, Schaffer J, Cerroni L, eds. *Dermatology*. [Philadelphia]: Elsevier, 2018 (ch. 120).

54. C. Epidermodysplasia verruciformis
The biopsy shows classic features of epidermodysplasia verruciformis (EDV). The finding of a blue-gray pallor of affected keratinocytes is classic in this condition. At higher power, in the inset, viral cytopathic changes can be noted. Alternating orthokeratosis and parakeratosis can be seen. Infection with human papilloma virus (HPV) 5 or 8 is typical. Actinic keratosis-like changes may also be present histologically, particularly in lesions from sun-exposed areas. Patients with EDV must be monitored for SCC development. Clinically EDV patients present with a tinea versicolor–like eruption that can be hypopigmented.
Tumors of follicular infundibulum (TFI) presents as skin-colored or hypopigmented macules or thin papules and can be multiple; however, they are usually not quite as numerous, and biopsy would show strands of keratinocytes with multifocal attachment to the epidermis. This pattern is not noted here. Idiopathic guttate hypomelanosis (IGH) is typically seen in adults and elderly patients, manifesting as hypopigmented oval guttate macules, typically on the shins and extensor forearms. Biopsy of IGH, though rarely performed, would show flattening of the dermoepidermal junction with reduction in melanin granules in basal and suprabasal keratinocytes. Pityriasis lichenoides chronica can present as hypopigmented lesions, but biopsy should show vacuolar interface dermatitis. Hypopigmented mycosis fungoides would show typical histologic findings of mycosis fungoides.
Bolognia J, Schaffer J, Cerroni L, eds. *Dermatology*. [Philadelphia]: Elsevier, 2018 (ch. 79).

55. C. Erdheim-Chester disease
Erdheim-Chester disease is a systemic histiocytosis that has skin involvement in approximately 25% of cases. Typical skin manifestations include brown-red to yellow papules and plaques and/or nodules, most commonly on the eyelids, scalp, neck, trunk, and/or axillae. Additional symptoms include fever, bone pain, exophthalmos, diabetes insipidus, and systemic lesions. Lesional histiocytes have *BRAFV600E* mutations. Over the past several years, BRAF inhibitors have been found to be an effective treatment. Histologically, a sea of monotonous, foamy histiocytes in the dermis are characteristic, as shown in the photomicrograph. Multinucleate giant cells and Touton giant cells can also be seen but are not prominent in this example.
The biopsy does not show a balloon cell melanoma. In melanoma, more aneuploidy, a high nuclear to cytoplasmic ratio, and prominent nucleoli would be expected. Fifty percent of melanomas also have *BRAFV600E* mutations, however. Although renal cell carcinoma cells can appear clear due to the presence of glycogen, cells are typically arranged in tubules with prominent blood vessels and also would be predicted to have a higher nuclear to cytoplasmic ratio than the cells pictured here. *BRAFV600E* mutations are not typical of renal cell carcinoma. Hand-Schüller-Christian is a form of Langerhans cell histiocytosis (LCH) that typically presents a triad of diabetes insipidus, bone lesions, and exophthalmos and is usually seen in children between 2–6 years of age. Macrophages in LCH are classically described as having a reniform (kidney-shaped) nucleus, which is not pictured in the photomicrograph. Xanthelasma affecting the scalp and neck would be very atypical and in this clinical context should raise concern for a histiocytosis, in this case Erdheim-Chester.
Bolognia J, Schaffer J, Cerroni L, eds. *Dermatology*. [Philadelphia]: Elsevier, 2018 (ch. 91).

56. B. Aggressive digital papillary adenocarcinoma
Histologic features of aggressive papillary digital adenocarcinoma include large blue nodules at low power. Higher-power examination reveals a composition of cells with very little visible cytoplasm arranged into papillary

structures with glandular spaces, hence the name. These features are shown here; the location on a finger is also a clue in this case. At 400x, cellular atypia, mitoses, and necrosis may be minimal, but there should be at least focally present large, hyperchromatic nuclei and mitoses. Decapitation secretion is also present on high power. The lesions are most commonly found on the hand and can metastasize. The tumor is often also referred to as papillary digital carcinoma.

Although there can be histologic overlap between aggressive digital papillary adenocarcinoma and hidradenoma papilliferum (HPAP), the digital location of this tumor is highly suspicious for the former. HPAP typically is most commonly a dermal-appearing nodule located on the vulva but can also be found on the breast, eyelid, or ear. At a histologic level, in HPAP, a more arborizing pattern of fronds is present and is sometimes described as being "mazelike." Decapitation secretion is also present. Atypia and mitoses should not be a prominent feature. Mucinous carcinoma shows blue islands of cells in a background of mucin (sometimes referred to as a "sea of snot") and often presents on the eyelids. These features are not seen here. Syringomas and desmoplastic trichoepitheliomas are not expected to occur on digits and show a paisley-tie pattern of tadpole-shaped duct with a red sclerotic stroma on biopsy.

Bolognia J, Schaffer J, Cerroni L, eds. *Dermatology*. [Philadelphia]: Elsevier, 2018 (ch. 111).

57. C. Leukocytoclastic vasculitis

The figure shows fibrinoid degeneration within a vessel wall and a dermal infiltrate composed of neutrophils and neutrophilic debris, features characteristic of leukocytoclastic vasculitis.

Histopathologic features of urticaria include a sparse-mixed infiltrate (including neutrophils and eosinophils) within the dermis, while Sweet syndrome shows a prominent dermal infiltrate composed of neutrophils and neutrophilic dust, often with upper dermal edema. Vascular damage or fibrinoid degeneration of the vascular walls is not a feature of either urticaria or Sweet syndrome. Intravascular lymphoma will show atypical lymphoid cells within the vascular lumina.

Bolognia J, Schaffer J, Cerroni L, eds. *Dermatology*. [Philadelphia]: Elsevier, 2018 (ch. 24).

58. D. Check peripheral blood flow cytometry and TCR clonality by V-beta

The biopsy shows changes reminiscent of a lobular panniculitis with "rimming" of individual adipocytes by atypical lymphocytes, a finding strongly suggestive of subcutaneous panniculitic T-cell lymphoma (SPTCL). Further support for a diagnosis of SPTCL could be achieved by demonstrating a T-cell clone in the blood and/or documenting the characteristic flow cytometric T-cell immunophenotypic changes: CD3+ CD4- CD8+ CD56- betaF1+. Demonstrating a T-cell clone in the biopsy using PCR could also help distinguish SPTCL from lupus.

The main histologic differential for SPTCL includes lupus panniculitis, in particular for patients with SLE; however, lupus panniculitis has a lobular histologic pattern with typical findings of lupus above the fat (interface change, lymphoid follicles). Such prominent rimming and presence of atypical lymphocytes would not be expected. Lipomembranous change is also a nice feature to support lupus panniculitis. There is an association of SPTCL with lupus, as in this case.

Treating for a lupus flare would be incorrect; given the diagnosis is not lupus panniculitis. Although OCPs can be a cause of erythema nodosum, this is not erythema nodosum. Erythema nodosum shows septal panniculitis with neutrophils in the acute phase or mononuclear cells, and granulomatous inflammation in the chronic phase.

Bolognia J, Schaffer J, Cerroni L, eds. *Dermatology*. [Philadelphia]: Elsevier, 2018 (ch. 120).

59. A. Porokeratosis

Pictured in the photomicrograph is a cornoid lamella, which is diagnostic of a porokeratosis. Porokeratosis of Mibelli can be a large solitary lesion, as in this case. Histologically, a coronoid lamella is a column of parakeratosis at a 45-degree angle that has dyskeratotic cells below, as pictured here. Lichenoid (present here) or psoriasiform changes can also be present.

None of the other diagnoses would be expected to have a cornoid lamella. Dermatophytes are not noted in the stratum corneum for tinea. There is no keratinocyte atypia as would be expected in squamous cell carcinoma.

Bolognia J, Schaffer J, Cerroni L, eds. *Dermatology*. [Philadelphia]: Elsevier, 2018 (ch. 109).

60. D. Reassure the patient

The biopsy shows chondrodermatitis nodularis helicis (CDNH). Histologic feature of CDNH, which are present in this case, include epidermal hyperplasia, a central overlying crust or ulcer, and an underlying fibrin core with granulation tissue. The presence of cartilage with degenerative changes (refer to * in figure) is another good clue to the diagnosis. Location at a site of pressure is also typical, commonly the helical and antihelical rim. No features of cutaneous squamous cell carcinoma, melanoma, or Merkel cell carcinoma are present.

Bolognia, Jean, Schaffer, Julie, Cerroni, Lorenzo, eds. Dermatology. [Philadelphia]: Elsevier, 2018 (ch. 88)

PROCEDURAL DERMATOLOGY

61. C. Genetic testing for *CDKN2A* mutation

This patient meets criteria for familial atypical multiple mole melanoma syndrome (FAMMM, also known as dysplastic nevus syndrome)—namely, greater than 50 melanocytic nevi, a history of histologically atypical nevi, and a family history of melanoma in a first- or second-degree relative. FAMMM syndrome is associated with markedly increased risk of cutaneous melanoma and several internal malignancies, most notably pancreatic cancer. FAMMM syndrome is caused by inherited mutation in the *CDKN2A* gene, a tumor suppressor that inhibits cellular proliferation. Formal genetic diagnosis of FAMMM syndrome in patients with clinical features of the syndrome is important to direct screening efforts in the individual and in family members. Screening biopsies of several nevi to screen for melanoma or atypia is not useful. Only lesions that are clinically suspicious for melanoma should be biopsied and treated. *MC1R* encodes the melanocortin-1 receptor, and germline variants in this gene are common, are associated with red hair and freckles, and confer an increased susceptibility to ultraviolet radiation and skin cancer in general. *MC1R* mutations are not associated with dysplastic nevus syndrome. BRAF encodes a serine/threonine kinase that promotes cellular growth in many tissues; somatic mutations in BRAF drive melanoma formation in about half of melanomas. BRAF mutations

are somatic, however, and are not inherited or germline mutations, so genetic testing for BRAF is not useful. While FAMMM syndrome is associated with pancreatic cancer, screening of asymptomatic patients with computed tomography scans has not been shown to be beneficial. Some centers advocate for screening with endoscopic ultrasound or cholangiopancreatography, but there are no official guidelines.
Bolognia J, Schaffer J, Cerroni L, eds. *Dermatology*. [Philadelphia]: Elsevier, 2018 (ch. 112 and 113).

62. C. 55 mg/kg
Tumescent anesthesia is often used for liposuction, hair transplant, or dermabrasion. It involves the infiltration of large volumes of dilute lidocaine (0.05–0.1% with 1:1,000,000 epinephrine) into the subcutaneous tissue. The anesthesia effect lasts several hours. In the subcutaneous fat, the lidocaine is absorbed much slower. The maximum dose is 55 mg/kg.
Bolognia J, Schaffer J, Cerroni L, eds. *Dermatology*. [Philadelphia]: Elsevier, 2018 (ch. 14).

63. E. Salicylic acid peel
Salicylic acid peel may cause tinnitus as a result of salicylism. Salicylic acid is a beta-hydroxy acid, which is both keratolytic and comedolytic. Glycolic acid, TCA, and Baker-Gordon peels have not been associated with tinnitus.
Bolognia J, Schaffer J, Cerroni L, eds. *Dermatology*. [Philadelphia]: Elsevier, 2018 (ch. 154).

64. C. Nd:YAG
Nd:YAG (1064 nm) is the safest option for hair removal in darker-pigmented skin types. Although diode is the most effective and usually safe in skin of color, Nd:YAG would be the safest option given the longer wavelength and less effect on melanin. Alexandrite, Ruby, and IPL are all best in skin types I–III given the shorter wavelength.
Bolognia J, Schaffer J, Cerroni L, eds. *Dermatology*. [Philadelphia]: Elsevier, 2018 (ch. 137).

65. B. Lavetor labii superioris alaeque nasi
The levator labii superioris alaeque (LLSAN) originates on the medial maxilla and then bifurcates and inserts into the medial orbicularis oris and nasal ala. Hyperactivity of this muscle may lead to excessive elevation of the upper lip on smiling, producing a "gummy smile." The LLSAN should be injected at the pyriform aperture/apical triangle of the upper lip with 1–2.5 units of onabotulinum toxin per side.
The nasalis muscle contributes to "bunny lines." The orbicularis oris is injected for the treatment of perioral rhytids. The zygomatic major should be avoided unless treating facial asymmetry. Injection of the depressor anguli oris treats downturn of the oral commissures.
Bolognia J, Schaffer J, Cerroni L, eds. *Dermatology*. [Philadelphia]: Elsevier, 2018 (ch. 159).

66. D. Sodium morrhuate
Sodium morrhuate is a detergent sclerosing agent with the highest risk of anaphylaxis. Other risks include pain, skin necrosis, and hyperpigmentation. Polidocanol and glycerin have the lowest risk of anaphylaxis. Anaphylaxis is rare with the use of sodium tetradecyl sulfate. Ethanolamine oleate has the highest risk for generalized urticaria.
Bolognia J, Schaffer J, Cerroni L, eds. *Dermatology*. [Philadelphia]: Elsevier, 2018 (ch. 155).

67. A. Breslow depth
B. Sentinel lymph node biopsy
For patients with intermediate-thickness melanoma (1.2–3.5 mm Breslow depth) in the Multicenter Selective Lymphadenectomy Trial-1 (MSLT-1) trial, sentinel lymph node biopsy status was the most significant predictor of disease recurrence and death from melanoma (hazard ratio of 2.64 and 2.40, respectively). Breslow depth was the next most significant predictor, with hazard ratio per 1 mm increase in depth of 1.62 for disease recurrence and 1.59 for death from melanoma. In this and other studies, male gender, primary tumor ulceration, and the presence of >1 mitosis per high-powered field were adverse prognostic indicators but were less significant.
Morton DL, Thompson JF, Cochran AJ, et al., MSLT Group. Final trial report of sentinel-node biopsy versus nodal observation in melanoma. *N Engl J Med*. 2014;370(7):599–609.

68. E. All of the above
The patient has field cancerization, marked by multiple cutaneous SCCs and multiple actinic keratoses within a sun-damaged field. This patient is at very high risk of subsequent SCCs. Treatments that decrease the burden of precursor lesions (actinic keratosis and squamous cell carcinoma in situ) are expected to decrease subsequent risk of SCC. This has been shown definitively for topical fluorouracil (decrease risk of SCC by 75% in first year) and oral niacinamide (decrease risk of 25%). Repeated cycles of photodynamic therapy have been shown in uncontrolled studies to decrease risk of subsequent SCCs in high-risk patients. The role of rigorous sun protection also must not be minimized, as randomized controlled trials of sunblock use have shown up to 40% reduction in subsequent SCCs. Other topical treatments for AKs, such as imiquimod and ingenol mebutate, are expected to decrease the risk of subsequent SCC but have not been studied specifically for SCC prevention.
Bolognia J, Schaffer J, Cerroni L, eds. *Dermatology*. [Philadelphia]: Elsevier, 2018 (ch. 108).

69. D. Perioral paresthesia
The maximum dose of lidocaine with epinephrine is 7 mg/kg. For a typical 70 kg (154 lb) patient, that is 350 mg, or 35 ml of 1% lidocaine. Without epinephrine, maximum dose is 5 mg/kg, or 28 ml of 1% lidocaine. This patient received 420 mg of lidocaine with epinephrine, so early signs of lidocaine toxicity are expected. The earliest signs of lidocaine toxicity are tongue/lip paresthesia with slurred speech, tinnitus, and blurred vision. Higher doses of lidocaine result in vomiting, tremors, and muscle spasms. Highest-level toxicity causes seizures and cardiac arrest.
Bolognia J, Schaffer J, Cerroni L, eds. *Dermatology*. [Philadelphia]: Elsevier, 2018 (ch. 143).

70. B. Tumor is noted at the deep surgical margin. Additional staged excision is required.
Moderately differentiated SCC is present at the deep aspect of the specimen, just beneath the extensive fibrosis, and scar tissue in the dermis. The epidermis and papillary dermis are unaffected. Because Mohs surgical specimens are processed *en face*, only the surgical margin is visualized on the slides. Thus any malignancy visible on Mohs intraoperative histology represents malignancy present at the surgical margin, and additional treatment is warranted to obtain complete excision. A decision to stop Mohs surgery with persistently positive margins may be occasionally indicated based on gross extension of the tumor over an extensive area or into critical structures,

but this determination cannot be made on the basis of a single histological slide.
Bolognia J, Schaffer J, Cerroni L, eds. *Dermatology.* [Philadelphia]: Elsevier, 2018 (ch. 150).

BASIC SCIENCE

71. C. *TP53*
The most commonly mutated protein in squamous cell carcinoma (SCC) is the tumor suppressor p53 (*TP53*). *BRAF* is commonly mutated in both benign melanocytic nevi as well as cutaneous melanoma. G Protein Subunit Alpha Q (*GNAQ*) is commonly mutated in blue nevi and uveal nevi. In addition, *GNAQ* is mutated in Sturge-Weber syndrome. Patched (*PTCH1*) is mutated in basal cell carcinoma, and *c-KIT* is commonly mutated in acral and mucosal melanoma.
Bolognia J, Schaffer J, Cerroni L, eds. *Dermatology.* [Philadelphia]: Elsevier, 2018 (chs. 107, 108, and 113).

72. B. Merkel cell carcinoma
Trichodysplasia spinulosa or viral-associated trichodysplasia (of immunosuppression) was found to be associated by a novel virus called trichodysplasia spinulosa-associated polyomavirus (TSPyV). Another polyomavirus, the Merkel cell virus (MCV), is involved in the pathogenesis of Merkel cell carcinoma (MCC). Squamous cell carcinoma (A) has been associated with human papilloma virus (HPV) subtypes 16 and 18 subtypes. Both Burkitt lymphoma (C) and Lipschütz ulcer (D) are associated with Epstein-Barr virus (EBV). Rosai-Dorfman (E) disease is a histiocytosis that is not associated with viral infections.
Bolognia J, Schaffer J, Cerroni L, eds. *Dermatology.* [Philadelphia]: Elsevier, 2018 (ch. 39 and 81).

73. B. Dorsal root ganglion
Varicella-zoster virus (VZV) enters the viral latency phase in the dorsal root or trigeminal ganglia where there is little to no viral replication. Upon reactivation, VZV begins to replicate and migrate from the dorsal root ganglion to cutaneous nerve fibers before infecting keratinocytes.
Bolognia J, Schaffer J, Cerroni L, eds. *Dermatology.* [Philadelphia]: Elsevier, 2018 (ch. 80).

74. D. Phosphorylation
Vemurafenib and dabrafenib are BRAF inhibitors used to treat patients with metastatic melanoma who harbor the V600E mutation. A number of cutaneous side effects may occur, including maculopapular, follicular, acneiform, keratosis pilaris-like eruptions (depicted in the figure), changing nevi, verrucous keratoses, squamous cell carcinomas, and erythema nodosum-like reactions. BRAF is a member of the RAF kinase family that functions in phosphorylation. The protein plays a role in regulating the MAP kinase/ERK signaling pathway.
Imatinib, a c-KIT and PDGF inhibitor, is used in the treatment of DFSP (fusion of *Col1A1-PDGFB*). Sirolimus is an inhibitor of the serine/threonine protein kinase mTOR (mammalian target of rapamycin). It has recently been used in the treatment of facial angiofibromas (topical formulations) and managing the sequelae of tuberous sclerosis complex. In addition, it is often used in the treatment of chronic GVHD and in posttransplantation recipients as an immunosuppressive drug with less potential for cutaneous carcinogenesis. Checkpoint inhibitors include anti-CTLA-4, anti-PD-1, and anti-PD-L1 agents. These drugs function by harnessing the immune response to target cancer. CTLA-4 is a checkpoint in lymphoid organs and functions to downregulate the immune response to promote tolerance of self and prevent autoimmunity. PD-1 is a checkpoint in peripheral tissues, and PD-L1 may be overexpressed by tumor cells in effort to evade the immune system. Checkpoint inhibitors block this immune suppression and restore T-cell activation.
Bolognia J, Schaffer J, Cerroni L, eds. *Dermatology.* [Philadelphia]: Elsevier, 2018 (ch. 21).

75. C. Inhibits *Smoothened*
Patched (*PTCH1*) is the most commonly mutated gene in basal cell carcinoma (70% of BCCs). Mutations in *PTCH1* as well as other genes in the hedgehog signaling pathway are responsible for hereditary basal cell nevus syndrome (Gorlin syndrome). Normally, *PTCH1* inhibits *Smoothened*, so when *PTCH1* is mutated in BCC, *Smoothened* is constitutively activated, resulting in *GL1* activation and cell growth. Vismodegib inhibits *Smoothened* to decrease activation of *GL1* and reduce cell growth.
Bolognia J, Schaffer J, Cerroni L, eds. *Dermatology.* [Philadelphia]: Elsevier, 2018 (chs. 107 and 108).

76. D. Anti-programmed cell death 1 (PD-1)
Squamous cell carcinoma rarely metastasizes (less than 5% of cases) but can be clinically aggressive and fatal once it does spread beyond the skin. In 2018, anti-PD-1 therapy (cemiplimab) was approved for advanced and metastatic SCC, which demonstrated superiority over traditional chemotherapy. This is the first and only immunotherapy currently approved for cutaneous SCC. Currently, there are two PD-1 inhibitors approved for metastatic melanoma (nivolumab, pembrolizumab), one PD-1 inhibitor approved for advanced cutaneous SCC (cemiplimab), and one PD-L1 inhibitor (avelumab) approved for metastatic MCC.
Bolognia J, Schaffer J, Cerroni L, eds. *Dermatology.* [Philadelphia]: Elsevier, 2018 (chs. 115 and 128).

77. E. Anti-interleukin 17A
Chronic plaque psoriasis is predominately a disease of the IL-23/IL-17 inflammatory pathway. The FDA approved "biologics" for psoriasis, including blocking antibodies against tumor necrosis factor alpha (TNFa), IL-23 p19, IL-23 p40, IL-17A, and IL-17 receptor. Blockade of IL-17 results in increased risk of cutaneous candidiasis, as IL-17 promotes antifungal immunity. Anti-IL-4a receptor is FDA approved for atopic dermatitis (dupilumab).
Bolognia J, Schaffer J, Cerroni L, eds. *Dermatology.* [Philadelphia]: Elsevier, 2018 (chs. 8 and 128).

78. B. Anti-interleukin 4 receptor alpha
Atopic dermatitis is mediated by Th2 cells and type 2 cytokines, such as IL-4, IL-13, and IL-22. The FDA-approved agent dupilumab is indicated for atopic dermatitis and blocks the IL-4 receptor alpha, thereby blocking both IL-4 and IL-13 signaling. A minority of patients develop dupilumab-mediated conjunctivitis (~10%). TNF–alpha blockers may cause paradoxical psoriasiform dermatitis and drug-induced lupus-like reactions. Anti-PD-1 agents may cause dermatitis, lichenoid reactions, psoriasis exacerbations, exanthems, leukoderma, granulomatous disease, immunobullous disease, and SJS.
Bolognia J, Schaffer J, Cerroni L, eds. *Dermatology.* [Philadelphia]: Elsevier, 2018 (chs. 12 and 128).

79. B. Collagen VII

This patient has epidermolysis bullosa acquisita (EBA), caused by circulating autoantibodies against collagen VII. Patients present with vesiculobullous lesions at sites of trauma (skin fragility) and milia-like scarring, which predominantly involves the extremities. Bullous SLE is also caused by circulating autoantibodies against collagen VII, but an elevated ANA would be present. Desmoglein-3 is targeted in pemphigus vulgaris. Desmocollin-1 is targeted by autoantibodies in subcorneal pustular dermatosis or IgA pemphigus. Bullous pemphigoid antigen 2 (collagen XVII or BP180) is targeted in bullous pemphigoid. Patients with bullous pemphigoid are typically elderly, have eosinophils on biopsy, and do not have positive ANA. Desmoplakin is targeted by autoantibodies in paraneoplastic pemphigus.

Bolognia J, Schaffer J, Cerroni L, eds. *Dermatology.* [Philadelphia]: Elsevier, 2018 (ch. 30).

80. D. Produced by living organisms or cells

Drugs referred to as "biologics" are those that are produced by living organisms or cells or contain components of living organisms. Monoclonal antibodies are made by living eukaryotic cells and then isolated, and thus are often referred to as "biologics." Biologics may be injected subcutaneously, intravenously, or intramuscularly. Traditional drugs are chemically synthesized. Either class of drug can bind receptors on cells, and the side effect profile depends on the target of the drug.

Bolognia J, Schaffer J, Cerroni L, eds. *Dermatology.* [Philadelphia]: Elsevier, 2018 (chs. 8 and 128).

GENERAL DERMATOLOGY

1. An otherwise healthy 26-year-old woman presents with fevers of 102°F, sore throat, and new painful lesions on her lower legs as shown. Appropriate first-line treatment is:

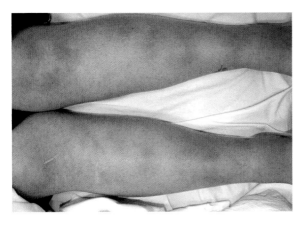

A. Intravenous methylprednisolone
B. Hydroxychloroquine
C. Valacyclovir
D. High-dose nonsteroidal antiinflammatory

2. A 12-year-old boy living in North Carolina presents with a 3-day history of fever up to 103°F associated with myalgias, headache, abdominal pain, and nausea/vomiting, associated with the eruption shown (see figure). What treatment should be started immediately?

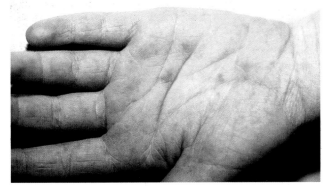

With permission from Ferri FF, in *Ferri's Clinical Advisor 2019*, 2019, Elsevier, 1208–1209.

A. Clarithromycin
B. Amoxicillin
C. Doxycycline
D. Chloramphenicol

3. A 76-year-old Caucasian woman presents to you with vulvar itching and the pictured findings on examination. Which of the following is an associated disease?

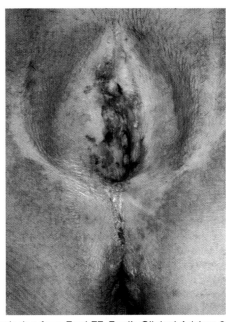

With permission from Ferri FF, *Ferri's Clinical Advisor 2019*, 2019, Elsevier, pp 820–820.e1.

A. Hepatitis C
B. Autoimmune thyroid disease
C. Monoclonal gammopathy
D. Bronchiolitis obliterans with organizing pneumonia

4. A young female presents with an asymptomatic eruption on her chest as pictured below. What is the first line treatment?

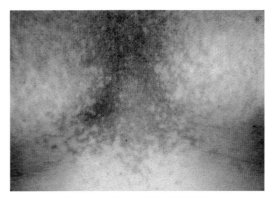

Courtesy Steven Binnick, MD.

A. Acitretin
B. Topical ketoconazole
C. Topical tazarotene
D. Minocycline
E. Oral fluconazole

5. A 68-year-old woman with a history of diabetes presents with the following eruption. She confirms leg swelling and pruritus and denies fevers or chills. There was no improvement with high-potency topical steroids. The rash does not improve 48 hours after starting cephalexin 500 mg four times daily. What is the next best step in management?

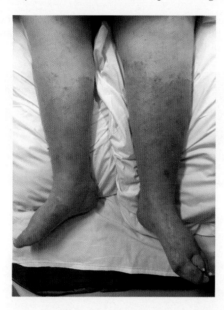

A. Change antibiotic to oral sulfamethoxazole-trimethoprim
B. Change antibiotic to oral terbinafine
C. Start topical clobetasol and encourage leg elevation
D. Biopsy for Hematoxylin and eosin and sterile tissue culture
E. Start topical terbinafine

6. A 45-year-old with a history of acute myeloid leukemia who recently underwent induction chemotherapy presents with the following disseminated firm lesions on the trunk and extremities. She is neutropenic and febrile. What is the most likely culprit?

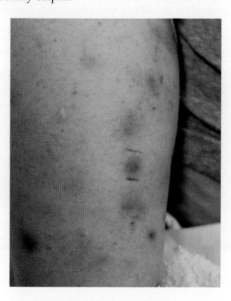

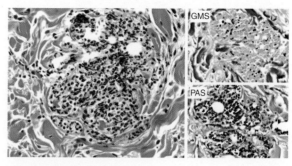

A. Varicella-zoster virus
B. *Cryptococcus neoformans*
C. *Candida albicans*
D. Aspergillus
E. *Pseudomonas aeruginosa*

7. A 57-year-old man without significant photodamage presents with this growth on his back. The gene that most likely mutated in this tumor has which of the following functions?

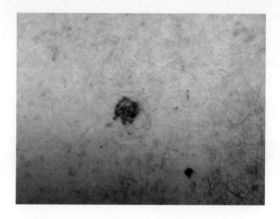

A. GTPase
B. Serine/threonine protein kinase
C. Transcription factor
D. Cell receptor tyrosine kinase

8. A 51-year-old woman patient presents with these lesions on the face and conchal bowls. Which of the following is the patient most at risk of developing within a long-standing lesion?

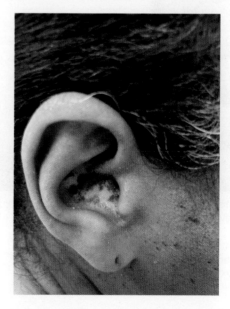

A. Melanoma
B. Basal cell carcinoma
C. Squamous cell carcinoma
D. Merkel cell carcinoma

9. This patient also has what associated condition?

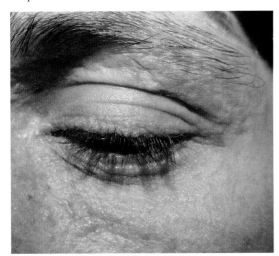

Courtesy of Dr. Eric W. Kraus.

A. Hoarseness
B. Arthritis
C. Blindness
D. Malignancy

10. A 50-year-old woman, originally from El Salvador, develops edematous, erythematous plaques and subcutaneous nodules on her legs 2 months after receiving a heart transplant for dilated cardiomyopathy. There were no recent changes in her immunosuppression. She also denies abdominal pain or diarrhea but does mention chronic constipation for years. Skin biopsy reveals intracellular amastigotes. What is the best treatment option?

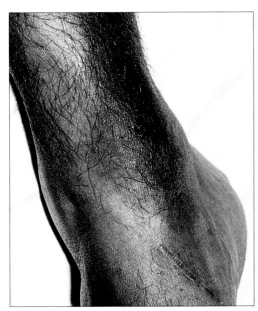

Reproduced from Peters W and Pasvol G (eds.), in *Tropical Medicine and Parasitology*, 5th edition, 2002, Mosby: London (image 169).

A. Prednisone
B. Nifurtimox
C. Sulfamethoxazole-trimethoprim
D. Amphotericin B
E. Bed rest and nonsteroidal antiinflammatory drugs

11. The patient below started a new medication prior to the development of this eruption. Which of the following medications is LEAST likely to be the culprit?

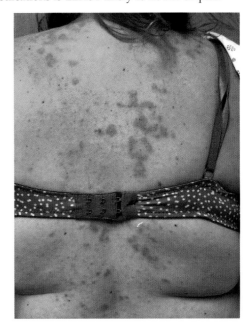

A. Proton pump inhibitor
B. Ibuprofen
C. Simvastatin
D. Amlodipine
E. Hydralazine

12. The patient reports an acute onset of this eruption. Which of the following statements about this condition is FALSE?

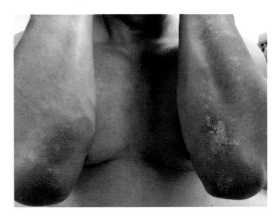

A. Biopsy will show plugged hair follicles, irregular hyperkeratosis, and alternating vertical and horizontal ortho and parakeratosis.
B. Treatment options include retinoids, methotrexate, and biologic agents.
C. May be associated with mutilating arthritis.
D. Commonly begins in the head and neck region and spreads caudally.
E. Can be associated with HIV infection or solid organ malignancy.

13. The patient reports recurring episodes of painful lesions lasting 2 to 3 days and associated with joint and abdominal pain. The diagnosis is:

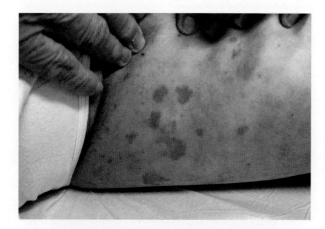

- **A.** Subacute cutaneous lupus erythematosus
- **B.** Urticarial vasculitis
- **C.** Tinea corporis
- **D.** Pityriasis rosea
- **E.** Urticaria with angioedema

14. Which of the following statements regarding this condition is true?

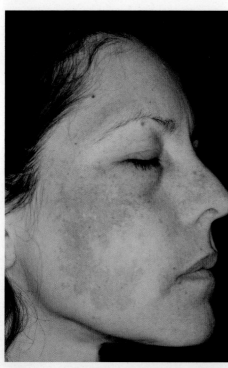

With permission from Sheth VM, Pandya AG, Melasma: a comprehensive update *Journal of the American Academy of Dermatology*, 2011, 65(4): 689–697.

- **A.** Increased expression of *KIT* and stem cell factor within the lesional epidermis and dermis, respectively, may play a role in pathogenesis of this condition.
- **B.** Has been reported to be triggered by ingestion of ammonium nitrate.
- **C.** Histology shows banana-shaped, yellow-brown deposits in the dermis.

- **D.** Amyloid deposits that stain positively with antikeratin antibodies are seen within the upper dermis.
- **E.** The systemic medication used to treat this condition is associated with risk of hemorrhagic strokes.

15. What may be associated with these findings?

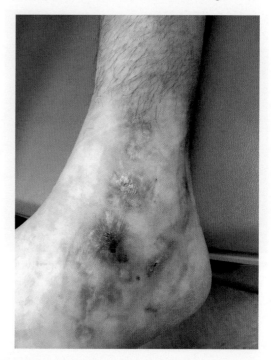

- **A.** Diabetes
- **B.** Cirrhosis
- **C.** End-stage renal disease
- **D.** Antithrombin III deficiency

16. The patient reports painful lesions of the oral mucosa without skin lesions. Which of the following statements regarding this condition is FALSE?

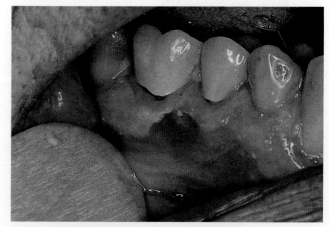

From James WD et al. in *Andrews' Diseases of the Skin*, 12th edition, 2016, Elsevier: Philadelphia (fig. 21-2).

- **A.** Most commonly associated with the initiation of vancomycin.
- **B.** Neonates of mothers with this condition may have a transient disease caused by maternal immunoglobulins that cross the placenta.

C. May be associated with initiation of captopril.

D. The antigens targeted by the autoantibodies in this condition are restricted to stratified squamous epithelia.

E. Monoclonal antibody targeting CD-20 has been successfully used as a treatment modality.

17. All of the following are features of this entity EXCEPT:

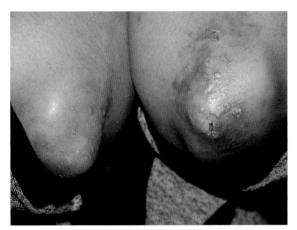

With permission from Chan LS, *Treatment of Skin Disease: Comprehensive Therapeutic Strategies*, 2018, Elsevier, 229–232.

A. Mucosal ulceration

B. Skin fragility

C. Linear deposits of C3 on the epidermal side of salt-split skin

D. Autoantibodies to collagen type VII

18. The elderly patient developed a pruritic scaly eruption after initiation of a new medication (see figure). Which of the following is the most likely culprit?

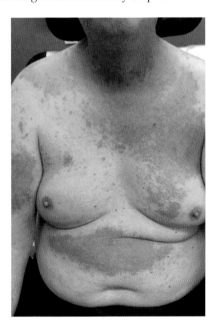

A. Trimethoprim/sulfamethoxazole

B. Penicillamine

C. Amlodipine

D. Hydralazine

E. Minocycline

19. Which of the following tests should be ordered initially in a 23-year-old male with no fevers, weight loss, or cough (choose all that apply)?

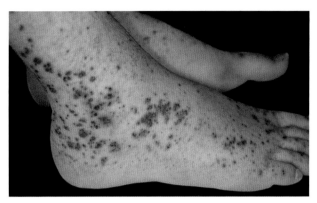

With permission from Habif TP, *Clinical Dermatology*, Elsevier, 2016 (fig. 18-17).

A. Complete blood count

B. Urinalysis

C. Basic metabolic panel

D. Serum protein electrophoresis

E. Antineutrophilic cytoplasmic antibody

20. Which of the following lab tests might be helpful in determining the underlying cause of this patient's eruption?

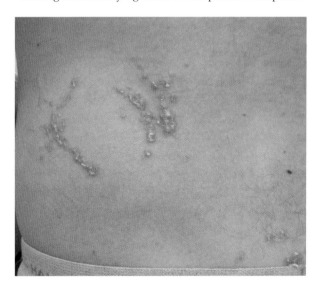

A. Glucose

B. Triglycerides

C. Vitamin D

D. CBC

21. A 72-year-old man was admitted with shortness of breath and bilateral lower extremity edema. On physician exam, the patient was noted to have macroglossia and the nail findings shown. Echocardiogram revealed restrictive cardiomyopathy. What is most likely associated?

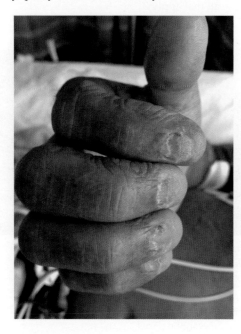

A. Plasma cell dyscrasia
B. Proximal muscle weakness
C. Galactorrhea
D. Hearing loss

22. This patient was started on oral therapy for treatment of his malignancy. He became fatigued and constipated and presented to the emergency department for evaluation. Labs revealed low T4. What is the most likely mechanism of action?

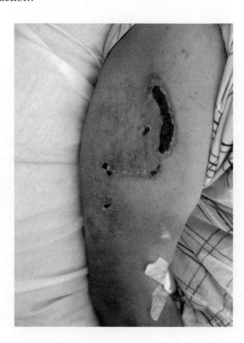

A. Decreased production of T4
B. Decreased secretion of TSH by the anterior pituitary
C. Inhibition of the RXR receptor
D. Increased deactivation of T4 to reverse T3

23. This 41-year-old female patient has failed topical corticosteroids, vitamin D analogues, and phototherapy. She has similar involvement on her scalp, lower back, and shins. She has a history of Crohn disease. Which systemic agent should be avoided?

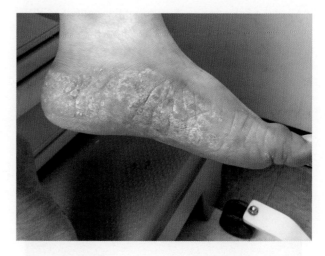

A. Adalimumab
B. Ixekizumab
C. Ustekinumab
D. Guselkumab

24. Administration of which of the following along with itraconazole will increase absorption?
A. Milk
B. Cola
C. Antacid
D. Proton pump inhibitor (PPI)

25. A 62-year-old man presents with a history of recurrent blisters on his scalp, face, and chest for 1 year. Identification of which autoantibody has the greatest risk of ocular involvement?

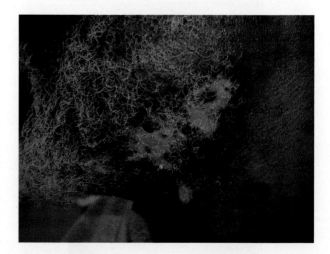

A. BP 180
B. Laminin 332
C. $\alpha_6\beta_4$ integrin
D. BP

26. What would you expect to see on biopsy of this condition?

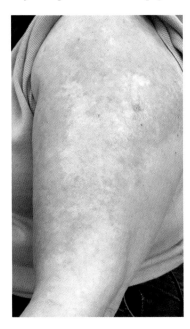

A. Spongiotic dermatitis with a mixed dermal inflammatory infiltrate
B. Interface dermatitis with vacuolar degeneration
C. Melanin in the upper dermis with increase in melanophages
D. Thickened collagen bundles with trapped eccrine glands

27. A 66-year-old gentleman presents to you with the following nail findings. The cause of the nail changes is attributed to:

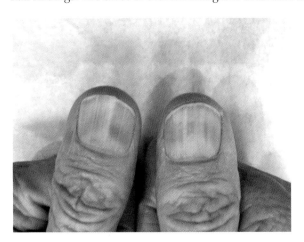

A. *Pseudomonas* infection of the nail
B. Melanoma
C. Chemotherapy
D. *Candida* infection of the nail
E. Oral retinoid

28. A hairdresser presents with eczematous patches and plaques on her bilateral hands and wrists. What is the most likely cause of her findings?
A. Ammonium persulfate
B. *p*-Phenylenediamine
C. Methacrylate
D. Propolis
E. *Lawsonia inermis*

29 A young woman presents with painful and pruritic papules with cold exposure on her bilateral feet as pictured. However, she reports no improvement with cold avoidance and warm clothing. What is best next-step treatment?

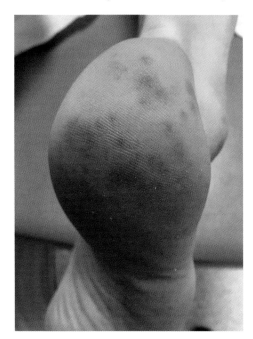

A. Nifedipine
B. Hydroxychloroquine
C. Topical corticosteroids
D. Aspirin
E. Topical nitroglycerin

30. A 28-year-old pregnant patient at 32-weeks gestation presents with the following eruption. What is the target of the autoantibodies found in this condition?

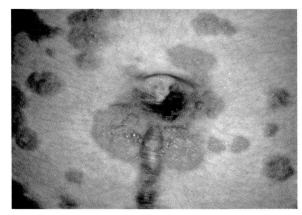

With permission from James WD, Berger TG, and Elston DM. Chronic blistering dermatoses, in *Andrews' Diseases of the Skin*, 12th edition, 2016, Elsevier, 451–470 (fig. 21.13).

A. Desmoglein 1
B. Desmoglein 3
C. BPAG1
D. BPAG2
E. Type VII collagen

31. An 85-year-old female developed the following on her bilateral shins. What underlying condition does the patient most likely have?

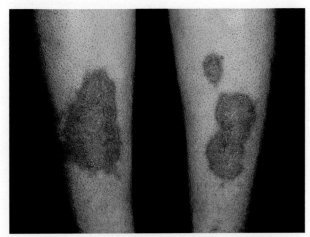

With permission from Chapman MS, Cutaneous manifestations of internal disease, in *Skin Disease: Diagnosis and Treatment*, 2018, Elsevier, 586–620.

A. Hypothyroidism
B. Systemic lupus erythematosus
C. Diabetes mellitus
D. Raynaud disease

32. A 56-year-old woman presents with the following eruption on the trunk and upper extremities. She has no history of autoimmune or vascular disease. Biopsy shows palisading histiocytes surrounding degenerated collagen. Which is the most likely medication culprit?

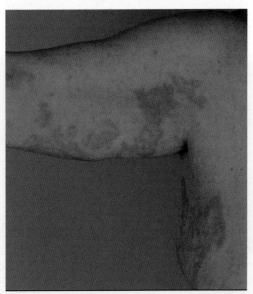

With permission from Rosenbach M, Reactive granulomatous dermatitis, in *Dermatologic Clinics*, 2015, volume 33, issue 3, 373–387, Elsevier Inc.

A. Sulfamethoxazole trimethoprim
B. Infliximab
C. Levetiracetam
D. Phenytoin

33. A 28-year-old woman developed significant pruritus and the following eruption on her elbows, knees, extensor forearms, and buttocks. A biopsy is performed along with a DIF. What are the most likely direct immunofluorescence findings?

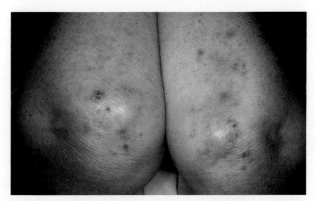

With permission from Kárpáti S, *Clinics in Dermatology*, 2012, volume 30, issue 1, 56–59.

A. Granular IgG and IgA deposition along the basement membrane
B. Negative DIF
C. Subcorneal IgA deposition
D. Granular IgA deposition within the dermal papillae

34. A 78-year-old man is hospitalized for congestive heart failure. He is started on several medications and develops the eruption pictured 2 weeks later. Biopsy shows subepidermal vesicles and neutrophils. A DIF shows linear deposition of IgA along the basement membrane. What is the most likely drug culprit?

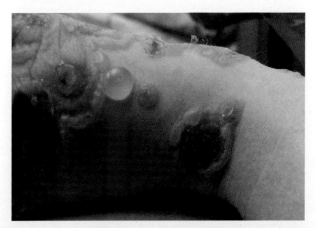

With permission from Korman NJ, *Treatment of Skin Disease: Comprehensive Therapeutic Strategies*, 2018, Elsevier, chapter 138, 451–453.

A. Furosemide
B. Captopril
C. Losartan
D. Metoprolol

35. An 83-year-old female with metastatic melanoma develops the following bullous eruption of her trunk and extremities. A biopsy is performed and shows subepidermal bullae with a mixed dermal inflammatory infiltrate with many eosinophils. DIF performed shows a fine, linear deposition of IgG and C3 along the basement membrane. Which medication is the most likely to be responsible?

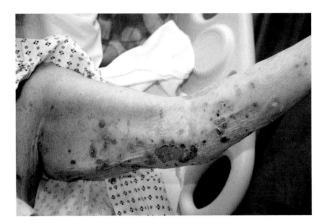

A. Pembrolizumab
B. Ipilimumab
C. Vemurafenib
D. Dacarbazine

36. This 81-year-old male presented with multiple large ulcerative and nodular nonmelanoma skin cancers of his face and trunk. Due to the number and size of the lesions, the patient was determined to be inoperable. He was subsequently treated with vismodegib. What is the molecular target of this medication?

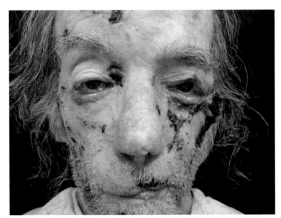

With permission from Gathings RM, Compassionate use of vismodegib and adjuvant radiotherapy in the treatment of multiple locally advanced and inoperable basal cell carcinomas and squamous cell carcinomas of the skin, *J Am Acad Dermatol*, 2013, Elsevier, 88–89 (fig. 1).

A. Tyrosine kinase
B. G-protein coupled receptor
C. Integral membrane protein receptor
D. Transcription factor

37. A 67-year-old man recently diagnosed with squamous cell carcinoma of the base of the mouth presents with the

eruption shown after starting an epidermal growth factor receptor inhibitor. What should be done next?

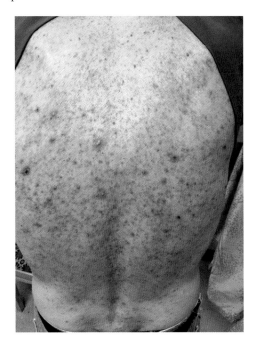

A. Perform a biopsy
B. Start isotretinoin
C. Start doxycycline
D. Start topical ivermectin

38. A 26-year-old male presents with the pictured eruption in his mouth. What is the most commonly associated underlying disease?

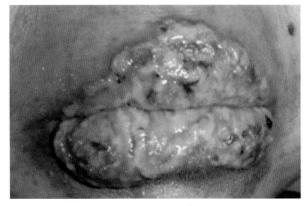

With permission from Hongmei Wang, Shufang Qiao, Xiujun Zhang, and Chun Liu, in *The American Journal of the Medical Sciences*, 2013, 345(2):168–171 (fig. 1A).

A. Acute leukemia
B. Hypothyroidism
C. Rheumatoid arthritis
D. Ulcerative colitis

39. An 84-year-old male with acute myeloid leukemia completed his second cycle of consolidation therapy 3 weeks ago. He was recently treated with granulocyte-colony stimulating factor to expedite peripheral blood count recovery. He presents with an eruption on the head, chest, and arms—representative lesion is depicted—with associated fever and arthralgias. Sterile tissue culture is negative. Which agent will likely result in prompt improvement of the rash?

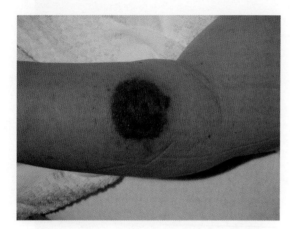

   A. High-dose oral corticosteroids
   B. Vancomycin
   C. Dapsone
   D. Cyclosporine

40. A 43-year-old man presents with the following vesicular eruption. Tzanck smear demonstrates the presence of multinucleate giant cells. What complication may be associated with the condition?

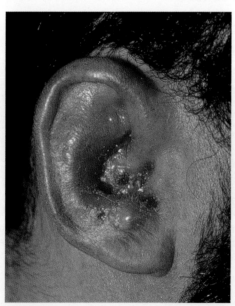

With permission from White GM and Cox NH (eds.), in *Diseases of the Skin: Color Atlas and Text*, 2nd edition, 2006, Mosby: St Louis.

   A. Ipsilateral facial palsy
   B. Keratitis
   C. Tinnitus
   D. Both A and C
   E. All of the above

PEDIATRIC DERMATOLOGY

41. A 24-year-old woman presents to the emergency department with a rash on her hands and feet. She is otherwise healthy, takes no medications, and works as a preschool teacher. She reports low-grade fevers for 2 days and myalgias. Otherwise she appears healthy. Examination is shown in the figure. What is the most likely underlying etiology?

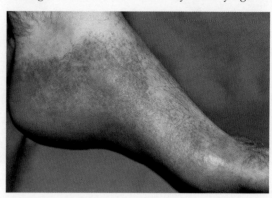

With permission from James WD, Berger T, Elston DM. Viral diseases, in *Andrews' Diseases of the Skin*, 12th ed., 2011, Elsevier, 360–413 (fig. 19-41).

   A. Enterovirus
   B. Mycoplasma
   C. Meningococcus
   D. Medication-induced
   E. Parvovirus B19

42. A 2-year-old boy is referred to your office for evaluation of a persistent rash for the past 3 weeks. The eruption involves the face and upper and lower extremities in a relatively symmetric distribution. What is the most likely etiology?

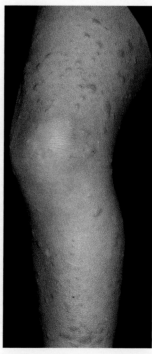

Courtesy of Curt Samlaska, MD.

A. Epstein-Barr virus infection
B. Varicella zoster virus infection
C. Noninfectious granulomas
D. Proliferation of histiocytes
E. Release of histamine

43. This infant is at increased risk for which of the following?

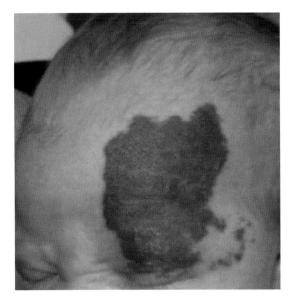

A. Seizures
B. Coarctation of the aorta
C. Glaucoma
D. Ulceration
E. Macrocephaly

44. While on the consult service, you are called to the medical intensive care unit to evaluate a 20-year-old male with hemophagocytic syndrome. His medical history is notable for frequent infections, and on examination you note that he has pale skin with silvery hair. Which of the following underlying diagnoses do you suspect?
A. Griscelli syndrome type I
B. Griscelli syndrome type II
C. Griscelli syndrome type III
D. Chédiak-Higashi syndrome
E. Elejalde syndrome

45. You are asked to see a 15-year-old boy who presented to the emergency room with an intractable nosebleed. On examination he has light skin and light eyes. You suspect an inherited disorder. What is the most likely cause of death in patients with this condition?
A. Cerebral hemorrhage
B. Cardiomyopathy
C. Progressive neurologic decline
D. Pulmonary fibrosis
E. Hemophagocytic syndrome

46. A young girl is brought to your office in July for evaluation of a sudden-onset, tender rash localized to the soles. She is otherwise healthy and, in fact, spent the weekend running around at her favorite amusement park. She denies any time spent in swimming pools. Examination is shown in the figure. What is the most likely diagnosis?

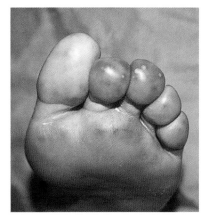

With permission from *Journal of the American Academy of Dermatology*, November 2002, 47(5 Supplement):S263–S265 (fig. 2).

A. Pernio
B. Pseudomonas "hot foot" syndrome
C. Idiopathic palmoplantar hidradenitis
D. Polyarteritis nodosa
E. Juvenile plantar dermatosis

47. This otherwise healthy 16-year-old boy presents with the below clinical and dermoscopic findings. Which of the following would be the best treatment option?

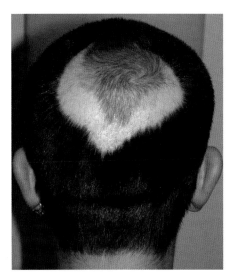

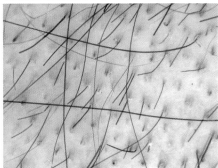

With permission from James WD, *Andrews' Diseases of the Skin Clinical Atlas*, 2018, Elsevier Inc., chapter 33, 517–541 (*left figure*); and Sperling LC, *Dermatology*, 2018, Elsevier Limited, chapter 69, 1162–1187 (*right figure*).

A. Oral griseofulvin at 10 mg/kg/day
B. Oral griseofulvin at 20 mg/kg/day
C. Habit reversal training
D. Doxycycline
E. Intralesional triamcinolone
F. Topical clindamycin

48. The most appropriate first step in treating this 10-year-old girl is:

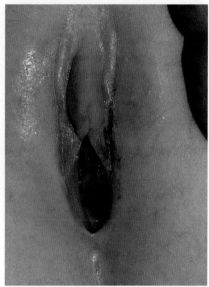

With permission from Murphy R, *Dermatologic Clinics*, 2010, volume 28, issue 4, 707–715.

A. Patch testing
B. Report suspected sexual abuse
C. Hydrocortisone 2.5% cream
D. Reassurance
E. Clobetasol 0.05% ointment

49. An infant presented with a firm, nontender subcutaneous nodule as pictured. Histology of the excised lesion would be expected to show which of the following?

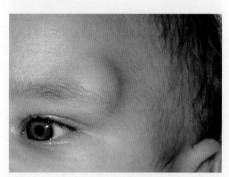

Courtesy Scott Bartlett, MD.

A. Stratified squamous epithelium with a granular layer, cyst wall containing mature adnexal structures
B. Stratified squamous epithelium without a granular layer, cystic space containing dense pink homogenized keratin
C. Mature adipocytes with small eccentric nuclei

D. Stratified squamous epithelium with a granular layer, cystic space containing laminated keratin

50. A 2-year-old previously healthy girl presents with recent onset of the below eruption after defervescing from a 4-day history of high fever complicated by febrile seizures. The causative agent in her illness has also been implicated in which of the following diseases?

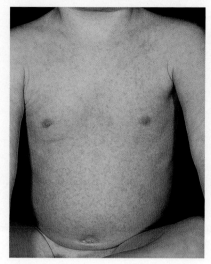

With permission from Dinulos JGH, *Exanthems and Drug Reactions Skin Disease: Diagnosis and Treatment*, 2018, Elsevier Inc., chapter 10, 282–305.

A. Papular purpuric gloves and socks syndrome
B. Drug reaction with eosinophilia and systemic symptoms
C. Kaposi sarcoma
D. Rheumatic fever
E. Oral hairy leukoplakia

DERMATOPATHOLOGY

51. This lesion is associated with which of the following?

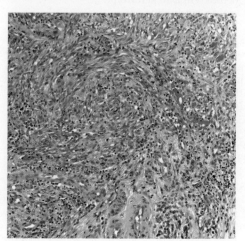

A. *Bartonella henselae*
B. Human herpes virus 8
C. Human papilloma virus
D. Polyoma virus

52. The histologic image below is most consistent with a diagnosis of:

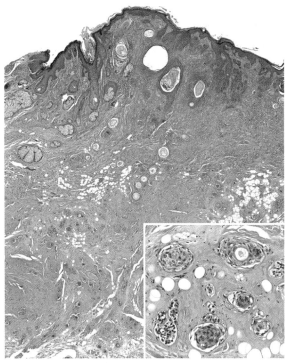

Courtesy, Lorenzo Cerroni, MD.

A. Hidrocystoma
B. Desmoplastic trichoepithelioma
C. Syringoma
D. Microcystic adnexal carcinoma
E. Chondroid syringoma

53. A teledermatology case is reviewed of a patient at a remote, rural location. The patient is 26-year-old healthy female who noted "bumps" on her chest and axillae. The bumps are described to be 12 in number, flesh-colored, deep-appearing, and 0.5–1.0 cm in size. The patient is also complaining of intermittent pain in her feet. Further questioning reveals that she has thickened skin on the feet and abnormal-appearing nails. The clinical photographs are never transmitted due to technical errors. However, a biopsy of one of the bumps is performed and the block is sent. The histology is shown in the figure. You request clinical photographs of the chest, axillae, hands, and feet. In addition, pictures of which body location and associated features would help establish the likely diagnosis?

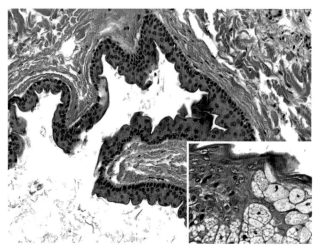

Courtesy, Lorenzo Cerroni, MD.

A. Oral mucosa, oral leukokeratosis
B. Eyes, aniridia
C. Eyes, heterochromia irides
D. Oral mucosa, oral cobblestoning
E. Legs and abdomen, lipoatrophy

54. A lesion is biopsied and shows the following histology. The correct diagnosis is:

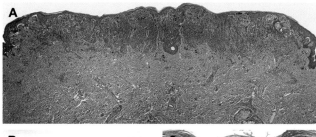
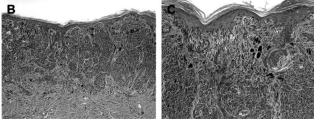

With permission from Ferrara, et al., *Dermatologic Clinics*, 2013, volume, 31, issue 4, 589–98, (fig. 2, p. 592).

A. Congenital-pattern melanocytic nevus
B. Malignant melanoma
C. Compound nevus
D. Spitz nevus
E. Combined nevus

55. A patient presents with multiple lesions on the buttocks. The histology is shown in the figure. If a systemic etiology is suspected, what test should be performed?

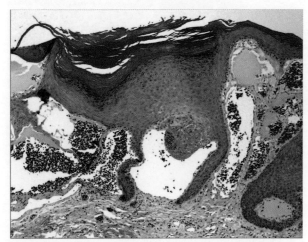

With permission from Sheth, et al., *Seminars in Diagnostic Pathology*, 2008, volume 25, issue 1, 1–16 (fig. 18, p. 13).

A. SPEP with IFE for POEMS syndrome
B. Genetic testing for Fabry disease
C. HIV testing for Kaposi sarcoma
D. Reassurance that this is a cherry hemangioma
E. Genetic testing for ataxia-telangiectasia

56. A patient presents with multiple red papules and nodules. A biopsy is performed. Which of the following studies would be indicated?

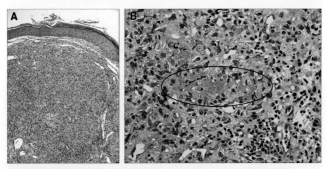

With permission from Sheth, et al., *Seminars in Diagnostic Pathology*, 2008, volume 25, issue 1, 1–16 (fig. 13, p. 10).

A. HIV testing
B. PCR of tissue to look for clonal T-cell population
C. Peripheral blood flow cytometry
D. QuantiFERON gold testing
E. Human herpesvirus-8 testing

57. A 25-year-old man presents with a 0.5-cm purple papule on the palmar right hand. It has been present for 3 months and is growing. Biopsy is performed and is shown in the figure. What other clinical features are associated with this lesion?

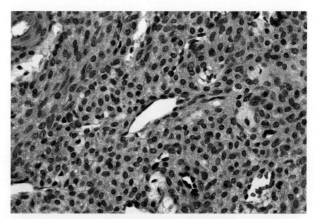

With permission from Andre, et al., Nail pathology, *Clinics in Dermatology*, 2013, volume 31 (fig. 19, p. 535).

A. Presence of arborizing vessels on dermoscopy
B. Temperature sensitivity elicited with ice cube or ice pack
C. Presence of central dilated follicle on dermoscopy
D. Positive Darier sign
E. Apple jelly color on dermoscopy

58. A 40-year-old woman presents with pink-red papules and plaques on the cheeks, nose, glabella, and forehead. A biopsy is performed. Given the suspected diagnosis, a CD123 stain is performed and is pictured in the figure. This pattern of CD123 staining supports which of the following diagnoses?

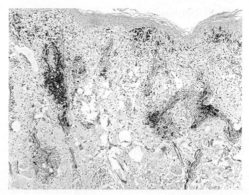

With permission from Brown, et al. *J Am Acad Dermatol*, 2013, volume 71 (fig. 3, p. 106).

A. Lupus erythematosus
B. Rosacea
C. Sweet's syndrome
D. Polymorphous light eruption
E. Leukemia cutis

59. S0X10 immunohistochemistry is performed on a specimen in the dermatopathology lab and is shown in the figure. This pattern is consistent with the following diagnosis:

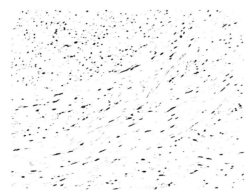

With permission from Nagarajan, et al., Use of new techniques in addition to IHC to diagnosis of melanocytic lesions, with emphasis on CGH, FISH, and mass spectrometry, *Dermatology (Actas Dermo-Silfiliograficas)*, 2017, volume 108 (fig. 2, p. 20).

A. Morpheaform basal cell carcinoma
B. Morphea
C. Desmoplastic melanoma
D. Scleredema
E. Scleromyxedema

60. A rapidly growing pigmented lesion with irregular borders, areas of clinical regression, and a blue-white veil is removed with an excisional biopsy due to concern for malignant melanoma. The biopsy is shown. Based on the histology, the dermatopathologist makes a diagnosis. Which of the following features must the dermatopathologist report in order for accurate pathologic staging by American Joint Committee on Cancer criteria to be performed?

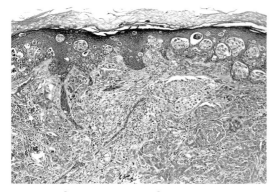

Courtesy, Lorenzo Cerroni, MD.

A. Clark level
B. Number of mitosis per high-power field
C. Presence or absence of ulceration
D. Whether or not the margins are involved
E. Presence or absence of BRAF mutation

PROCEDURAL DERMATOLOGY

61. A 67-year-old woman with a history of atrial fibrillation and prior embolic stroke presents in consultation for management of a primary basal cell carcinoma of the nasal tip. She has been on stable warfarin therapy for 18 months. Which of the following is the most appropriate management of her perioperative anticoagulation?

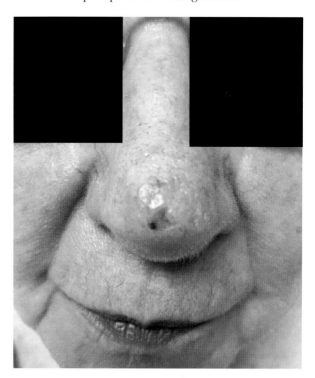

A. Proceed with Mohs surgery without alteration of anti-coagulation regimen, as long as the prothrombin time is within the therapeutic range.
B. Stop warfarin for 2 days then proceed with Mohs surgery and resume warfarin 24 hours after Mohs surgery.
C. Hold warfarin and initiate bridging therapy with low-molecular-weight heparin. After 5 days, proceed with Mohs surgery while omitting low-molecular-weight heparin 12 hours before and 12 hours after surgery.
D. Transition from warfarin to a direct oral anticoagulant (e.g., direct factor Xa inhibitor) and proceed with Mohs surgery.
E. The patient is not a good surgical candidate because of increased bleeding risk. Refer for radiation treatment while continuing warfarin therapy.

62. A 63-year-old man presents with eroded red plaque as shown on the scrotum. The lesion has been slowly progressive over 15 months. Biopsy reveals large clear cells with abundant cytoplasm and nuclear atypia in the epidermis with scatter into the upper spinous layer of the epidermis. Which of the following additional diagnostic tests are indicated prior to treatment?

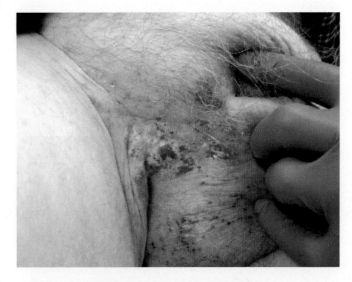

A. Genetic testing for *CDKN2A* mutation
B. Genetic testing for *MLH1/MSH2* mutations
C. Colonoscopy
D. Chest/abdomen/pelvis computed tomography scan
E. Bone scan nuclear medicine test

63. A 67-year-old woman presents for consideration of Mohs surgery for the infiltrative basal cell carcinoma shown. What anatomic structure is at risk of significant injury during surgical extirpation of the tumor?

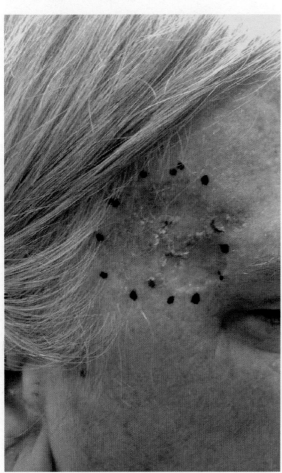

A. Superficial temporal artery
B. Facial artery
C. Auriculotemporal nerve
D. Supraorbital nerve
E. Temporal nerve

64. Which of the following is the optimal laser for removing a green tattoo?
   A. Nd:YAG
   B. Nd:YAG frequency-doubled
   C. Ruby
   D. Alexandrite
   E. Pulse dye laser

65. Which of the following sclerosants has the lowest risk for telangiectatic matting?
   A. Sodium tetradecyl sulfate
   B. Sodium morrhuate
   C. Polidocanol
   D. Glycerin
   E. Ethanolamine oleate

66. Injection of which anatomic site with filler has the highest risk for blindness?
   A. Temple
   B. Glabella
   C. Nasolabial fold
   D. Tear trough
   E. Forehead

67. Which of the following characteristics of hyaluronic acid fillers increases longevity?
   A. Cross-linking
   B. G′
   C. Viscosity
   D. Concentration
   E. None of the above

68. A 78-year-old man presents with this slowly progressing lesion on the fingernail for the last 12 months. Biopsy confirms malignancy. What is the most common malignant tumor of the nail unit?

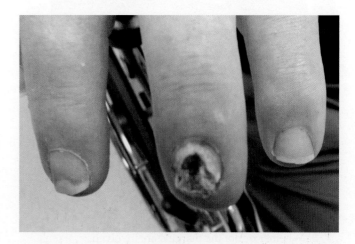

A. Basal cell carcinoma
B. Squamous cell carcinoma
C. Malignant melanoma
D. Aggressive digital papillary adenocarcinoma
E. Giant cell tumor of the tendon sheath

69. During cutaneous photodynamic therapy with either amino-levulinic acid or methyl aminolevulinate, what is the active compound that absorbs visible light?
   A. Methyl aminolevulinate
   B. Porphobilinogen
   C. Uroporphyrinogen
   D. Protoporphyrin IX
   E. Heme

70. A 72-year-old man presents with this 1.7 centimeter defect on the cutaneous lower eyelid after Mohs surgical removal of a basal cell carcinoma. When performing a Mustarde rotation flap, what is the primary tissue reservoir that is utilized for reconstruction of this defect?

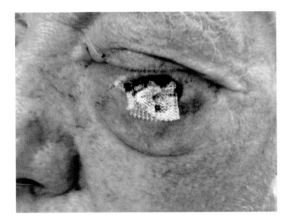

   A. Upper eyelid
   B. Lower eyelid
   C. Temple and lateral cheek
   D. Medial cheek
   E. Nasal sidewall

BASIC SCIENCE

71. A 60-year-old man comes to the office with a painful new rash. Direct immunofluorescence shows intercellular membrane staining. What type protein is targeted in this disease?

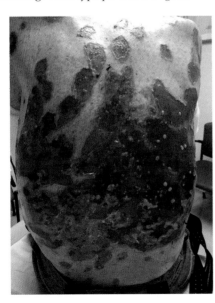

   A. G-protein coupled receptor
   B. Calcium-dependent adhesion molecule

   C. Nuclear transcription factor
   D. Intracellular kinase
   E. Receptor tyrosine kinase

72. A normal-appearing child with severe eczema and elevated IgE levels presents with frequent viral infections as shown. Genetic testing is most likely to show a deficiency in which gene?

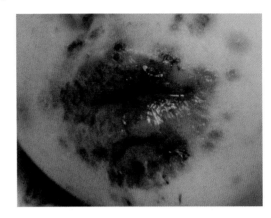

   A. Signal transducer and activator of transcription 3 (*STAT3*)
   B. Dedicator of cytokinesis 8 (*DOCK8*)
   C. Interleukin-1 receptor antagonist
   D. Transglutaminase
   E. Cyclin-dependent kinase inhibitor 2A (*CDKN2A*)

73. Corneocytes are keratinocytes that form the stratum corneum. What is the primary component of the cornified envelope on corneocytes?
   A. Lamellar bodies
   B. Phospholipids
   C. Complex carbohydrates
   D. Cross-linked proteins
   E. Ribonucleic acids

74. The lesion shown was positive for human papillomavirus (HPV). How do HPV proteins transform keratinocytes into cancer cells?

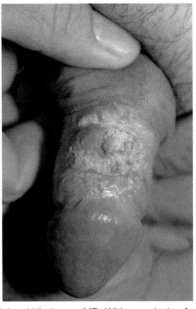

Courtesy Reinhard Kirnbauer, MD. With permission from Bolognia, in *Dermatology*, 4th edition, 2017, 1394 (ch 79, fig. 79–24).

A. Activate oncogenes
B. Inhibit tumor suppressors
C. Activate tumor suppressors
D. Inhibit oncogenes
E. Keratinocyte cytolysis

75. A 45-year-old man had onabotulinumtoxinA injected into the orbicularis oculi to reduce rhytides. What is the mechanism of action of onabotulinumtoxinA?
A. Cleaves SNAP-25 protein
B. Blocks acetylcholine receptor
C. Inhibits endocytosis
D. Activates acetylcholinesterase
E. Blocks ion-voltage sodium channels

76. A 6-year-old boy presents with the following eruption. The immune cell predominately implicated in this rash is the cause of what other dermatological disease?

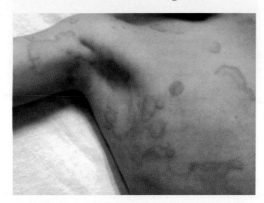

A. Lupus pernio
B. Mycosis fungoides
C. Acral melanoma
D. Urticaria pigmentosa
E. Eosinophilic fasciitis

77. The gene complex most strongly associated with this rash is *HLA-Cw6*. What is the function of HLA proteins?

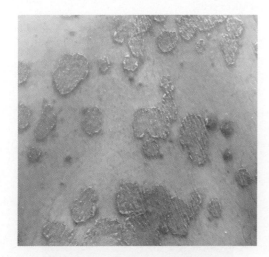

A. Stimulate B cells to produce antibodies
B. Present peptides to T cells
C. Detect microbial pathogens
D. Degrade foreign proteins
E. Promote self-tolerance

78. Muckle-Wells syndrome is often referred to as an autoinflammatory disease due to its defect in the innate immune system. What key feature distinguishes adaptive from innate immunity?
A. Recognizes pathogens
B. Produces cytokines
C. Eliminate pathogens
D. Enhanced secondary response
E. Stimulate other immune cells

79. A patient with chronic idiopathic urticaria started on omalizumab to control her symptoms. How does omalizumab treat this disease?

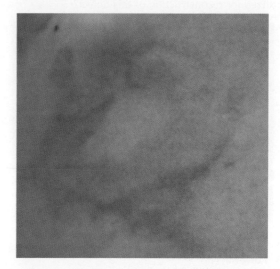

A. Inhibits eosinophil migration
B. Stabilizes mast cells
C. Inhibits cyclooxygenase
D. Binds to circulating IgE
E. Blocks histamine

80. The patient presents with an intensely pruritic rash as shown. Other family members have a similar rash. At what anatomic location does this infestation occur?

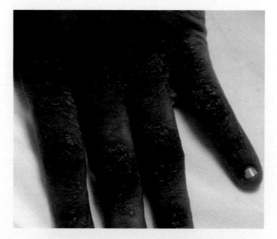

A. Sebaceous gland
B. Dermal-epidermal junction
C. Hair follicular infundibulum
D. Papillary dermis
E. Epidermis

GENERAL DERMATOLOGY

1. D. High-dose nonsteroidal antiinflammatory
Poststreptococcal erythema nodosum (EN), a septal panniculitis, commonly presents on the lower legs in healthy young individuals. Streptococcal infection is the most common infectious cause of erythema nodosum. Coccidiomycosis, viral upper respiratory tract infections, and bacterial gastroenteritis (Yersinia most commonly) are also associated with EN. Inflammatory bowel disease, use of oral contraceptives, and sarcoidosis are other associations. Treatment includes potassium iodide and high-dose nonsteroidal antiinflammatories, which are considered first-line therapy. Compression and leg elevation are also indicated. Tumor necrosis factor-alpha inhibitors have been used to treat recalcitrant EN, although they may be associated with the development of paradoxical panniculitis. Intravenous steroids, hydroxychloroquine, and valacyclovir are not indicated.
Bolognia J, Schaffer J, Cerroni L, eds. *Dermatology.* [Philadelphia]: Elsevier, 2018 (ch. 100).

2. C. Doxycycline
This child is presenting with a classic case of Rocky Mountain spotted fever (RMSF), caused by a tick bite (*Dermacentor variabilis*), with subsequent infection by *Rickettsia rickettsii*. Patients typically present after an incubation period of 2–14 days with high-grade fever, headache, myalgias, and gastrointestinal symptoms. The rash of RMSF typically begins on day 3–5 of the illness with pink macules on the wrists and ankles that develop into papules, which subsequently spread to the trunk. Petechiae and purpura develop eventually. The rash may not occur in 15% of patients. Given the severity of the disease, doxycycline is the treatment of choice for both children and adults, with the exception of non-life-threatening disease in pregnant women who may consider treatment with chloramphenicol. This is in contrast to Lyme disease in children under age 8, where amoxicillin is preferred over doxycycline.
Bolognia J, Schaffer J, Cerroni L, eds. *Dermatology.* [Philadelphia]: Elsevier, 2018 (ch. 76).

3. B. Autoimmune thyroid disease
Lichen sclerosus is a chronic inflammatory disease that commonly affects the anogenital region. Pruritus is the most prevalent symptom, but patients can experience pain and dyspareunia or be completely asymptomatic. Patients require long-term follow-up given their increased risk of scarring and development of squamous cell carcinoma. Classic findings are seen here including ivory white atrophic plaques, fusion of the labia and purpura, and hemorrhage/purpura in the setting of active disease. Other autoimmune disorders may be associated, including thyroid disease. Vulvar lichen planus may be associated with hepatitis C infection. Paraneoplastic pemphigus, which may also affect the genitals, is associated with bronchiolitis obliterans with organizing pneumonia. Monoclonal gammopathies are unrelated to lichen sclerosis.
Bolognia J, Schaffer J, Cerroni L, eds. *Dermatology.* [Philadelphia]: Elsevier, 2018 (ch. 73).

4. D. Minocycline
The patient pictured has confluent and reticulated papillomatosis (CARP). CARP typically presents at puberty and is more common in females and darker skin types. It presents as red or brown rough, keratotic plaques in a reticulated pattern within the intermammary region. The differential diagnosis includes tinea versicolor, extensive acanthosis nigricans, Darier disease, and prurigo pigmentosa. Minocycline 100 mg twice daily for 6 weeks is the treatment of choice for CARP, with a 50% response rate. Topical and oral retinoids are also treatment options.
Bolognia J, Schaffer J, Cerroni L, eds. *Dermatology.* [Philadelphia]: Elsevier, 2018 (ch. 109).

5. B. Change antibiotic to oral terbinafine
Tinea pedis is a superficial mycotic infection of the feet. Common causative dermatophytes include *T. rubrum*, *E. floccosum*, *T. mentagrophytes*, and *T. interdigitale*. Note the thickened yellow nails suggestive of onychomycosis, which is frequently associated with chronic tinea pedis. Extension of the infection onto the dorsal feet and distal legs is consistent with tinea corporis. Also note the active scaly border at the proximal edge and the papulonodular inflammation within involved areas on the legs, suggestive of perifollicular invasion (Majocchi granuloma).
Systemic antifungals including terbinafine, griseofulvin, fluconazole (B), or intraconazole are indicated over topical antifungals for patients with Majocchi granuloma. Systemic agents should also be considered in those with diabetes, immunocompromised hosts, or with moccasin-type tinea pedis. Majocchi granuloma is less responsive to topical antifungals (E).
Bolognia J, Schaffer J, Cerroni L, eds. *Dermatology.* [Philadelphia]: Elsevier, 2018 (ch. 77).

6. C. *Candida albicans*
Candida albicans is the most common cause of both systemic and localized candida infection, while *Candida tropicalis* is more likely to disseminate to the skin. Disseminated candidiasis is often seen in neutropenic patients with hematologic malignancies including leukemia. Clinically, lesions are firm papulonodules and pustules on the trunk and extremities. They typically have light centers but can occasionally appear hemorrhagic or ecthyma gangrenosum-like. Systemic sites of involvement include the liver, spleen, muscle, kidney, retina, and heart valves. Patients are often severely ill with a sepsis-like presentation. Gomori methenamine silver and periodic acid–Schiff stains will highlight yeast structures.
Cryptococcus neoformans (B) is the causative pathogen of cryptococcosis. Common cutaneous presentations include ulceration, cellulitis, and molluscoid lesions. Histologically, *C. neoformans* will have a characteristic gelatinous capsule that will appear as a clearing around individual yeast. Histological examination of *Aspergillus* (D) will demonstrate septate hyphae with 45-degree branching. Disseminated zoster (A) would not be Periodic acid–Schiff positive and would show viral cytopathic changes.
Bolognia J, Schaffer J, Cerroni L, eds. *Dermatology.* [Philadelphia]: Elsevier, 2018 (ch. 77).

7. B. Serine/threonine protein kinase
The frequency of a given genetic alteration seen in melanomas depends on the location on the body as well as the degree of ultraviolet light exposure. Melanomas that arise within intermittently sun-exposed skin (i.e., without chronic sun damage) are more likely to have *BRAF* mutations. The somatic mutation in *BRAF* that leads to a substitution of glutamic acid (E) for valine (V) at codon 600 (i.e., V600E) has been utilized in the development of target therapies such as vemurafenib and other BRAF inhibitors. The function of *BRAF* is that of a protein kinase via the mitogen-activated protein kinase (MAPK) pathway. The MAPK pathway regulates cell migration, proliferation, and growth. *NRAS* is a GTPase that is also part of the MAPK pathway and is mutated in some melanomas. KIT

mutations and/or amplifications are seen in 30%–40% of chronically sun-damaged, mucosal, or acral lentiginous melanomas. The *KIT* receptor on the cell surface is a receptor tyrosine kinase. Ligand binding to the *KIT* receptor activates the MAPK signaling pathway.
Bolognia J, Schaffer J, Cerroni L, eds. *Dermatology.* [Philadelphia]: Elsevier, 2018 (ch. 113).

8. C. Squamous cell carcinoma
The patient has discoid lupus erythematosus (DLE). These lesions classically present as discoid plaques with dyspigmentation, notably peripheral hyperpigmentation and central hypopigmentation with follicular plugging and atrophy. Hypertrophic plaques may develop as well. In rare circumstances, squamous cell carcinoma can develop in lesions of DLE. Other skin cancers are not associated with DLE.
Bolognia J, Schaffer J, Cerroni L, eds. *Dermatology.* [Philadelphia]: Elsevier, 2018 (ch. 41).

9. A. Hoarseness
Lipoid proteinosis is an autosomal recessive disease (mutation in extracellular matrix protein-1 [ECM1] protein) that results in deposition of hyaline material in the skin. Cutaneous findings include blistering on the face and extremities, waxy thickened skin, beaded eyelid papules, alopecia of eyebrows and eyelashes, warty papules on extensor extremities, and thickened cobblestoned lips or mucosa. Other findings include hoarseness, dysphagia, memory loss, dystonia, amygdala dysfunction, mental retardation, and corneal ulcers. The other options are not associated with this disease.
Bolognia J, Schaffer J, Cerroni L, eds. *Dermatology.* [Philadelphia]: Elsevier, 2018 (ch. 48).

10. B. Nifurtimox
This patient has reactivation of chronic American trypanosomiasis (Chagas disease) following cardiac transplant and immunosuppression. American trypanosomiasis is caused by *Trypanosoma cruzi* and transmitted by the triatomine (*Reduviidae*) bug. It is endemic in many areas of Central and South America. Clinical manifestations are separated into acute and chronic phases of the disease. During acute infection, patients may develop a chagoma, local inflammation, and edema at the bug bite site and port of parasite entry. This often occurs on the face, causing unilateral periorbital and palpebral edema, referred to as the Romaña sign. While most patients have spontaneous resolution, approximately 30% will develop chronic infection with heart and gastrointestinal (GI) involvement. Chronic Chagas disease may present with congestive heart failure, arrhythmias, heart block, megacolon, and megaesophagus. Reactivation occurs in immunocompromised patients with chronic Chagas disease following organ and bone marrow transplant, as well as inpatients with HIV/AIDS. Reactivated Chagas disease may be severe, presenting with new erythematous nodules and plaques favoring the lower extremities. Skin biopsy of these lesions will show the presence of intracellular amastigotes. There are two established treatments for Chagas disease: nifurtimox and benznidazole.
Bolognia J, Schaffer J, Cerroni L, eds. *Dermatology.* [Philadelphia]: Elsevier, 2018 (ch. 83).

11. E. Hydralazine
The picture shows subacute cutaneous lupus erythematosus (SCLE) with truncal oval and annular scaly plaques. All of the listed medications have been reported as possible triggers for drug-induced SCLE with the exception of hydralazine. Hydralazine can cause drug-induced systemic lupus erythematosus (SLE), not drug-induced SCLE. Drug-induced SCLE is indistinguishable from idiopathic SCLE on clinical, histologic, or laboratory features. Anti-Ro/SSA and/or anti-La/SSB are positive. The most commonly implicated medications that trigger SCLE are calcium channel blockers, Angiotensin-converting enzyme inhibitors, terbinafine, TNF-alpha inhibitors, antiepileptics, proton pump inhibitors, nonsteroidal antiinflammatory drugs, and thrombocyte inhibitors.
Bolognia J, Schaffer J, Cerroni L, eds. *Dermatology.* [Philadelphia]: Elsevier, 2018 (ch. 41).

12. C. May be associated with mutilating arthritis
The picture demonstrates classic features of pityriasis rubra pilaris (PRP), with follicular papules coalescing into orange-red plaques. Pathology demonstrates plugged dilated follicles with alternating pattern of orthokeratosis and parakeratosis ("checkerboard" pattern). Systemic retinoids are considered first-line treatment, but biologic therapy is also another option. The most common form of PRP, the classic adult subtype, begins in the head and neck regions and advances caudally. PRP can be associated with HIV infection or internal malignancy, including renal cell, bronchogenic, and hepatocellular carcinomas. Unlike psoriasis and multicentric reticulohistiocytosis, PRP has not been associated with mutilating arthritis. The differential includes psoriasis, but the clinical clue in the Kodachrome is the presence of follicular scaly papules.
Bolognia J, Schaffer J, Cerroni L, eds. *Dermatology.* [Philadelphia]: Elsevier, 2018 (ch. 9).

13. B. Urticarial vasculitis
Urticarial vasculitis presents with urticarial lesions that are often painful rather that pruritic, last greater than 24 hours, and often heal with hyperpigmentation. Low complement levels are associated with more severe disease and systemic involvement. The pathophysiology involves immune complex deposition (type III hypersensitivity) resulting in leukocytoclastic vasculitis. The other entities are considered in the clinical differential diagnosis. SCLE is usually photodistributed and lacks purpura and hyperpigmentation. Tinea corporis may present with annular lesions with active scaly edge but not with systemic symptoms. Pityriasis rosea presents with papulosquamous lesions along the lines of cleavage, often with trailing scale, and would not result in painful lesions. The lesions of true urticaria last less than 24 hours.
Bolognia J, Schaffer J, Cerroni L, eds. *Dermatology.* [Philadelphia]: Elsevier, 2018 (ch. 18).

14. A. Increased expression of *KIT* and stem cell factor within the lesional epidermis and dermis, respectively, may play a role in pathogenesis of this condition
The photograph shows the classic appearance of melasma: hyperpigmented macules and/or patches of the face, which are often symmetric and with a "moth-eaten" appearance of the edges. Increased expression of *KIT* and stem cell factor within the lesional epidermis and dermis, respectively, may play a role in pathogenesis of this condition. On the contrary, loss of pigmentation in conditions such as piebaldism and vitiligo harbor *KIT* mutations. Erythema dyschromicum perstans, not melasma, has been associated with the ingestion of the fertilizer ammonium nitrate. The histology of exogenous ochronosis related to application of hydroquinone demonstrates the banana-shaped, yellow-brown deposits in the dermis. Exogenous ochronosis appears clinically as blue, brown, or black

mottled macules in areas of hydroquinone application. Choice (D) describes the histopathologic findings of macular amyloidosis, not melasma. Tranexamic acid is a systemic medication used to treat melasma. Tranexamic acid has been associated with increasing the risk of thrombotic events such as pulmonary embolism and ischemic strokes, not hemorrhagic strokes.
Bolognia J, Schaffer J, Cerroni L, eds. *Dermatology.* [Philadelphia]: Elsevier, 2018 (ch. 67).

15. D. Antithrombin III deficiency
Livedoid vasculopathy classically presents with painful punched-out ulcerations on the lower legs (especially over the ankles) and may have a surrounding livedo reticularis. Healing with atrophic ivory white scars (atrophie blanche) is typical. Some patients may have an identifiable hypercoagulable proclivity (i.e., factor V Leiden, antithrombin III deficiency, hyperhomocysteinemia, antiphospholipid antibodies, altered fibrinolysis, or platelet activation). Evaluation for a hypercoagulable state may identify such individuals. Lesions that mimic livedoid vasculopathy can be seen in patients with idiopathic and lupus-associated antiphospholipid syndrome. Treatment with antiplatelet and anticoagulant agents is standard.
Diabetes may be associated with leg lesions, including diabetic dermopathy (hyperpigmented atrophic macules) and necrobiosis lipoidica (yellow-translucent plaques that may ulcerate).
Cirrhosis may be associated with jaundice, pruritus, spider angiomas, telangiectasias, palmar erythema, dilated abdominal wall veins, and gynecomastia. End-stage renal disease may be associated with xerosis, pruritus, acquired perforating dermatosis, pseudoporphyria, and calciphylaxis. The ulcers of calciphylaxis are typically more necrotic, stellate ulcers that usually occur at fatty sites.
Bolognia J, Schaffer J, Cerroni L, eds. *Dermatology.* [Philadelphia]: Elsevier, 2018 (ch. 23).

16. A. Most commonly associated with the initiation of vancomycin
Pemphigus vulgaris is an autoimmune blistering disease caused by IgG autoantibodies to desmoglein 1 and desmoglein 3. Neonates of mothers with this condition may have a transient disease caused by maternal IgG that crosses the placenta. Pemphigus vulgaris may be associated with initiation of certain medications, specifically penicillamine and captopril. Desmoglein 1 and desmoglein 3 are restricted to stratified squamous epithelia. Rituximab is a monoclonal antibody to CD-20 used in the treatment of pemphigus that depletes the antibody-producing B cells. Linear IgA bullous dermatosis (LABD) and not pemphigus vulgaris is associated with vancomycin. While oral findings are seen in 80% of LABD cases, they do not occur in isolation without concurrent skin involvement.
Bolognia J, Schaffer J, Cerroni L, eds. *Dermatology.* [Philadelphia]: Elsevier, 2018 (ch. 29).

17. C. Linear deposits of C3 on the epidermal side of salt-split skin
Epidermolysis bullosa acquisita is a rare acquired autoimmune blistering disorder due to production of antibodies to type VII collagen leading to a subepidermal split. Patients can have variable presentation, resembling bullous pemphigoid or mucous membrane pemphigoid, or have more severe disease closely resembling dystrophic EB. Skin fragility, blisters, erosions, and scarring particularly at trauma-prone surfaces are characteristic findings of this

mechanobullous disorder. The presence of milia may be a diagnostic clue. DIF commonly shows a linear pattern of IgG on the basement membrane zone, but C3, IgA, and IgM deposition may occur as well. In a salt-split skin preparation, the deposits are on the dermal side of the cleavage (floor) as opposed to the epidermal side (roof) as seen in bullous pemphigoid. EBA can be difficult to manage, as it is often treatment refractory.
Bolognia J, Schaffer J, Cerroni L, eds. *Dermatology.* [Philadelphia]: Elsevier, 2018 (ch. 30).

18. C. Amlodipine
The photograph demonstrates an eczematous eruption. Calcium channel blockers are the pharmacologic class most strongly associated with development of chronic eczematous eruptions in the elderly population. The differential diagnosis for diffuse chronic eczematous eruptions in the elderly should include contact dermatitis, asteatotic dermatitis, scabies, eczematous presentation of bullous pemphigoid, and mycosis fungoides. It is important to consider eczematous drug eruptions as well.
Summers EM, Bingham CS, Dahle KW, Sweeney C, Ying J, Sontheimer RD. Chronic eczematous eruptions in the aging further support for an association with exposure to calcium channel blockers. *JAMA Dermatol.* 2013;149(7): 814–818.

19. A. CBC
B. Urinalysis
C. Basic metabolic panel
The figure demonstrates palpable purpura of cutaneous small vessel vasculitis (CSVV). CSVV can be isolated to the skin, be skin predominant with internal organ involvement, or be a cutaneous manifestation of a systemic vasculitis. Once diagnosis of CSVV is confirmed, basic laboratory testing should include a CBC, urinalysis, and basic metabolic panel (BMP). Additional tests (including SPEP and ANCAs) may be checked based on suspicion of an underlying disorder and guided by review of systems. In this scenario, a healthy 23-year-old male without a cough is unlikely to have a monoclonal gammopathy or medium vessel ANCA-positive vasculitis. It is important to consider costs of diagnostic workup. Urinalysis and renal function in particular are important, as the kidneys tend to be more commonly involved than other internal organs.
Bolognia J, Schaffer J, Cerroni L, eds. *Dermatology.* [Philadelphia]: Elsevier, 2018 (ch. 24).

20. C. Vitamin D
Calcinosis cutis is a result of local or systemic calcium dysregulation in the skin. The cause of calcinosis cutis is broadly divided into five categories: dystrophic, metastatic, iatrogenic, idiopathic, or mixed. Dystrophic calcinosis occurs when preexisting damage to the skin results in calcium deposition, such as with autoimmune connective tissue disease for example. Metastatic calcification is a result of systemic metabolic disorder (e.g., advanced kidney disease, sarcoidosis, hyperparathyroidism, etc.). Iatrogenic calcinosis cutis is due to medical therapy or testing, while in idiopathic calcinosis no cause is identified. There are some cases that are classified as mixed.
In determining the underlying cause, laboratory workup is often helpful and should include serum calcium and phosphate levels (to determine the calcium phosphate product), parathyroid hormone, vitamin D3, and 24-hour urinary calcium excretion. Lab abnormalities are seen most often in metastatic causes of calcification, but normal values do not exclude these disorders.

Bolognia J, Schaffer J, Cerroni L, eds. *Dermatology*. [Philadelphia]: Elsevier, 2018 (ch. 50).

21. A. Plasma cell dyscrasia

This constellation of findings is seen in primary systemic amyloidosis, which is associated with plasma cell dyscrasias. The presenting symptoms of primary systemic amyloidosis are varied but include fatigue, weight loss, dyspnea, and oral cavity changes such as macroglossia. Purpura, petechia, and ecchymosis are often seen after minor trauma, especially on the eyelids, neck, and anogenital region. There may be waxy, translucent infiltrative purpuric papules in these areas as well. Less common cutaneous features include nail dystrophy due to amyloid in the matrix that resembles nail lichen planus with longitudinal ridging and thinning as pictured here.

Dermatomyositis with polymyositis is associated with proximal muscle weakness. The nail findings commonly seen in dermatomyositis include periungual telangiectasias and cuticle hypertrophy. Cardiac disease, when present, is usually asymptomatic and most commonly presents as arrhythmias or conduction defects. Acromegaly, which results from excessive growth hormone, is associated with macroglossia and cardiomegaly. Thick, hard nails may be associated. Hunter syndrome (mucopolysaccharidosis type II) is an X linked recessive disorder that results in accumulation of glycosaminoglycans in various organ systems, such as the heart, liver, and spleen. Clinically, macroglossia, cardiomyopathy, severe skeletal abnormalities, and progressive neurological decline with overall reduced life expectancy are associated.

Bolognia J, Schaffer J, Cerroni L, eds. *Dermatology*. [Philadelphia]: Elsevier, 2018 (chs. 42, 47, 48).

22. B. Decreased secretion of thyroid-stimulating hormone by the anterior pituitary

The patient has mycosis fungoides as depicted in the Kodachrome. Bexarotene is an oral retinoid used in the treatment of cutaneous T-cell lymphoma. Among the known side effects of bexarotene is central hypothyroidism, which is seen in about 40% of treated patients. This effect is thought to be mediated via suppression of the secretion of the β-subunit of TSH in the anterior pituitary. As a result of this known side effect, free T4 levels should be monitored in any patient receiving bexarotene and thyroid hormone replacement therapy given as needed.

Bolognia J, Schaffer J, Cerroni L, eds. *Dermatology*. [Philadelphia]: Elsevier, 2018 (ch. 126).

23. B. Ixekizumab

This patient has psoriasis that is unresponsive to standard therapies, therefore systemic treatment is indicated. Ixekizumab is an IL-17A blocker Food and Drug Administration (FDA) approved for the treatment of psoriasis. IL-17 blockers are associated with new onset and/or exacerbation of inflammatory bowel disease (IBD) and therefore best avoided in this patient with Crohn disease. Adalimumab is a TNF-alpha inhibitor that is FDA approved for the treatment of psoriasis as well as Crohn disease. Ustekinumab is a monoclonal antibody that targets IL-12 and IL-23. Ustekinumab is FDA approved for the treatment of psoriasis as well as Crohn disease. Guselkumab is a monoclonal antibody that targets IL-23 and is FDA approved for the treatment of psoriasis. This medication is not known to exacerbate underlying IBD.

Bolognia J, Schaffer J, Cerroni L, eds. *Dermatology*. [Philadelphia]: Elsevier, 2018 (ch. 128).

24. B. Cola

The azole oral antifungals are commonly utilized in dermatology and have multiple potential drug interactions. Itraconazole and ketoconazole require an acid milieu for adequate absorption, therefore medications such as H2 blockers, proton pump inhibitors, sucralfate, and didanosine significantly interfere with their absorption. Conversely, administration of itraconazole or ketoconazole with carbonated cola beverages helps acidify the stomach (pH < 3) and thereby increase their absorption. As an alternative, fluconazole and voriconazole do not require an acid milieu for their absorption.

Bolognia J, Schaffer J, Cerroni L, eds. *Dermatology*. [Philadelphia]: Elsevier, 2018 (ch. 131).

25. C. $\alpha_6\beta_4$ integrin

Mucous membrane (cicatricial) pemphigoid is a chronic autoimmune blistering disorder that affects skin and mucous membranes and has a tendency to lead to scarring. The two most frequent sites of involvement are the oral and conjunctival mucosa. Conjunctival involvement occurs overall in about 40% of cases and can ultimately lead to blindness. The ocular involvement starts as nonspecific symptoms of chronic conjunctivitis such as burning, soreness, foreign-body sensation, or mucous production. Chronic inflammation can progress to scar tissue formation with symblepharon, ankyloblepharon, trichiasis, and/or entropion and eventual blindness.

Cicatricial pemphigoid is divided into four subgroups. The first group has autoantibodies directed against laminin 332. This subgroup has an overall increase risk of associated malignancy. The second subgroup is termed ocular mucous membrane pemphigoid, because these patients have predominately or exclusively ocular disease. Ocular mucous membrane pemphigoid is characterized by autoantibodies directed against the β_4 subunit of the $\alpha_6\beta_4$ integrin. The largest subgroup is the third, with clinical involvement of both skin and mucosa. This subgroup has autoantibodies directed against the same target antigens as in bullous pemphigoid, namely the C-terminal portion of BP180. The fourth group is heterogeneous, and it is unclear if damage is due to autoantibody-mediated response to the proteins in the basement membrane.

Bolognia J, Schaffer J, Cerroni L, eds. *Dermatology*. [Philadelphia]: Elsevier, 2018 (ch. 30).

26. D. Thickened collagen bundles with trapped eccrine glands

The Kodachrome illustrates indurated, hyperpigmented to violaceous sclerotic plaques on the upper arm, characteristic of morphea. The histopathology of morphea depends on the stage of the lesion (early inflammatory or late sclerosis); classically thickened dermis and perivascular infiltrate of lymphocytes and plasma cells may be seen, while advanced disease results in thickened collagen bundles and trapped eccrine glands.

Spongiotic dermatitis with mixed dermal inflammatory infiltrate characterizes an acute contact dermatitis in which erythema, vesicles, or scale would be clinically evident. In cutaneous lupus, histopathology reveals a lymphohistiocytic interface dermatitis with vacuolar degeneration, periadnexal inflammation, and follicular plugging. Clinically patients with subacute cutaneous lupus present with a photosensitive dermatitis that is typically annular or papulosquamous in morphology. Postinflammatory pigmentary alteration clinically manifests as hyper- or hypopigmentation after an inflammatory skin condition. On pathology there is an increase in melanin in the upper

dermis and upper dermal vessels, which is located primarily in macrophages (melanophages).
Bolognia J, Schaffer J, Cerroni L, eds. *Dermatology.* [Philadelphia]: Elsevier, 2018 (chs. 14, 41, 100).

27. C. Chemotherapy
Chemotherapeutic agents may cause both longitudinal and transverse melanonychia. Psoralens, hydroxyurea, and zidovudine are also causes of melanonychia. Other nail changes from chemotherapy include Beau's lines, onycholysis (taxanes associated with hemorrhagic onycholysis), leukonychia, splinter hemorrhages (tyrosine kinase inhibitors and vascular endothelial growth factor receptor inhibitors), and pyogenic granuloma-like lesions (epidermal growth factor receptor inhibitors).
Pseudomonas infection of the nail causes green discoloration due to pyocyanin. Candida infection may result in chronic paronychia in addition to irritant dermatitis. Melanoma may cause longitudinal melanonychia, not transverse as in this patient. Oral retinoids may cause multiple changes, including nail fragility, paronychia, and periungual pyogenic granulomas.
Bolognia J, Schaffer J, Cerroni L, eds. *Dermatology.* [Philadelphia]: Elsevier, 2018 (ch. 71).

28. B. *p*-Phenylenediamine
p-Phenylenediamine (PPD) is a potent sensitizer found in hair dye. Hairdressers can present with allergic contact dermatitis of the hands, wrists, eyelids, and nose.
Ammonium persulfate is found in hair bleach. It may cause contact urticaria and a generalized histamine reaction. Methacrylate is found in artificial nails and may cause dermatitis on the hands or eyelids. Propolis is made by bees from resinous exudates of plants and most notably causes an allergic contact dermatitis of the lips, as it may be used in lip balms. *Lawsonia inermis* is natural henna and does not commonly cause an allergic contact dermatitis.
Bolognia J, Schaffer J, Cerroni L, eds. *Dermatology.* [Philadelphia]: Elsevier, 2018 (ch. 14).

29. A. Nifedipine
Pernio is pictured here with acral distributed purpuric papules, which may have overlying dry scale. In a double-blind, placebo-controlled trial, nifedipine was found to be effective in the treatment of pernio, with an approximately 70% response rate. There are only anecdotal reports supporting the use of topical steroids and topical nitroglycerin in the treatment of pernio. Hydroxychloroquine should be considered in chilblains lupus. Aspirin may be effective in erythromelalgia.
Bolognia J, Schaffer J, Cerroni L, eds. *Dermatology.* [Philadelphia]: Elsevier, 2018 (ch. 88).

30. D. BPAG2
Patients with pemphigoid gestationis have autoantibodies of the IgG1 subclasses directed against the hemidesmosomal protein BPAG2 (BP180; collagen XVII), as seen in classical bullous pemphigoid. Pemphigoid gestationis presents with abrupt onset typically in the second or third trimester of urticarial or vesicular plaques on the trunk and abdomen, particularly around the umbilicus, which rapidly generalizes. Direct immunofluorescence reveals linear C3 > IgG. There is increased risk for premature delivery and small-for-gestational-age neonates. Desmoglein 1 and 3 autoantibodies are found in pemphigus vulgaris. BPAG1 (BP230) is a member of the plakin family, and autoantibodies to this protein may be found in patients with bullous pemphigoid. Type VII collagen is the

target in epidermolysis bullosa acquisita and bullous systemic lupus erythematosus.
Bolognia J, Schaffer J, Cerroni L, eds. *Dermatology.* [Philadelphia]: Elsevier, 2018 (ch. 27).

31. C. Diabetes mellitus
The figure depicts necrobiosis lipoidica diabeticorum (NLD). The pathogenesis is unknown, but there is a correlation with diabetes mellitus, which may be found in approximately 15%–65% of patients. While thyroid dysfunction is also associated with this condition, it is less frequent than diabetes. The clinical presentation is typically yellow/red-brown plaques on the distal shins, often with central atrophy. Ulceration may occur.
Pretibial myxedema, associated with Graves disease (hyperthyroidism), presents as indurated waxy plaques on the distal anterior lower extremities secondary to mucin deposition with a peau d'orange appearance. Skin lesions of SLE may be annular, but the distribution is usually on the head and neck. NLD is not associated with Raynaud.
Bolognia J, Schaffer J, Cerroni L, eds. *Dermatology.* [Philadelphia]: Elsevier, 2018 (ch. 91).

32. B. Infliximab
The eruption shown in the vignette is drug-induced interstitial granulomatous dermatitis or institutional granulomatous drug reaction (IGDR). The most common causes are calcium channel blockers, TNF-alpha inhibitors, and HMG-CoA reductase inhibitors. The rash is characterized by erythematous plaques, which are often annular and distributed on the trunk, medial thighs, axillae, and buttocks. Reactive granulomatous dermatitis may also present with palpable cords or nodules. The other choices are not classical causes of IGDR but may cause other drug hypersensitive reactions such as DRESS, SJS, or morbilliform drug eruptions.
Bolognia J, Schaffer J, Cerroni L, eds. *Dermatology.* [Philadelphia]: Elsevier, 2018 (ch. 91).

33. D. Granular IgA deposition within the dermal papillae
The patient above has dermatitis herpetiformis, with extensor vesicles and erosions that are classically pruritic. It is a cutaneous manifestation of gluten sensitivity or Celiac disease. Patients produce IgA antiendomysial antibodies that are directed against tissue transglutaminase. DIF findings include granular IGA deposition in the dermal papillae. The treatment is gluten restriction, and dapsone may help control dermatologic symptoms.
Bolognia J, Schaffer J, Cerroni L, eds. *Dermatology.* [Philadelphia]: Elsevier, 2018 (ch. 31).

34. B. Captopril
The patient has drug-induced linear IgA bullous dermatosis (LABD). There are multiple drugs associated with LABD, most commonly vancomycin. Cephalosporins, penicillins, ACEIs (particularly captopril), and NSAIDs are other common causes. Furosemide is a classical cause of drug-induced bullous pemphigoid; however, the clinical features (annular vesicular plaques with string of pearls) and histologic/immunofluorescence features (linear IgA) point toward LABD.
Bolognia J, Schaffer J, Cerroni L, eds. *Dermatology.* [Philadelphia]: Elsevier, 2018 (ch. 31).

35. A. Pembrolizumab
Bullous eruptions have been recently described as an immune-related adverse event (irAE) associated with checkpoint inhibitor therapy, in particular anti-programmed death 1 (PD-1) and programmed death ligand 1 (PD-L1)

therapy. Other common drug causes of bullous pemphigoid include furosemide, spironolactone, NSAIDs, ACEIs, TNF alpha inhibitors, antibiotics, and potassium iodide. Unlike most common cutaneous irAE (i.e., lichenoid, maculopapular, pruritus, vitiligo) to checkpoint inhibitors, bullous eruptions may be severe and frequently result in interrupted cancer therapy.
Bolognia J, Schaffer J, Cerroni L, eds. *Dermatology.* [Philadelphia]: Elsevier, 2018 (ch. 30).

36. **B.** G-protein coupled receptor
Vismodegib targets the G-protein coupled receptor smoothened (SMO). SMO is a G -protein receptor that is a critical part of the Sonic Hedgehog signaling pathway. In normal cells, the patched protein, a 12-span transmembrane protein receptor (protein product of human *PTCH* gene), constitutively inhibits SMO, a seven-pass transmembrane G-protein receptor. When Sonic Hedgehog binds the patched protein, SMO is released from inhibition and leads to downstream activation of Gli, a transcription factor that mediates proliferation and tumorigenesis. Vismodegib is a smoothened inhibitor that functions to regulate the Sonic Hedgehog pathway for treatment of patients with nevoid basal cell carcinoma syndrome or locally advanced BCCs deemed inoperable. Common side effects include dysgeusia, alopecia, fatigue, and muscle cramps.
Bolognia J, Schaffer J, Cerroni L, eds. *Dermatology.* [Philadelphia]: Elsevier, 2018 (ch. 107).

37. **C.** Start doxycycline
The patient has an EGFR inhibitor–associated acneiform (papulopustular) eruption. Treatment is determined based on the grade of eruption—determined by body surface area of involvement and impact on quality of life. Grade 1 (<10% BSA) eruptions are managed with topical agents (hydrocortisone, clindamycin), while grade 2 (10%–30% BSA) eruptions frequently require oral tetracycline therapy. Of the answer choices, the most appropriate first-line treatment based on this grade 2 rash is oral doxycycline. Isotretinoin can be considered in refractory cases, but may be limited by its tendency to cause xerosis and retinoid dermatitis. Culture is recommended to evaluate for antibiotic resistance, but biopsy is not indicated unless there are atypical features or the rash fails to respond to recommended therapy.
Bolognia J, Schaffer J, Cerroni L, eds. *Dermatology.* [Philadelphia]: Elsevier, 2018 (ch. 36).

38. **D.** Ulcerative colitis
The Kodachrome depicts pyostomatitis vegetans, a rare pustular eruption of the oral mucosa associated with inflammatory bowel disease. It is characterized by a chronic, vegetative eruption of the labial and buccal mucosa, with snail-track-like pustules. The differential includes paraneoplastic pemphigus, Behçet disease, major aphthae, as well as infectious entities such as herpes labialis/gingivostomatitis.
Bolognia J, Schaffer J, Cerroni L, eds. *Dermatology.* [Philadelphia]: Elsevier, 2018 (ch. 26).

39. **A.** High-dose oral corticosteroids.
The patient has Sweet syndrome, which is often associated with fever and leukocytosis and less commonly with myalgia and arthralgia. Drug-induced Sweet syndrome is commonly associated with granulocyte-colony stimulating factor, antibiotics, antihypertensives, contraceptives, immunosuppressants, retinoids, and NSAIDs. Other triggers of Sweet syndrome include infection, malignancy (particularly acute myeloid leukemia, gammopathy, and

myelodysplasia), inflammatory bowel disease, and autoimmune disorders. Prompt response to systemic corticosteroids is typical and part of the diagnostic criteria.
Bolognia J, Schaffer J, Cerroni L, eds. *Dermatology.* [Philadelphia]: Elsevier, 2018 (ch. 26).

40. **D.** Both A and C
Ramsay-Hunt syndrome is due to reactivation of latent varicella-zoster virus within the geniculate ganglion of the facial nerve. Cutaneous findings typically reveal grouped vesicles of the external auditory canal. The tympanic membrane, anterior two-thirds of the tongue, and hard palate may also be affected. Neurological complications include ear pain, ipsilateral facial paralysis, loss of taste in the anterior two-thirds of the tongue, and, rarely, tinnitus, hearing loss, or vertigo (D).
Keratitis is a complication of herpes zoster affecting the ophthalmic division of the trigeminal nerve. Hutchinson sign, which refers to the presence of cutaneous lesions on the nasal tip, is associated with a higher risk of ocular complications, including conjunctivitis, keratitis, uveitis, acute retinal necrosis, and optic neuritis. Ophthalmologic consultation should promptly be obtained.
Bolognia J, Schaffer J, Cerroni L, eds. *Dermatology.* [Philadelphia]: Elsevier, 2018 (ch. 80).

PEDIATRIC DERMATOLOGY

41. **E.** Parvovirus B19
The clinical image depicts edema and erythema with petechiae of the foot with sharp demarcation at the ankle. The vignette describes a young adult with exposure to children and symptoms of myalgias. Taken together, a diagnosis of papular purpuric gloves and socks syndrome is favored. The most likely underlying etiology is parvovirus B19 infection.
Coxsackievirus infection typically presents with vesicles and papules on the palms and soles as well as oral mucosa (hand-foot-mouth disease). Mycoplasma infection is a common cause of erythema multiforme, which typically presents with targetoid lesions on the palms and soles, or mycoplasma-associated mucositis, which manifests predominantly with mucosal erosions. Purpuric lesions on the palms can be seen with meningococcemia, a life-threatening emergency, but the patient is not ill-appearing. Serum-sickness-like reaction can present with edema and erythema of the hands, but the patient has no prior antibiotic exposure.
Bolognia J, Schaffer J, Cerroni L, eds. *Dermatology.* [Philadelphia]: Elsevier, 2018 (ch. 81).

42. **A.** Epstein-Barr virus infection
The clinical image and vignette suggest a diagnosis of Gianotti-Crosti syndrome (papular acrodermatitis of childhood). This entity typically affects young children (median age 2 years old; most cases appear before the age of 4). Historically the eruption was seen in the setting of Hepatitis B virus infection, but with advances in vaccination, the most common cause today is infection with Epstein-Barr virus (EBV). The eruption resolves spontaneously but over a prolonged time-course of 1–2 months.
Primary varicella would present more acutely, and the vignette does not describe transient lesions as would be expected in urticaria. The image does not depict sarcoidosis or Langerhans cell histiocytosis.
Bolognia J, Schaffer J, Cerroni L, eds. *Dermatology.* [Philadelphia]: Elsevier, 2018 (ch. 80).

43. B. Coarctation of the aorta
This patient has a large segmental infantile hemangioma and is at risk for PHACE(S) syndrome, an acronym coined for a spectrum of anomalies associated with such lesions: *P, p*osterior fossa and other structural brain malformations; *H, h*emangioma; *A, a*rterial anomalies of cervical and cerebral vessels; *C, c*ardiac defects (especially *c*oarctation of the aorta); *E, e*ye anomalies; and *S, s*ternal defects and *s*upraumbilical raphe. Seizures and glaucoma are associated with Sturge-Weber syndrome, which is associated with capillary malformations involving the forehead area (A, C); highest risk sites for ulceration include the lip, anogenital area, and skin folds (D).
Bolognia J, Schaffer J, Cerroni L, eds. *Dermatology*. [Philadelphia]: Elsevier, 2018 (chs. 103 and 104).

44. B. Griscelli syndrome type II
The vignette describes a patient with silvery hair, immunodeficiency, and hemophagocytic syndrome, all characteristic features of Griscelli syndrome (GS) type II. Griscelli type I features neurologic symptoms, whereas type III has mild, mainly cutaneous features. Patient's with Chédiak-Higashi syndrome often develop hemophagocytic syndrome but also present with severe neurologic dysfunction, and death typically occurs by age 10. Elejalde syndrome patients have severe neurologic dysfunction, akin to GS1 patients.
Bolognia J, Schaffer J, Cerroni L, eds. *Dermatology*. [Philadelphia]: Elsevier, 2018 (ch. 66).

45. D. Pulmonary fibrosis
The vignette describes a patient with Hermansky-Pudlak syndrome, an autosomal recessive disorder that features oculocutaneous albinism, a bleeding diathesis, and lysosomal accumulation of ceroid lipofuscin. The condition is common in individuals of Puerto Rican descent, and the leading cause of death among these patients is pulmonary fibrosis. Extensive ecchymoses, cardiomyopathy, and renal failure can also occur. The other answers are not features of this syndrome.
Bolognia J, Schaffer J, Cerroni L, eds. *Dermatology*. [Philadelphia]: Elsevier, 2018 (ch. 66).

46. C. Idiopathic palmoplantar hidradenitis
The vignette and clinical image support a diagnosis of idiopathic palmoplantar hidradenitis. The disease is primarily seen in children following rigorous physical activity. Patients suddenly develop multiple tender nodules on the soles more commonly than the palms. A biopsy shows neutrophilic infiltrate of the sweat glands.
Juvenile plantar dermatosis has a characteristic "glazed" appearance, which is not seen here, and associated with atopic dermatitis. While the remaining choices are in the differential diagnosis for idiopathic palmoplantar hidradenitis, the history is most suggestive of this entity. Presentation in July makes pernio less likely, and the patient has not been exposed to swimming pools, decreasing the likelihood of pseudomonas hot-foot syndrome. Cutaneous polyarteritis nodosa, a medium-vessel vasculitis, typically manifests with livedo reticularis, erythematous papules, nodules, plaques, or ulcerative lesions.
Bolognia J, Schaffer J, Cerroni L, eds. *Dermatology*. [Philadelphia]: Elsevier, 2018 (ch. 39).

47. C. Habit reversal training
Trichotillomania is a disorder in which self-induced plucking or breakage of the hair results in patchy alopecia of the scalp, eyebrows, eyelashes, and/or pubic region. Often the alopecic patches have irregular borders, unusual shapes, erosions, and hairs of varying lengths. Trichotillomania may be associated with stress or a personality disorder. The Diagnostics and Statistics Manual for Mental Health Disorders, Fifth edition (DSM-5) classifies trichotillomania under "obsessive-compulsive and related disorders," but many patients who chronically pull their hair do not meet all of the DSM-5 criteria. Confirmation of the diagnosis can be accomplished by creating a hair growth window in which a specific area is repeatedly shaved and normal-density hair regrows, as the hairs are too short to manipulate. Treatment for trichotillomania includes habit reversal training/behavioral modification therapy, hypnosis, psychotherapy, and pharmacologic therapy. If pharmacologic treatment is planned, clomipramine is the recommended first-line medication.
Griseofulvin is a first-line therapy for tinea capitis. Doxycycline is used to treat a number of alopecias, including central centrifugal cicatricial alopecia, acne keloidalis, dissecting cellulitis of the scalp, and folliculitis decalvans. Intralesional triamcinolone is frequently used to treat localized alopecia areata. Topical clindamycin is a treatment option for folliculitis decalvans.
Bolognia J, Schaffer J, Cerroni L, eds. *Dermatology*. [Philadelphia]: Elsevier, 2018 (ch. 69).

48. E. Clobetasol 0.05% ointment
Lichen sclerosus (LS), previously known as lichen sclerosus et atrophicus, is a chronic inflammatory skin disease that affects the epidermis and superficial dermis, leading to characteristic ivory-white patches of scarlike atrophy. In approximately 85% of patients, the anogenital area is affected, with a smaller fraction of patients exhibiting extragenital involvement. The peak incidence in women is during the fifth and sixth decades, with a second peak in prepubertal girls between the ages of 8 and 13. In women and girls, the ivory-white shiny or wrinkled patches often extend circumferentially around the vulva to the perineum and perianal areas in a "figure of eight" configuration. The fragility of the dermal-epidermal junction may lead to development of purpura or hemorrhagic bullae within affected areas, which may occur with little or no trauma. For this reason, in children LS may be confused with sexual abuse.
LS may be asymptomatic, but it is often accompanied by severe pruritus and soreness. LS may also be complicated by fissures, dysuria, dyspareunia, or pain with defecation. Untreated disease may result in irreversible scarring, including burying of the clitoris and fusion or loss of the labia minora with narrowing of the introitus. In addition, both men and women are at increased risk of developing genital squamous cell carcinomas (SCCs) in areas of LS. In boys and men, lichen sclerosus of the penis (balanitis xerotica obliterans) often leads to phimosis. Circumcision may be a first-line treatment for phimosis due to LS, though recurrence is possible. First-line treatment for vulvar LS is ultrapotent topical steroids, such as clobetasol propionate, which are safe and highly effective in the treatment of genital LS for all age groups. Appropriate treatment is often a 3-month course of daily or twice-daily application followed by tapering of frequency of application for maintenance. Low-potency topical steroids such as hydrocortisone are not appropriate first-line treatment. In addition, cream bases contain alcohol and are more likely to cause stinging and burning than ointment bases. Importantly, there is evidence that vulvar SCC appears to develop primarily in untreated or infrequently treated lesions of vulvar LS, highlighting the importance of long-term treatment of this chronic disease.

Bolognia J, Schaffer J, Cerroni L, eds. *Dermatology*. [Philadelphia]: Elsevier, 2018 (chs. 44 and 73).

49. A. Stratified squamous epithelium with a cyst wall containing mature adnexal structures

Dermoid cysts are the result of entrapment of ectodermal tissue along fusion planes during embryogenesis. They present as firm, nontender, noncompressible subcutaneous nodules that are generally 1–4 cm in diameter. Dermoid cysts are most commonly found around the eyes, frequently on the upper lateral forehead near the eyebrow. They may also be found on the nose, scalp, neck, sternum, sacrum, or scrotum. Midline lesions are much more likely to have intracranial extension than do periocular lesions, and imaging is recommended for midline lesions prior to surgical excision, which is the treatment of choice.

The other options are the histopathologic descriptions of a trichilemmal (pilar) cyst (B), lipoma (C), and epidermoid cyst (D).

Bolognia J, Schaffer J, Cerroni L, eds. *Dermatology*. [Philadelphia]: Elsevier, 2018 (ch. 64).

50. B. Drug reaction with eosinophilia and systemic symptoms

Roseola infantum (aka exanthem subitum or sixth disease) is a common febrile disease and cause of viral exanthem in infants and young children. Patients present with high fever that lasts for 3–5 days, which may be complicated by febrile seizures. As the fever subsides, an exanthem develops, which is composed of pink-red macules and papules primarily on the trunk, neck, and proximal extremities. The lesions may be surrounded by a white halo and last for 1–2 days. Patients may also exhibit red papules on the soft palate called Nagayama spots. Roseola infantum is caused by human herpesvirus-6 which has also been implicated in drug reaction with eosinophilia and systemic symptoms/drug-induced hypersensitivity syndrome (DRESS/DIHS), as there may be viral reactivation, and in pityriasis rosea.

Papular purpuric gloves and socks syndrome is most commonly due to parvovirus B19 infection, which also causes fifth disease (also known as erythema infectiosum) in children. Kaposi sarcoma is caused by HHV-8, which is also associated with multicentric Castleman disease and primary effusion lymphoma. Rheumatic fever is a complication of group A beta-hemolytic streptococcal infection, which also causes scarlet fever, poststreptococcal glomerulonephritis, and several streptococcal skin infections. Oral hairy leukoplakia is caused by Epstein-Barr virus (HHV-4), which is also a causative agent in infectious mononucleosis, extranodal NK/T-cell lymphoma, and nasopharyngeal carcinoma.

Bolognia J, Schaffer J, Cerroni L, eds. *Dermatology*. [Philadelphia]: Elsevier, 2018 (ch. 80).

DERMATOPATHOLOGY

51. B. Human herpes virus 8

The figure illustrates a proliferation of spindle cells with slitlike vascular spaces that contain extravasated red blood cells. There is an infiltrate containing plasma cells and hemosiderin deposition (lower right corner). Kaposi sarcoma (KS) may present in the patch stage with an increased number of dermal vessels that have dilated or slitlike lumens. The plaque and nodular stages show a more prominent proliferation of spindle cells. Lesions from all stages of KS show nuclear staining for HHV-8 using immunohistochemistry.

Bartonella henselae causes bacillary angiomatosis, which is characterized histologically by a nodular capillary proliferation containing colonies of purple bacilli. Verruca would stain positive for human papillomavirus. Polyoma virus may be found in Merkel cell carcinoma.

Bolognia J, Schaffer J, Cerroni L, eds. *Dermatology*. [Philadelphia]: Elsevier, 2018 (ch. 114).

52. D. Microcystic adnexal carcinoma

The diagnosis is microcystic adnexal carcinoma (MAC). This lesion is deeply infiltrative and poorly circumscribed, which is concerning and is a central clue to the diagnosis. A biphasic pattern of epithelial structures is typical of MAC, where superficial follicular (pilar) keratinization can be seen with ductal differentiation in deeper portions (shown in high power in the inset). Other clues to the diagnosis of MAC when present include perineural extension and lymphoid aggregates. MAC most commonly presents as a plaque on the chin/cutaneous lip.

There are overlapping features between MAC and benign entities, including syringoma and desmoplastic trichoepithelioma (DTE), which have a paisley-tie or tad-pole pattern of epithelial structures with red sclerotic stroma between them. Syringoma and DTE, however, are smaller, more clearly circumscribed, and have a round shape at low power. Syringomas tend not to have horn cysts, though DTEs do. Morpheaform BCC is also in this histologic differential, but these do not usually have a paisley-tie pattern, and more specific features of BCC are likely to be evident. Hidrocystomas are simple cysts lined by cuboidal cells. Chondroid syringomas (mixed tumors) have a sweat duct component with cartilaginous differentiation in the stroma hence "mixed tumor."

Bolognia J, Schaffer J, Cerroni L, eds. *Dermatology*. [Philadelphia]: Elsevier, 2018 (ch. 111).

53. A. Oral mucosa, oral leukokeratosis

Pictured in the photomicrograph is a steatocystoma. The most characteristic histologic features include: wavy, eosinophilic cuticle sometimes referred to as having a shark-tooth-like appearance, and presence of sebaceous glands in the cyst wall (shown in the high-power inset). Vellus hairs may be seen within the cyst cavity as well. This patient has a steatocystoma confirmed by histology, multiple other lesions that also sound like steatocystomas (steatocystoma multiplex), painful keratoderma, and nail dystrophy. Based on this collection of findings it would be reasonable to consider a diagnosis of pachyonychia congenita (PC). In pachyonychia, congenital oral leukokeratosis may also be present. Pictures of all of these features would help confirm or refute this potential diagnosis. Three cardinal manifestations of PC are: toenail dystrophy, focal keratoderma, and plantar pain (usually heels). Wedge-shaped subungual hyperkeratosis leading to "omega" nails is characteristic. Other features include steatocystomas (as shown here), angular cheilitis, and natal teeth, among others. PC results from mutations in keratins 6, 16, or 17.

Oral cobblestoning is seen in Cowden disease. Heterochromia iridis is most common in Waardenburg syndrome. Lipoatrophy and aniridia are not features of PC.

Bolognia J, Schaffer J, Cerroni L, eds. *Dermatology*. [Philadelphia]: Elsevier, 2018 (ch. 58).

54. D. Spitz nevus

At low power Spitz nevi have a "raining down pattern," with nests oriented in a vertical fashion along the rete ridges; this is nicely illustrated in this case. Melanocytes within the nests of Spitz nevi are also commonly described as having vertical orientation and are generally large, spindled, and epithelioid in appearance. Hyperkeratosis, hypergranulosis, and pseudoepitheliomatous hyperplasia may be commonly noted on biopsy. Features that reassure the pathologist of a Spitz nevus (and not a melanoma) are the sharp definition of the edge of the lesion laterally, symmetry from left to right, and "maturation" from top to bottom of the lesion. Buckshot scatter can be seen in the center of lesions and is considered okay even in typical Spitz nevi.

A compound nevus would not have this pattern. Congenital nevi have typical features of nevi (symmetric on low power, bland cytology, maturation) but can also aggregate around hair follicles and in nerves and can even be present in and around blood vessel walls or show a single-file interstitial pattern. Melanoma should be asymmetric at low power, lack maturation, and on high power have more cellular pleomorphism, high nuclear:cytoplasmic ratio, prominent nucleoli, and often mitoses. Combined nevi have components of two different nevus types, most commonly banal nevi (i.e., compound or intradermal plus blue nevus).

Bolognia J, Schaffer J, Cerroni L, eds. *Dermatology*. [Philadelphia]: Elsevier, 2018 (ch. 112).

55. **B.** Genetic testing for Fabry disease

The biopsy shows an angiokeratoma. Histologic features include hyperkeratosis and acanthosis associated with ectatic, thin-walled vessels that are in contact with the epidermis (in fact, they often look like they are in the epidermis in angiokeratomas). Patients with Fabry syndrome can have many angiokeratomas or "angiokeratoma corporis diffusum" in which angiokeratomas are often found/accentuated in a bathing trunk distribution. The number of angiokeratomas in Fabry can vary and may be few or numerous.

POEMS syndrome may be suspected in patients developing many cherry hemangiomas and/or glomeruloid hemangioma(s) in the correct clinical context. A diagnosis of glomeruloid hemangioma should always make you think of POEMS syndrome. POEMS is characterized by a *m*onoclonal gammopathy and sensorimotor *p*olyneuropathy, *o*rganomegaly, *e*ndocrinopathy, and *s*kin changes (most commonly diffuse hyperpigmentation, induration, hypertrichosis, and hyperhidrosis). However, the photomicrograph is neither a glomeruloid hemangioma nor cherry angioma. Cherry angiomas typically lack the hyperkeratosis and acanthosis and, rather than dilated thin-walled vessels, show groups of small vessels that are variably dilated and have pink, hyalinized vessel walls.

The photomicrograph does not show Kaposi sarcoma, which would have a vascular proliferation in the dermis. This is not simply a telangiectasia; in ataxia telangiectasia, telangiectasias are most common on the conjunctivae, face, and ears.

Bolognia J, Schaffer J, Cerroni L, eds. *Dermatology*. [Philadelphia]: Elsevier, 2018 (ch. 63).

56. **A.** HIV testing

Bacillary angiomatosis (BA) is shown here. Histologically, BA is a vascular lesion. Pictured in panel (B), which helps establish a diagnosis of BA, is the presence of an amorphous collection (inside oval) of organisms within the vascular lesion. Other clues to the diagnosis of BA are the presence of clusters of neutrophils, which also is a clue to a bacterial infection. BA is usually caused by the Gram-negative bacilli *Bartonella henselae* and *quintana*. Clinically,

lesions present as red to purple "vascular-appearing" papules, nodules, or ulcers. BA usually occurs in HIV+ patients with CD4 counts <100, and checking for HIV is the most appropriate diagnostic test here. BA can also affect the respiratory tract, bones, lymph nodes, and GI tract.

HHV8 is seen in Kaposi sarcoma, not BA. Checking QuantiFERON gold for latent tuberculosis would not be indicated. This is not a T-cell neoplasm, so PCR and flow cytometry are not indicated.

Bolognia J, Schaffer J, Cerroni L, eds. *Dermatology*. [Philadelphia]: Elsevier, 2018 (ch. 74).

57. **B.** Temperature sensitivity elicited with ice cube or ice pack

The biopsy shows a glomus tumor. Glomus tumors most commonly present on the hand, including the nail bed (subungual) and palm. They are typically red to blue papules or plaques that are characteristically tender to touch and may have associated paroxysmal pain in response to temperature changes and/or pressure.

Histologically glomus tumors show well-circumscribed proliferations composed of sheets and/or clusters of uniform glomus cells (as shown in high power in the photomicrograph). Glomus cells are monotonous and they all appear the same. Glomus cells have a characteristic round shape with a central nucleus and pale eosinophilic cytoplasm. There may be a variable number of small vessels; those cases with increased vessel density may be referred to as glomangiomas.

Arborizing vessels are seen in basal cell carcinoma (BCC). The histology seen here is not typical of BCC. Glomus tumors are not typically associated with dilated follicles. Apple jelly color on dermoscopy can be seen in granulomatous disorders. Darier sign, or urtication with gentle stroking, can be seen in mastocytosis but is not a feature of a glomus tumor.

Bolognia J, Schaffer J, Cerroni L, eds. *Dermatology*. [Philadelphia]: Elsevier, 2018 (ch. 114).

58. **A.** Lupus erythematosus

The photomicrograph shows positive CD123 staining. When positive, CD123 staining supports the diagnosis of a connective tissue disease, including lupus erythematosus. CD123 marks plasmacytoid dendritic cells, which are abundant in connective tissue diseases. In order to be positive, CD123 must mark clusters of cells (defined as 20 or more closely associated cells) rather than just scattered individual cells. Large clusters of CD123+ cells are present in this case, easily meeting these criteria.

Although sparse background CD123+ staining may be seen in other disorders (and in normal skin), including those listed, large clusters of CD123+ cells would not be expected in any of these other disorders. Lack of CD123+ staining could support any of the following disorders if the correct histologic features were noted, including a dense infiltrate of pleomorphic blue cells (leukemia cutis), superficial dermal edema and perivascular lymphoid infiltrate (polymorphous light eruption), and nodular and/or diffuse infiltrate of neutrophils with papillary dermal edema (Sweet syndrome).

Bolognia J, Schaffer J, Cerroni L, eds. *Dermatology*. [Philadelphia]: Elsevier, 2018 (ch. 41).

59. **C.** Desmoplastic melanoma

SOX10 is a melanocyte transcription factor present in the nucleus of melanocytic cells and is used to identify lesions of melanocytic origin. When SOX10 staining is positive (as shown), a nuclear pattern is seen. Most desmoplastic melanomas express SOX10, confirming the diagnosis in this case.

Histologically, desmoplastic melanoma can be subtle, where tumor cells may be present singly or in small clusters (as in this case) and often have a fascicular or "spindled" morphology in a background of a dense fibrous stroma (the stroma cannot be appreciated here due to absence of eosin staining). SOX10 nicely highlights the melanoma cells in this case.

The other diagnoses would not be expected to have SOX10 positive cells in the dermis.

Bolognia J, Schaffer J, Cerroni L, eds. *Dermatology.* [Philadelphia]: Elsevier, 2018 (ch. 113).

60. C. Presence or absence of ulceration

The diagnosis is malignant melanoma. According to the American Joint Committee on Cancer, 8th edition (AJCC8) the most recent melanoma staging released in 2017, the most important factor in T staging is the tumor thickness. The other central histologic feature needed for correct T staging with AJCC 8 is presence or absence of histologic (not clinical) ulceration, which is the correct answer. The Clark level (anatomic level of invasion) is no longer used in melanoma staging. Mitotic counts were removed from T staging in AJCC 8. Although the dermatopathologist must also comment on the involvement (or not) of the margins, this consideration is not part of the formal staging criteria. Presence or absence of *BRAF* mutation (one of the most common oncogenic mutations in cutaneous melanoma) is not part of the AJCC staging criteria but is often checked in advanced melanomas, given its therapeutic implications.

Bolognia J, Schaffer J, Cerroni L, eds. *Dermatology.* [Philadelphia]: Elsevier, 2018 (ch. 113).

PROCEDURAL DERMATOLOGY

61. A. Proceed with Mohs surgery without alteration of anticoagulation regimen, as long as the prothrombin time is within the therapeutic range.

Anticoagulant therapy with warfarin or direct oral anticoagulants (apixaban, rivaroxaban, dabigatran) does increase the bleeding risk around Mohs surgery by 2- to10-fold, depending on the study. However, the absolute risk of bleeding complications with these medications remains low (<10%), and the consequences of postoperative bleeding are minor. By contrast, the risk of systemic embolism, while very low, can result in irreversible functional impairment or death. Thus systemic anticoagulants are continued without modification during the vast majority of Mohs procedures, even those involving more complex reconstruction. For patients at even higher bleeding risk (multiple anticoagulants, history of prior bleeding, or with anticipated extensive reconstruction), interruption of anticoagulation may be considered in conjunction with the patient's internist or cardiologist. In cases of warfarin interruption, the medication must be held for 3–5 days prior to surgery to achieve normalization of coagulation parameters and an additional 3–7 days are expected after resumption of therapy before the patient is fully anticoagulated again.

Bolognia J, Schaffer J, Cerroni L, eds. *Dermatology.* [Philadelphia]: Elsevier, 2018 (ch. 151).

62. C. Colonoscopy

This presentation and biopsy are diagnostic of extramammary Paget disease (EMPD). The disease has been associated with simultaneous colon or bladder cancer in an unknown fraction of patients. Although the disease usually presents as an intraepidermal malignancy, colonoscopy and urethral cystoscopy are recommended to rule out colorectal or urothelial carcinoma. In the absence of other symptoms, computed tomography is not required for intraepidermal EMPD. *CDKN2A* mutations are found in melanoma. *MLH1/MSH2* mutations are found in Muir-Torre syndrome.

Bolognia J, Schaffer J, Cerroni L, eds. *Dermatology.* [Philadelphia]: Elsevier, 2018 (ch. 73).

63. E. Temporal nerve

The temporal branch of the facial nerve (cranial nerve VII) passes across the anatomic temple just superficial to the superficial musculoaponeurotic system (SMAS) fascia. Because there is very little subcutaneous adipose in this area, the nerve it at high risk of injury during cutaneous surgery. The temporal nerve supplies motor fibers to the ipsilateral frontalis muscle, and nerve injury results in ipsilateral brow ptosis. The frontal branch of the superficial temporal artery also passes through this area, but due to the presence of numerous collateral vessels, ligation of this artery has minimal effect. The facial artery courses superomedially from the angle of the mandible, across the lower cheek, to the lateral alar base where it becomes the angular artery. The auriculotemporal nerve and supraorbital nerve are sensory branches of cranial nerve V1. The auriculotemporal nerve supplies the skin of the preauricular cheek, superior auricle, and temporal scalp; injury of this nerve in the temple is unlikely. The supraorbital nerve exits the supraorbital foramen and supplies the forehead and frontal scalp over the mid eyebrow.

Bolognia J, Schaffer J, Cerroni L, eds. *Dermatology.* [Philadelphia]: Elsevier, 2018 (ch. 142).

64. C. Ruby

The optimal laser wavelength for removing green tattoo ink is the QS ruby laser (694 nm). QS alexandrite (755 nm) may also fade green ink. Nd:YAG (1064 nm) may be used to remove black, blue, or brown ink. Nd:YAG frequency-doubled (532 nm) may treat brown, yellow, white, red, or violet tattoos. Pulse dye laser (595 nm) treats vascular lesions.

Bolognia J, Schaffer J, Cerroni L, eds. *Dermatology.* [Philadelphia]: Elsevier, 2018 (ch. 137).

65. D. Glycerin

Telangiectatic matting, nests of fine telangiectasia, can occur around veins that have been previously treated with sclerotherapy or surgical intervention. Obesity, pregnancy, estrogen-containing medications are all risk factors. Sodium tetradecyl sulfate, sodium morrhuate, polidocanol, and ethanolamine oleate are all detergents, which have the highest risk of telangiectatic matting. The risk of this complication may be reduced by using an appropriate volume and concentration and using low pressure when injecting as well as discontinuing oral contraceptives prior to treatment. Glycerin has a lower risk of matting, and injection into the matting can be used as a treatment of this complication.

Bolognia J, Schaffer J, Cerroni L, eds. *Dermatology.* [Philadelphia]: Elsevier, 2018 (ch. 155).

66. B. Glabella

Blindness has been reported as a complication from filler injected into every facial cosmetic subunit. Blindness results from retrograde embolization of the filler into the

ocular vessels. Occlusion of the supratrochlear and supra-orbital arteries can lead to occlusion of the central retinal artery. Visual complications may present with immediate unilateral vision loss, ocular pain, headache, nausea, or vomiting. The highest risk site is the glabella, followed by the nasal region, nasolabial fold, and forehead.
Bolognia J, Schaffer J, Cerroni L, eds. *Dermatology.* [Philadelphia]: Elsevier, 2018 (ch. 158).

67. **A.** Cross-linking
The cross-linking of hyaluronic acid (HA) fillers increases durability and allows the filler to be more resistant to degradation. G′ represents the elastic modulus of the filler in response to shear forces. A higher G′ leads to increased resistance to movement, decreased spread after placement, and increased volume support after injection. The viscosity is how well the filler flows. The concentration refers to the concentration of both free HA and cross-linked HA. Understanding the properties of various fillers is important in facial rejuvenation and volumizing procedures.
Bolognia J, Schaffer J, Cerroni L, eds. *Dermatology.* [Philadelphia]: Elsevier, 2018 (ch. 158).

68. **B.** Squamous cell carcinoma
SCC is the most common malignant tumor of the nail unit, including invasive SCC, SCC in situ, and epithelioma cuniculatum (verrucous carcinoma). Complications include metastasis and digital loss. The second most common malignant tumor of the nail is malignant melanoma. Basal cell carcinoma of the nail unit and aggressive digital papillary adenocarcinoma are rare malignant nail tumors. Giant cell tumor of the tendon sheath is a benign tumor that is often treated with surgical excision and may present on the nail unit.
Bolognia J, Schaffer J, Cerroni L, eds. *Dermatology.* [Philadelphia]: Elsevier, 2018 (ch. 71).

69. **D.** Protoporphyrin IX
The prodrug (aminolevulinic acid [ALA] or methyl aminolevulinate [MAL]) enters the cell and is metabolized in the heme synthesis pathway, through the intermediates porphobilinogen, uroporphyrinogen, coproporphyrinogen, protoporphyrinogen IX, and finally protoporphyrin IX. Normally protoporphyrin IX is metabolized by the enzyme ferrochelatase to heme, but the enzyme is overwhelmed by the quantity of ALA/MAL added to the system during PDT. Protoporphyrin IX thus accumulates to high levels and absorbs visible light, generating free radicals and cytotoxicity.
Bolognia J, Schaffer J, Cerroni L, eds. *Dermatology.* [Philadelphia]: Elsevier, 2018 (ch. 135).

70. **C.** Temple and lateral cheek
The Mustarde rotation flap recruits skin and soft tissue from the reservoir of skin laxity on the temple and lateral cheek. This tissue is mobilized via an arcing incision from the lateral canthus superiorly and laterally onto the temple and extending as far as required to the sideburn or preauricular cheek (or occasionally onto the infra-auricular neck). As this large reservoir of skin and soft tissue rotates into place, it can restore vertical height to the lower lid with the primary tension vector in the horizontal direction, preventing downward tension and ectropion of the lower lid.
Bolognia J, Schaffer J, Cerroni L, eds. *Dermatology.* [Philadelphia]: Elsevier, 2018 (ch. 147).

BASIC SCIENCE

71. **B.** Calcium-dependent adhesion molecule
Desmoglein-3 (Dsg-3) is the target of autoantibodies in pemphigus vulgaris. Dsg-3 is a member of the calcium-dependent adhesion (cadherin) family of molecules responsible for keratinocyte-keratinocyte binding. Patched1 (PTCH1) is an example of a G-coupled receptor. BRAF is a member of the MAP kinase signaling pathway and functions as an intracellular signal transduction kinase. The glucocorticoid receptor is a type of nuclear transcription factor, and the epidermal growth factor receptor is a type of receptor tyrosine kinase.
Bolognia J, Schaffer J, Cerroni L, eds. *Dermatology.* [Philadelphia]: Elsevier, 2018 (ch. 28 and 29).

72. **B.** Dedicator of cytokinesis 8 (DOCK8)
DOCK8 deficiency is also known as autosomal recessive hyperimmunoglobulin E syndrome. Similar to autosomal dominant hyperimmunoglobulin E syndrome (Job syndrome), caused by activating mutations in STAT3, DOCK8 deficiency also has elevated levels of IgE, eosinophilia, and dermatitis. However, patients with DOCK8 deficiency do not have craniofacial abnormalities and are more susceptible to viral infections, including human papillomavirus, molluscum contagiosum, and herpes virus (herpes simplex infection is shown). Deficiency of interleukin-1 receptor antagonist (DIRA) presents with pustular eruption in infancy. Defects in transglutaminase (TGM1) results in lamellar ichthyosis. CDKN2A loss is associated with familial melanoma.
Bolognia J, Schaffer J, Cerroni L, eds. *Dermatology.* [Philadelphia]: Elsevier, 2018 (ch. 60).

73. **D.** Cross-linked proteins
Corneocytes are terminally differentiated keratinocytes that lack nuclei and organelles. They contain a specialized cornified envelope composed of cross-linked proteins, such as loricrin, involucrin, envoplakin, and periplakin that is highly insoluble. Lamellar bodies are organelles within the stratum granulosum composed of lipids that extrude their contents to form the intercellular lipids within the stratum corneum.
Bolognia J, Schaffer J, Cerroni L, eds. *Dermatology.* [Philadelphia]: Elsevier, 2018 (ch. 56).

74. **B.** Inhibit tumor suppressors
Human papillomavirus proteins E6 and E7 inhibit tumor suppressors p53 and Rb, respectively. Therefore E6 and E7 are viral oncogenes. HPV does not cause cell lysis of keratinocytes. High-risk HPV subtypes (e.g., 16, 18) are associated with the development of squamous cell carcinoma.
Bolognia J, Schaffer J, Cerroni L, eds. *Dermatology.* [Philadelphia]: Elsevier, 2018 (ch. 79).

75. **A.** Cleaves SNAP-25 protein
OnabotulinumtoxinA (Botox) is a type A botulinum toxin that cleaves SNAP-25 on presynaptic neurons, preventing fusion and exocytosis of synaptic vesicles carrying acetylcholine. All types of botulinum toxin cleave members of the SNARE protein family, including SNAP-25, syntaxin, and VAMP/synaptobrevin, which prevents fusion of exocytic vesicles with the presynaptic neuronal membrane. Thus, acetylcholine is not released into the synaptic cleft and is unavailable to bind to acetylcholine receptors on postsynaptic cells.
Bolognia J, Schaffer J, Cerroni L, eds. *Dermatology.* [Philadelphia]: Elsevier, 2018 (ch. 159).

76. D. Urticaria pigmentosa
Urticaria is caused by activation of mast cells and basophils by allergens, resulting in release of histamine, prostaglandins, and leukotrienes. Urticaria pigmentosa is a form cutaneous mastocytosis or collection of mast cells in the skin. Lupus pernio is a clinical presentation of sarcoidosis (granulomatous disorder of macrophages). Mycosis fungoides is a variant of cutaneous T-cell lymphoma. Eosinophilic fasciitis is an autoimmune disease of mixed inflammatory cells and with eosinophilic infiltration of fascia.
Bolognia J, Schaffer J, Cerroni L, eds. *Dermatology*. [Philadelphia]: Elsevier, 2018 (ch. 18).

77. B. Present peptides to T cells
The gene complex most highly associated with psoriasis is HLA-Cw6. Human leukocyte antigens (HLA) are part of the major histocompatibility complex (MHC) that presents peptides to T cells. The T-cell receptor (TCR) recognizes peptides bound to MHC. T cells stimulate B cells to produce antibodies by a number of cytokines (choice A); Toll-like receptors (TLRs) are the classical type of pattern recognition receptors expressed on many immune and nonimmune cells that detect conserved motifs on bacteria, viruses, and fungi (choice C); antigen-processing pathway shuttles proteins into lysosomes for protein degradation that can then be loaded onto MHC class molecules for antigen presentation (choice D); many cells and cytokines can promote self-tolerance, such as regulatory T cells (choice E).
Bolognia J, Schaffer J, Cerroni L, eds. *Dermatology*. [Philadelphia]: Elsevier, 2018 (chs. 4 and 8).

78. D. Enhanced secondary response
Adaptive immunity is most notably distinguished from the innate immune system due to immunological memory, where the second immune response to the same antigen is more robust. Both innate and adaptive immune components can recognize pathogens, produce cytokines, eliminate pathogens, and stimulate other cells of the immune system.
Bolognia J, Schaffer J, Cerroni L, eds. *Dermatology*. [Philadelphia]: Elsevier, 2018 (ch. 4).

79. D. Binds to circulating IgE
Omalizumab is a monoclonal antibody that binds circulating IgE to prevent binding of IgE to the high-affinity IgE receptor on mast cells, basophils, and dendritic cells. Mepolizumab is a novel monoclonal antibody directed against IL-5, which is crucial for eosinophilic differentiation, and is used in the treatment of various eosinophilic disorders such as asthma and eosinophilic granulomatosis with polyangiitis. NSAIDs may inhibit cyclooxygenase. Cromolyn sodium is an example of a mast cell stabilizer.
Bolognia J, Schaffer J, Cerroni L, eds. *Dermatology*. [Philadelphia]: Elsevier, 2018 (chs. 18 and 128).

80. E. Epidermis
The rash shown is scabies, which presents with intensely pruritic papules and burrows. Scabies is caused by epidermal invasion of the mite *Sarcoptes scabiei var. hominis*, which lives its entire life within the epidermis.
Bolognia J, Schaffer J, Cerroni L, eds. *Dermatology*. [Philadelphia]: Elsevier, 2018 (ch. 84).

GENERAL DERMATOLOGY

1. A 73-year-old is started on an antibiotic for upper respiratory tract infection. He develops a symmetric pruritic rash localized to the axillae and anogenital skin. What is the most common drug culprit?

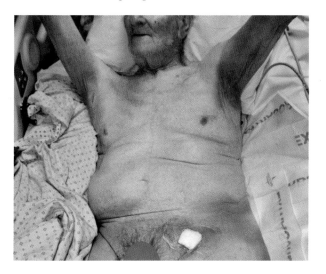

   A. Amoxicillin
   B. Trimethoprim-sulfamethoxazole
   C. Doxycycline
   D. Azithromycin

2. A 32-year-old female presents to the emergency department with a painful eruption in the groin as pictured. She has no other mucosal lesions or cutaneous findings. She recalls having a similar eruption 3 years prior after taking the same medication that she took last night. Which agent is LEAST likely to be responsible for her eruption?

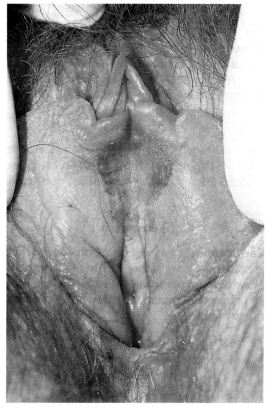

With permission from Edwards L, *Obstetric and Gynecologic Dermatology*, 2008, Elsevier, 217–239 (fig. 20.20).

   A. Pseudoephedrine
   B. Oral contraceptive
   C. Ibuprofen
   D. Acetaminophen

3. A 57-year-old male with history of epilepsy develops the following eruption 4 weeks after initiation of carbamazepine. The patient has associated fever and cervical lymphadenopathy, as well as peripheral eosinophilia of 18%. You

diagnose his underlying eruption and tell his primary team to stop carbamazepine. What is the most likely other organ system to be affected?

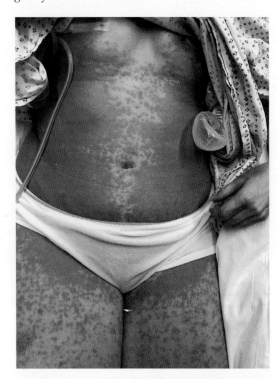

A. Thyroid
B. Liver
C. Heart
D. Kidney

4. A primiparous 27-year-old pregnant female develops the following pruritic eruption at 36-weeks gestation. What is the associated risk to the fetus?

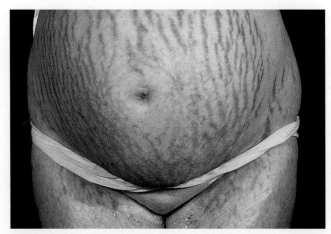

With permission from Ambros-Rudolph CM, in *Obstetric and Gynecologic Dermatology*, 2008, Elsevier, chapter 6, 49–55.

A. Stillbirth
B. Fetal distress
C. Intrauterine growth restriction
D. No effect on the fetus

5. A 69-year-old male presents to your clinic for a full body skin exam. He states that he has noticed mild itching and a rash on his scrotum. The findings are pictured. You recommend all the following EXCEPT:

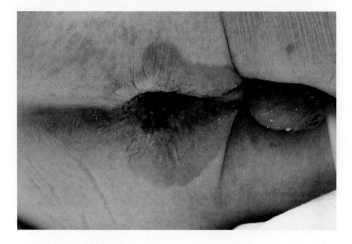

A. Chest x-ray
B. Colonoscopy
C. Cystoscopy
D. Prostate examination

6. An 85-year-old female presents with increased fatigue, weight loss, and the cutaneous findings shown below. What is your diagnosis?

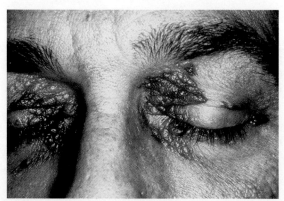

With permission from Fitzpatrick JE, in *Dermatology Secrets Plus*, 2016, Elsevier, 141–148 (fig. 16-2)

A. Sarcoidosis
B. Xanthelasma
C. Primary systemic amyloidosis
D. Nodular amyloidosis

7. What is the diagnosis?

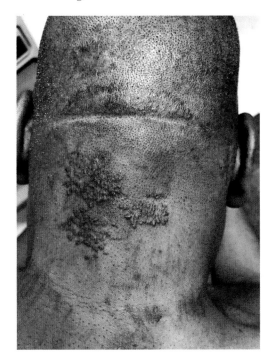

A. Acne keloidalis nuchae
B. Sarcoidosis
C. Elastosis perforans serpiginosa
D. Granuloma annulare
E. Disseminate and recurrent infundibulofolliculitis

8. What is the diagnosis?

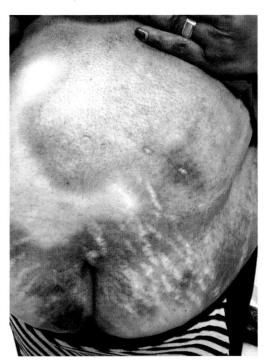

A. Morphea
B. Erythema chronicum migrans
C. Calciphylaxis
D. Nephrogenic systemic fibrosis

9. The patient has this recurrent eruption not responsive to antibiotics. He gives a history of monthly mouth ulcers, fevers, and painful nodules on his lower legs. Which listed systemic manifestations is most likely?

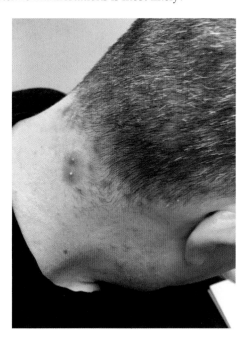

A. Pulmonary fibrosis
B. Photosensitivity
C. Hyperostosis
D. Pulmonary artery aneurysm

10. Which of the following would NOT be present on dermoscopy?

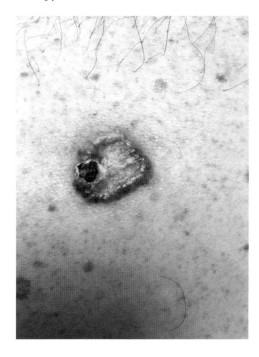

A. Leaflike structures and spoke-wheel areas
B. Blue-gray ovoid nests and globules
C. Pigment network
D. Arborizing vessels

11. What is the best next step? Select all that apply.

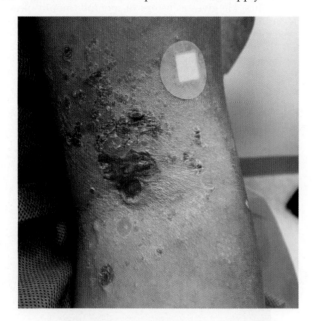

A. Oral cephalexin
B. Bacterial culture
C. Valacyclovir
D. Topical steroids

12. What is the cause of the following eruption?

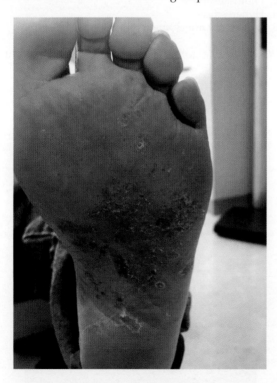

A. Fungal infection
B. Bacterial infection
C. Gene mutation
D. Medication

13. A 17-year-old man presents 2 weeks after starting 0.5mg/kg isotretinoin with worsening acne and the following examination. Which of the following recommendations are indicated (select all that apply)?

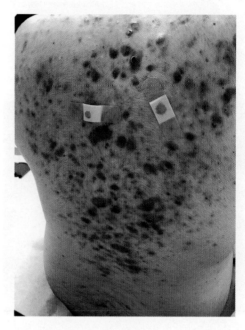

A. Initiate oral corticosteroids
B. Hold isotretinoin
C. Increase isotretinoin to 1 mg/kg
D. Discontinue anabolic steroid supplements
E. Bacterial culture
F. Referral for radiation therapy

14. Which medication can cause this eruption?

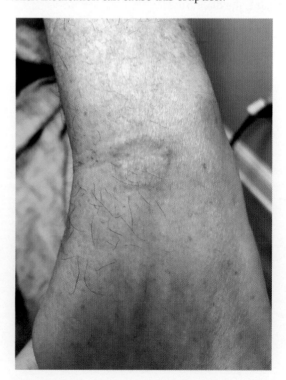

A. Adalimumab
B. Furosemide
C. Lisinopril
D. Terbinafine

15. A 71-year-old woman presents with this CK20 positive/ TTF-1 negative, rapidly growing tumor on her right shin. Physical exam reveals a 2.3 cm ulcerated red nodule. Negative expression of which of the following is associated with more aggressive tumor behavior?

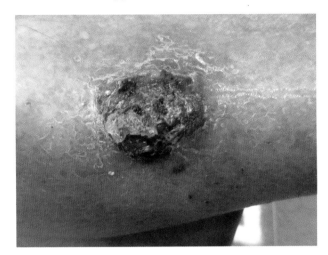

A. p63
B. S100
C. Polyomavirus
D. CK7

16. A 21-year-old man presents with this eruption for 6 years. The distribution includes the face, chest, axilla, lower legs (seen here), and feet. His father has similar papules. Which of the following is NOT associated with this condition?

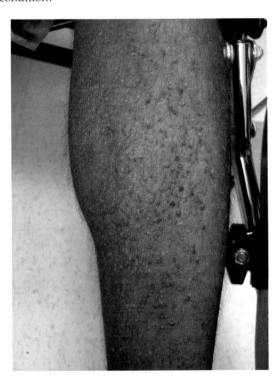

A. Spiked focal keratoderma
B. White papules on the hard palate
C. Salivary gland obstruction
D. Macrocephaly

17. Which of the following herbal supplements is associated with an increased risk of bleeding?
A. Ginseng
B. Goldenseal
C. Ginkgo
D. *Glycyrrhiza glabra*

18. A 67-year-old man receiving chemotherapy for acute myelogenous leukemia develops this eruption. Treatment with valacyclovir is initiated. What treatment-associated complication is he at increased risk for?

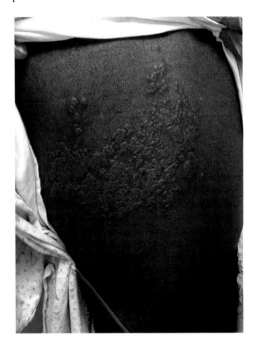

A. Thrombotic thrombocytopenic purpura
B. Liver failure
C. Dissemination of infection
D. Acute respiratory distress syndrome

19. What is the most likely diagnosis?

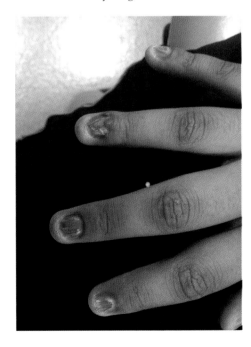

A. Systemic sclerosis
B. Psoriasis
C. Lichen planus
D. Onychomycosis

20. A 43-year-old woman undergoes patch testing for persistent allergic contact dermatitis on her face and neck. Patch testing reveals a positive reaction to balsam of Peru. Allergy to which spice can be observed in patients with allergy to balsam of Peru?
    A. Nutmeg
    B. Cloves
    C. Turmeric
    D. Cardamom

21. A 46-year-old woman reports sudden onset of multiple lesions occurring on the arms, legs, and buttocks. This clinical presentation has been associated with which of the following?

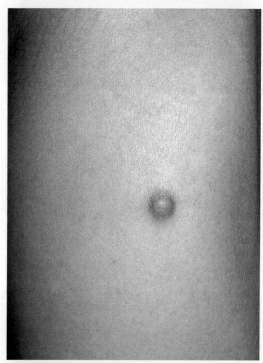

With permission from Huang P-Y, Chu C-Y, Hsiao C-H, *Journal of the American Academy of Dermatology*, 2007, Elsevier.

A. Systemic lupus erythematosus
B. Hematologic malignancy
C. HIV
D. Pregnancy
E. All of the above

22. Which of the following statements regarding this condition is FALSE?

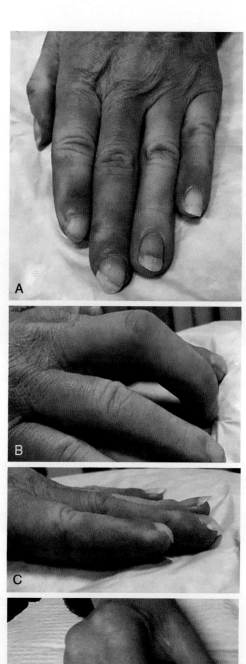

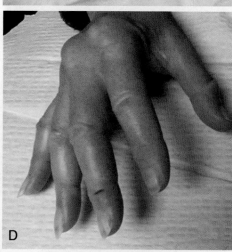

With permission from Pearson DR, Werth VP, Pappas-Taffer L, *Clinics in Dermatology*, 2018, volume 36, issue 4, 459–474.

A. Pulmonary arterial hypertension is more common in patients with limited cutaneous systemic sclerosis than in patients with diffuse cutaneous systemic sclerosis.

B. Anticentromere antibody is more commonly seen in patients with limited cutaneous systemic sclerosis than in patients with diffuse cutaneous systemic sclerosis.

C. Tendon friction rubs are more commonly seen in patients with limited cutaneous systemic sclerosis than in patients with diffuse cutaneous systemic sclerosis.

D. Anti-RNA polymerase III antibody is more common in patients with diffuse cutaneous systemic sclerosis than in patients with limited cutaneous systemic sclerosis.

E. Antitopoisomerase I (Scl-70) antibody is more commonly seen in patients with diffuse cutaneous systemic sclerosis than in patients with limited cutaneous systemic sclerosis.

23. A 34-year-old woman with the following skin finding was started on hydroxychloroquine. Which of the following medications does NOT have a potential interaction with hydroxychloroquine?

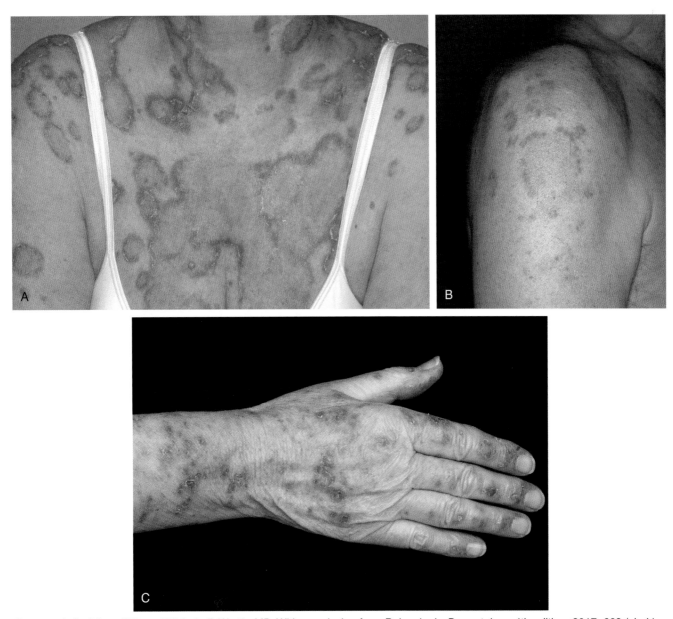

Courtesy Lela A Lee, MD, and Victoria P. Werth, MD. With permission from Bolognia, in *Dermatology*, 4th edition, 2017, 668 (ch 41, fig. 41-8). Courtesy Lorenzo Cerroni, MD. With permission from Bolognia, in *Dermatology*, 4th edition, 2017, 668 (ch 41, fig. 41-8).

A. Ziprasidone
B. Tamoxifen
C. Digoxin
D. Atenolol
E. Amiodarone

24. A sheepherder presents with the following solitary lesion. He reports mild fever and malaise. This condition is most likely caused by which of the following?

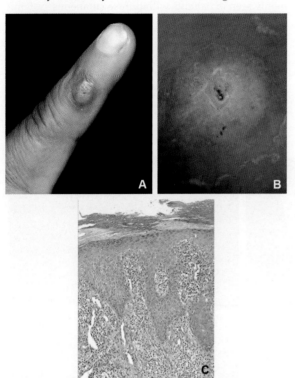

With permission from Chavez-Alvarez S, Barbosa-Moreno L, et al. *J Am Acad Dermatol*. 2016 May;74(5):e95–e96.

  A. Herpesvirus
  B. Parapoxvirus
  C. Gram-positive spore-forming rod
  D. Paramyxovirus
  E. Papovavirus

25. A patient develops the following eruption starting on the axillae and face. Which of the following medication was the patient most likely started on several days prior?

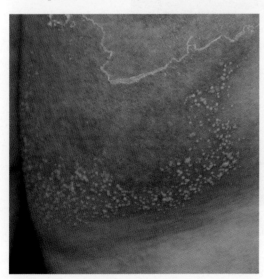

Courtesy Giuseppe Micali, Department of Dermatology, University of Catania, Italy.

  A. Ciprofloxacin
  B. Trimethoprim/sulfamethoxazole
  C. Penicillin
  D. Hydralazine
  E. Allopurinol

26. All of the following medications have been associated with this condition EXCEPT:

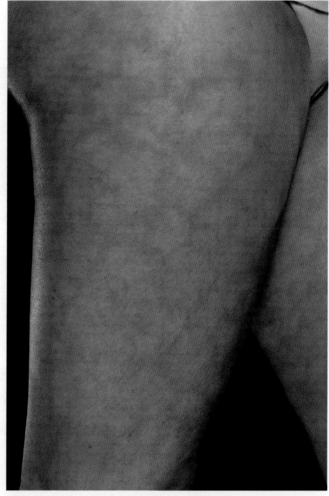

With permission from Katugampola RP, Finlay AY, *Treatment of Skin Disease: Comprehensive Therapeutic Strategies*, Elsevier, 2018, 457–459.

  A. Amantadine
  B. Quinidine
  C. Minocycline
  D. Trimethoprim/sulfamethoxazole

27. Which of the following organisms is most commonly responsible for this finding in the axilla?

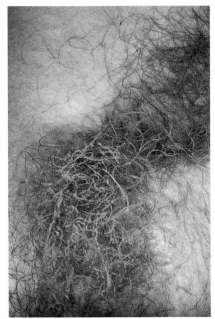

With permission from Habif TP, in Hair diseases, *Clinical Dermatology*, 2016, Elsevier, 923–959 (fig. 24-37).

A. *Piedraia hortae*
B. *Corynebacterium tenuis*
C. *Kytococcus sedentarius*
D. *Trichosporon asahii*
E. *Corynebacterium minutissimum*

28. A middle-aged male developed these lesions on his feet after returning from a trip to the Amazon rainforest, where he admits to walking barefoot. What is the causative agent?

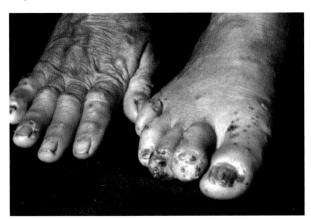

With permission from Cestari TF, Pessato S, *Clinics in Dermatology*, 2007, volume 25, issue 2, 158–164.

A. *Dermatobia hominis*
B. *Cordylobia anthropophaga*
C. *Cochliomyia hominivorax*
D. *Ancylostoma braziliense*
E. *Tunga penetrans*

29. Which of the following medications is most likely to have been associated with the onset of this condition?

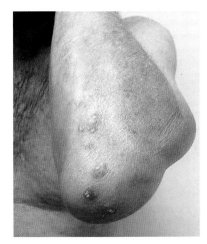

Courtesy Robert Micheletti, MD.

A. Montelukast
B. Hydralazine
C. Minocycline
D. Penicillamine
E. Leflunomide

30. A 20-year-old man presents with this finding. Biopsy demonstrates pseudoepitheliomatous hyperplasia; suppurative and granulomatous inflammation; and round yeast forms with broad-based budding and thick, double-contoured walls. Which other organ is most likely to be involved?

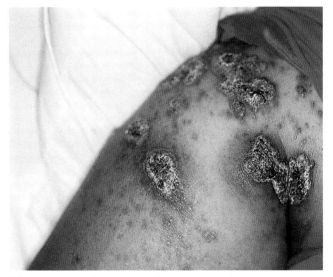

With permission from Norton SA, *Dermatological Signs of Systemic Disease*, 2017, Elsevier, 277–284.

A. Liver
B. Lymphatic system
C. Heart
D. Lungs
E. Kidneys

31. A 60-year-old male presents with weight gain, constipation, bradycardia, fatigue, and cold intolerance. All of the following cutaneous findings are associated with this condition EXCEPT:

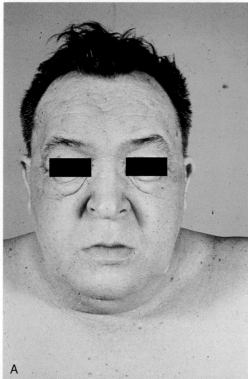

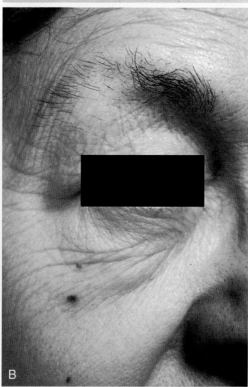

With permission from Ferri FF, *Ferri's Clinical Advisor 2019*, 2019, Elsevier, 761–762.e2.

A. Madarosis
B. Yellowish discoloration of the skin
C. Palmoplantar keratoderma
D. Trichomegaly
E. All of the above can occur in association with this condition

32. This finding is most commonly associated with which of the following?

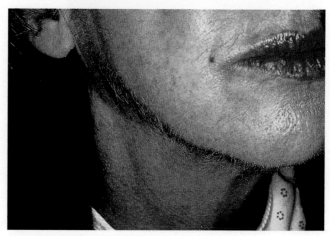

With permission from Antonovich DD, Thiers BH, Callen JP, *Cancer of the Skin*, 2011, Elsevier.

A. Myeloma
B. Breast cancer
C. Lung carcinoma
D. Melanoma

33. This finding is most likely associated with what other condition?

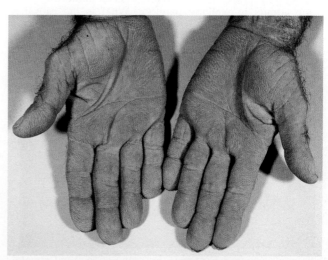

With permission from Cowen EW, Callen JP, *Dermatological Signs of Systemic Disease*, 2017, Elsevier, 131–140.

A. Cutaneous squamous cell carcinoma
B. Lung carcinoma
C. Melanoma
D. Hepatic carcinoma
E. Pancreatic carcinoma

34. This patient presents with fevers, headache, ocular pain, myalgias, arthralgias, nausea, bleeding gums, and bloody stool. Which of the following is the likely vector for this condition?

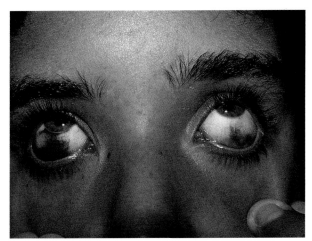

With permission from Lupi O, Mosquito-borne hemorrhagic fevers, in *Dermatologic Clinics*, volume 29, issue 1, 2011, 33–38.

A. *Phlebotomus papatasii*
B. Culex mosquito
C. *Aedes aegypti*
D. *Lutzomyia verrucosum*
E. *Xenopsylla cheopis*

35. A 20-year-old man presents with a penile erosion that is nontender and has been present for 18 days. Nontender bilateral inguinal lymphadenopathy is also noted. What is the most likely diagnosis?

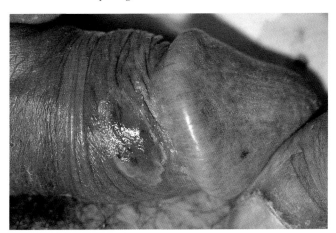

With permission from James WD, Berger TG, Elston DM, *Andrews' Diseases of the Skin,* 2016, Elsevier, 343–358.e3.

A. Primary syphilis
B. Chancroid
C. Herpes simplex
D. Lymphogranuloma venereum
E. HIV

36. A patient presents with painful vesicles in a dermatomal distribution on the forehead and on the tip of his nose. She is diagnosed with ophthalmic zoster by the ophthalmologist. Which nerve branch is involved?

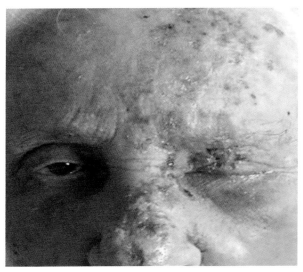

With permission from Vij A, Bergfeld WF, *Clinics in Dermatology*, 2015, volume 33, issue 2, 217–226.

A. Ophthalmic
B. Mandibular
C. Infraorbital
D. Zygomatic
E. Temporal

37. This condition is associated with which of the following human papilloma virus types?

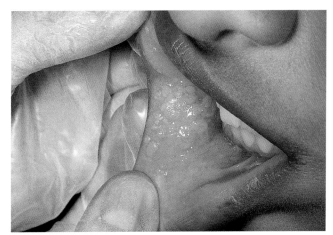

With permission from Paller AS, Mancini AJ, *Hurwitz Clinical Pediatric Dermatology*, 2016, Elsevier, 360–381.e3.

A. 3
B. 4
C. 7
D. 10
E. 13

38. An HIV-positive man presents with these lesions on the face, back, and hands. The virus responsible for these lesions is also implicated in what other condition?

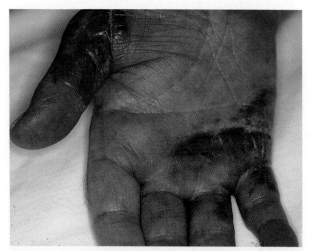

With permission from Schwartz RA, Micali G, Nasca MR, and Scuderi L, in Kaposi sarcoma: A continuing conundrum, *Journal of the American Academy of Dermatology*, 2008, 59(2):179–206.

A. Pityriasis rosea
B. Angiosarcoma
C. Primary effusion lymphoma
D. Bacillary angiomatosis
E. Pyogenic granuloma

39. Which of the following conditions is most likely associated with this cutaneous finding?

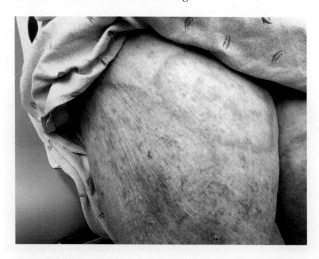

A. Hypertension
B. Ulcerative colitis
C. Congestive heart failure
D. Diabetes

40. This patient with a pruritic eruption on the face was found on patch testing to have a significant allergic reaction to formaldehyde and quaternium-15. Which of the following foods is most likely to cause systemic contact dermatitis in this patient?

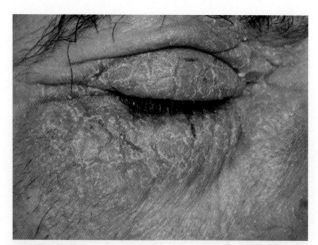

With permission from González-Muñoz P, Conde-Salazar L, Vañó-Galván S, Allergic contact dermatitis caused by cosmetic products, in *Dermatology* (*Actas Dermo-Sifiliográficas*, English Edition), 2014, volume 105, issue 9, 822–832.

A. Prunes
B. Mangos
C. Artificially sweetened, low-calorie drinks
D. Strawberries
E. Cheese

PEDIATRIC DERMATOLOGY

41. Which of the following is most likely to be a complication of the rash shown?

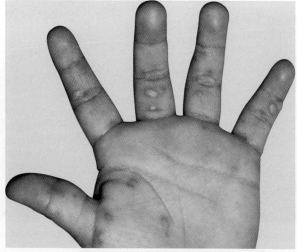

With permission from Kollipara R, *Dermatological Signs of Systemic Disease*, 2017, chapter 31, 262–270.

A. Hypothyroidism
B. Subacute sclerosing panencephalitis
C. Onychomadesis
D. Herpes simplex encephalitis
E. Aplastic anemia

42. The most appropriate step for management of this otherwise healthy infant is:

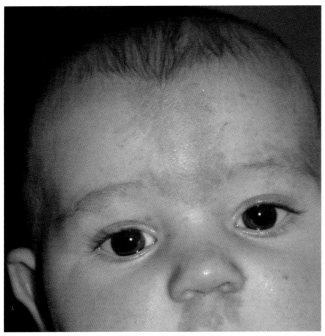

With permission from James WD, *Andrews' Diseases of the Skin Clinical Atlas*, 2018, Elsevier, chapter 28, 405–435.

A. Magnetic resonance imaging with gadolinium
B. Ophthalmology referral
C. Laryngoscopy
D. Pulsed dye laser
E. Reassurance

43. This child, whose mother is similarly affected, is most likely at increased risk for which of the following?

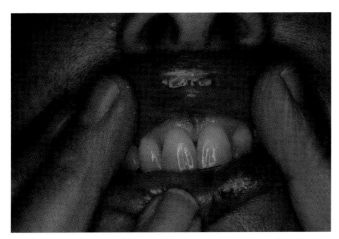

With permission Bhate C, *Treatment of Skin Disease: Comprehensive Therapeutic Strategies*, 2018, Elsevier, chapter 188, 621–623. All rights reserved.

A. Pulmonic stenosis
B. Gastrointestinal polyps
C. Electrocardiogram defects
D. Multiple skin cancers
E. Deafness

44. A healthy 11-year-old female presents with an abrupt onset of this rash. What laboratory value is most likely to be elevated?

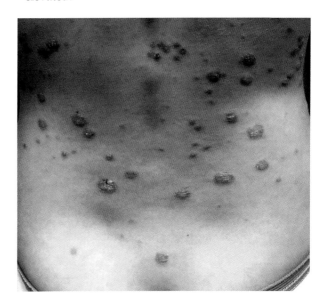

A. Anti-DNase B
B. Atypical lymphocyte count
C. Antihistone antibody
D. Aldolase
E. Anti-dsDNA

45. A 14-year-old girl with corneal scarring, microstomia, joint contractures, and the below skin findings is at the highest risk of mortality from which of the following?

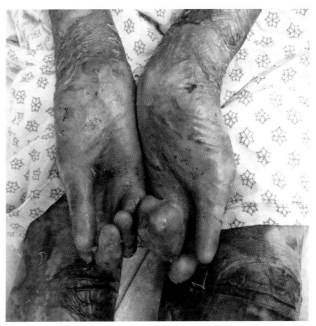

With permission from James WD, *Andrews' Diseases of the Skin Clinical Atlas*, 2018, Elsevier, chapter 27, 379–404.

A. Metastatic squamous cell carcinoma
B. Chronic renal failure
C. Bacterial sepsis
D. Dilated cardiomyopathy

46. A 9-year-old girl presents to you for multiple subcutaneous nodules of the head, neck, and trunk. Excision of five nodules was performed, and histopathology of four of the nodules revealed cysts containing laminated keratin with a cyst wall composed of stratified squamous epithelium, including a granular layer. Histopathologic examination of the fifth nodule showed a similar cyst that also contained basophilic and shadow cells. The mother volunteers that a recent x-ray revealed a mandibular osteoma. What additional finding is most likely present in this patient?
A. Sebaceous adenoma
B. Trichilemmomas
C. Bifid ribs
D. Congenital hypertrophy of the retinal pigment epithelium
E. Multiple oral papillomas

47. An otherwise healthy 13-year-old girl presents with a 6-month history of the skin lesion shown. Which two of the following are the most appropriate next steps?

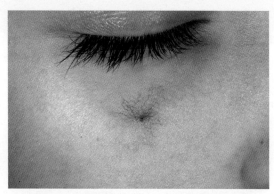

With permission from Habif TP, *Clinical Dermatology*, 2016, Elsevier, chapter 23, 901–922.

A. Transthoracic contrast echocardiography
B. Reassurance
C. MRI of the brain
D. Pregnancy test
E. Liver ultrasound
F. Discussion of pulsed dye laser therapy
G. Complete blood count
H. Liver function tests

48. The boy pictured may also have which of the following?

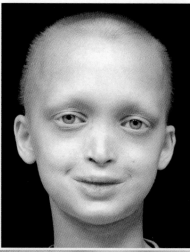

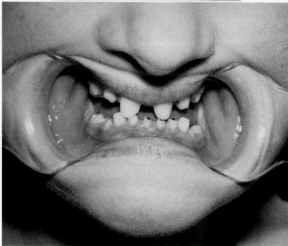

Courtesy Scott Bartlett, MD.

A. Premature atherosclerosis
B. Short, thickened fingernails
C. Recurrent fevers during infancy
D. Angiokeratoma corporis diffusum

49. This child was born with normal-appearing hair at birth but now has the clinical and microscopic hair findings shown. These abnormalities are most likely to be associated with which of the following?

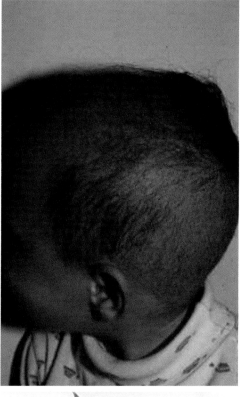

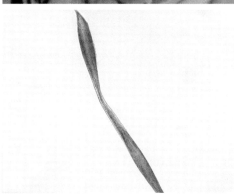

With permission from Cheng AS, Bayliss S. The genetics of hair shaft disorders, in *Journal of the American Academy of Dermatology*, 2008, volume 59, issue 1, 1–22.

A. Traumatic heat styling
B. Basal cell carcinomas
C. Mental retardation and diffuse hypopigmentation
D. Ichthyosis linearis circumflexa and severe atopy
E. Perifollicular erythema and follicular hyperkeratosis

50. A 7-month-old girl presents with this eruption involving the diaper area. The remainder of her skin is clear. She is otherwise healthy and meeting her developmental milestones. What is the most appropriate management?

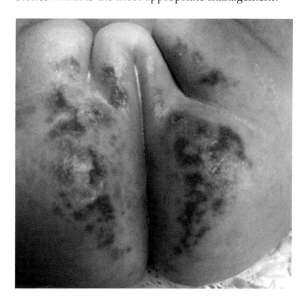

A. Refer to Child Protective Services for evaluation for possible child abuse
B. Skin biopsy
C. Check zinc levels
D. Start low-potency topical corticosteroid plus barrier cream
E. Begin amoxicillin

DERMATOPATHOLOGY

51. A 56-year-old man comes in for a pruritic skin eruption. A biopsy is performed and shown below. Based on this diagnosis, targeting which cytokine(s) would offer a reasonable treatment strategy for this patient?

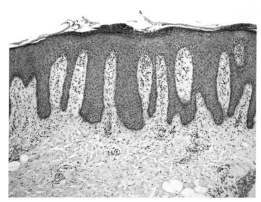

With permission from Ghoreschi, et al., in *Clinics in Dermatology*, 2007, volume 25 (fig. 1, p. 575).

A. IL-31
B. IL-23 and/or IL-27
C. IL-23
D. IL-4 and/or IL-13
E. IL-4

52. A 64-year-old man presents with hypertrichosis of the cheeks, sclerodermoid plaques on the chest, and vesicles and erosions on the dorsal hands. A biopsy is performed and the results are shown. A direct immunofluorescence of perilesional skin is negative. Which of the following laboratory tests would be most important in evaluating a potential underlying etiology of the skin lesions?

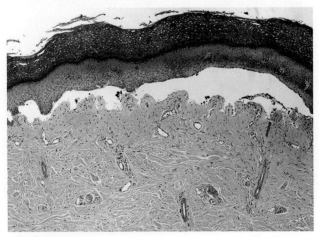

With permission from Trofymenko, et al., *Clinical Gastroenterology and Hepatology*, 2017, volume 15 (fig. 1, p. A37).

A. Serum protein electrophoresis (SPEP) with IFE
B. Serum collagen VII antibodies
C. Serum ferritin level
D. Serum ceruloplasmin level
E. Serum BP180 and BP230 antibodies

53. A 1-year-old male presents with a widespread eruption of salmon-colored papules and plaques with scale and islands of sparing. Upon closer inspection there is follicular prominence, a waxy palmoplantar keratoderma, and prominent facial involvement. A biopsy is performed to help confirm the suspected diagnosis. Based on the biopsy findings and the clinical presentation, exome sequencing is ordered. The genomics lab should be directed to prioritize evaluation of which of the following genes?

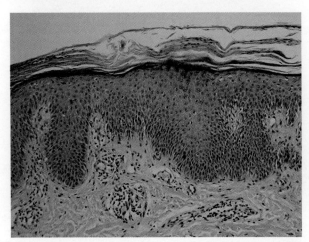

With permission from Muller et al., *J Am Acad Dermatol*, 2008, volume 59 (fig. 2, p. S66).

A. Keratin 10
B. *ABCA12*
C. *STS*
D. *CARD14*
E. HLA-B27

54. A 50-year-old man with metastatic melanoma is started on vemurafenib. Three months later the patient notes the development of multiple keratotic papules on his back, shoulder, and upper arms. The largest lesion is biopsied and the result is shown. The development of these lesions are largely reduced with the addition of which medication?

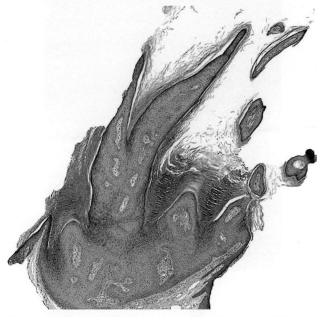

With permission from Ko, et al., *J Am Acad Dermatol*, 2013, volume 69 (fig. 2, p. e96).

A. Urea 40% cream
B. Trametinib
C. Acitretin
D. Nicotinamide
E. 5-Fluorocuracil cream

55. A 30-year-old patient with no prior medical history comes in for a total body skin examination. He states that his father recently died from mesothelioma at age 50, prompting the patient to "get everything checked out," including his skin. The patient has approximately 30 scattered nevi, 6 of which are pink, dome-shaped papules, as pictured.

This representative lesion is biopsied, and the biopsy findings are shown. Special stains confirm the cells to be of melanocytic origin. In this case, the astute dermatologist would suspect the following diagnosis and refer the patient to the following specialist for further evaluation:

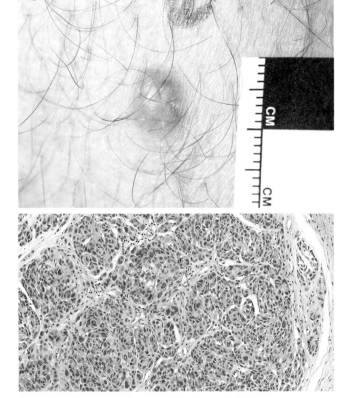

With permission from Clarke and Merchant, *Diagnostic Histopathology*, 2018, volume 24, 338–340.

A. BAP1 syndrome—ophthalmology
B. Familial atypical multiple mole melanoma syndrome—gastroenterology
C. Peutz-Jeghers—gastroenterology
D. Carney complex—cardiology
E. Cutaneous mosaic disorder—no referral required

56. A 1-centimeter plaque is biopsied from the arm of a 56-year-old woman. The dermatopathologist suspects a diagnosis of Merkel cell carcinoma and orders an immunostain to confirm the diagnosis. The results of the immunostain are shown. Based on the staining pattern and the suspected diagnosis, what stain did the dermatopathologist order?

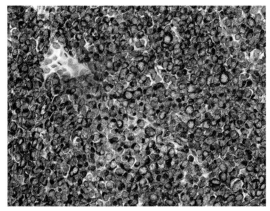

With permission from Daoud, et al., *Seminars in Diagnostic Pathology*, 2013, volume 30, 234–244.

A. Polyoma virus
B. CK20
C. CD20
D. INSM1
E. CD30

57. A 35-year-old male presents with a ulcerated plaque on the penis. A biopsy is obtained and the following pattern is noted. The correct diagnosis is:

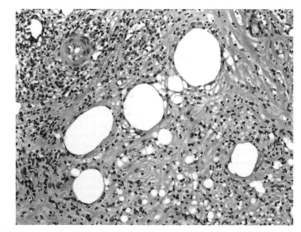

With permission from Gomez-Armayones, et al., *Dermatology (Actas Dermo-Sifilograficas)*, 2014, volume 105 (fig. 3, p. 598).

A. Chancroid
B. Herpes simplex virus
C. Invasive squamous cell carcinoma
D. Syphilitic chancre
E. Paraffinoma

58. A 79-year-old man with a history of multiple basal cell and squamous cell carcinomas presents with an 1.2-cm brown patch on his left cheek. The man is reluctant to have another biopsy performed, and so the dermatologist decides to perform clinical confocal microscopy (see image). The dermatologist is worried about lentigo maligna based on which of the following features demonstrated on confocal microscopy?

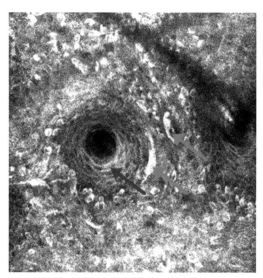

With permission from Star et al., *Dermatologic Clinics*, 2016, volume 34 (fig. 5, p.424).

A. Pagetoid spread of atypical cells
B. Microscopic ulceration
C. Obliteration of adnexal structures
D. Large dendritic-shaped cells around a hair follicle
E. Perineural invasion by large dendritic melanocytes

59. A 6-year-old female presents with papules on the buttocks and lower legs. A biopsy is performed and shows the following pattern (see figure). Presuming a complete history and physical examination have already been performed, which two tests are most urgent?

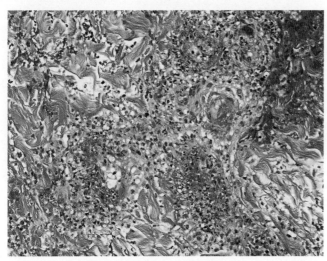

Courtesy David F Fiorentino, MD.

A. Urinalysis and stool guaiac
B. Liver function tests and creatinine
C. Serum complement levels and complete blood count
D. Antinuclear antibody (ANA) and erythrocyte sedimentation rate (ESR)
E. Creatinine and pulmonary function tests

60. A 36-year-old man presents with a few papules and a 1-cm plaque. A biopsy is performed and shows the following pattern. Based on the diagnosis, what lab test should be ordered by the clinician?

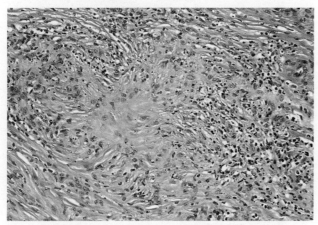

With permission from Brinster NK, in *Dermatopathology: High-Yield Pathology*, 2011, Elsevier, 139 (fig. 3).

A. *TSC1* and *TSC2* genetic testing
B. Urinalysis
C. T-cell receptor (TCR) gene rearrangement testing
D. SPEP and IFE
E. *PTEN* and *AKT* genetic testing

PROCEDURAL DERMATOLOGY

61. Which of the following is not a component of a Jessner's peel?
A. Resorcinol
B. Ethanol
C. Lactic acid
D. Glycolic acid
E. Salicylic acid

62. When repairing these defects from a Mohs surgery removal of one SCC and one BCC, in what tissue plane should undermining be performed?

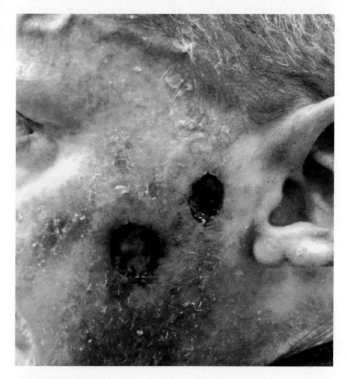

A. Deep reticular dermis
B. Junction of dermis and subcutaneous adipose
C. Deep subcutaneous adipose superficial to the fascia
D. Submuscular/fascial plane
E. Deep to fascia overlying periosteum

63. A 60-year-old man presents with the squamous cell carcinoma shown in the photo. Mohs surgery is performed and perineural invasion is noted within a large nerve tracking inferiorly from the tumor. Clear margins are not obtained, and the patient is referred to otolaryngology for continuing excision of the tumor. Which of the following is the potential course of perineural extension of this tumor?

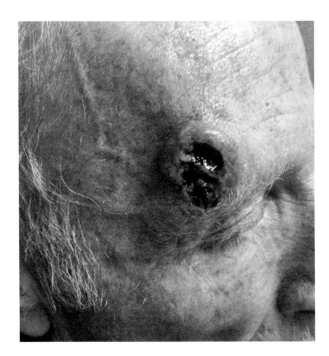

A. Supraorbital nerve tracking to facial nerve and geniculate ganglion
B. Supraorbital nerve tracking to ophthalmic nerve and trigeminal ganglion
C. Supratrochlear nerve tracking to ophthalmic nerve and trigeminal ganglion
D. Temporal nerve tracking to facial nerve and geniculate ganglion
E. Temporal nerve tracking to ophthalmic nerve and trigeminal ganglion

64. A 58-year-old man presents with this lesion on the trunk (dermoscopy pictured). A biopsy confirms the diagnosis of melanoma in situ. What is the appropriate next step in the diagnostic workup?

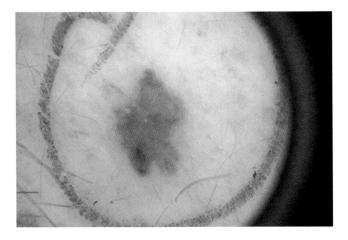

A. Chest radiograph
B. Chest/abdomen/pelvis computed tomography scan
C. Sentinel node biopsy
D. Genetic testing for *CDKN2A* mutation
E. Nothing, proceed directly to wide local excision

65. A 58-year-old woman with a history of mitral valve prolapse and mitral regurgitation presents for excision of a basal cell carcinoma on left upper arm. What is the appropriate perioperative antibiotic prophylaxis against infective endocarditis?
A. Oral cephalexin 2000 mg once, 1 hour prior to surgery
B. Oral cephalexin 500 mg twice daily for 5 days beginning the morning of surgery
C. Oral clindamycin 600 mg once, 1 hour prior to surgery
D. Oral clindamycin 300 mg twice daily for 5 days beginning the morning of surgery
E. No antibiotics are indicated.

66. All of the following statements are true regarding the complication shown below after sclerotherapy EXCEPT:

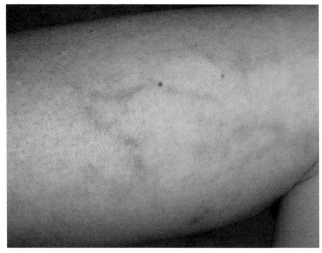

With permission from Bolognia, in *Dermatology*, 4th edition, 2017, 2620 (ch 155, fig. 155-11).

A. This occurs in 10%–30% of patients.
B. This will resolve in 95% of patients.
C. This occurs with both hypertonic saline and detergent sclerosants.
D. This is exclusively a result of hemosiderin deposition.
E. It can be minimized by treating feeder veins prior to distal vessels.

67. A 59-year-old man presents with a biopsy-confirmed nodular basal cell carcinoma of the left upper back, measuring 0.8 x 1.2 centimeters. What is the expected cure rate if the lesion is treated with electrodesiccation and curettage?
A. 40%
B. 65%
C. 80%
D. 95%
E. 99%

68. A 66-year-old man presents with the nasal tip and ala defect shown after complete extirpation of a recurrent basal cell carcinoma with Mohs surgery. Which of the following reconstructive options will provide robust vascular support for a cartilage graft?

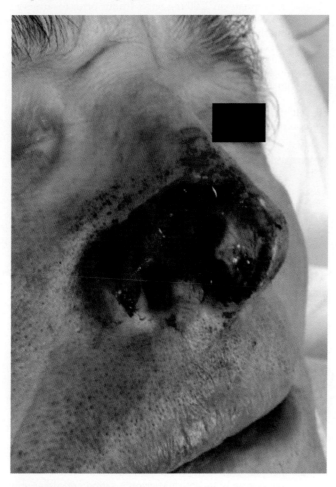

A. Single-stage local flap placed over cartilage graft
B. Staged interpolation flap placed over cartilage graft
C. Full-thickness skin graft placed over cartilage graft
D. Delayed full-thickness skin graft placed over cartilage graft
E. Split-thickness skin graft placed over cartilage graft

69. What is the preservative added to saline, which can decrease the pain associated with botulinum toxin injections?
A. Benzalkonium chloride
B. Benzyl alcohol
C. DMDM hydantoin
D. None; preservative-free saline is less painful

70. Treatment with botulinum toxin for glabellar rhytides is contraindicated in patients with all of the following neurological diseases EXCEPT:
A. Myasthenia gravis
B. Multiple sclerosis
C. Eaton-Lambert syndrome
D. Amyotrophic lateral sclerosis

71. A patient presents with the linear lesion shown since birth. Biopsy shows an epidermal nevus. What is developmental event that leads to this type of lesion?

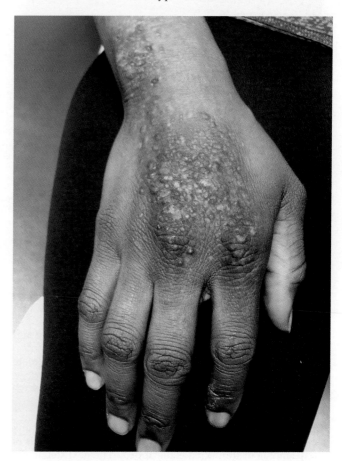

A. Germ cell mutation
B. Postzygotic mutation
C. Ultraviolet-induced mutation
D. Chromosomal inactivation
E. Oocyte mutation

72. Patients with Waardenburg syndrome can present with piebaldism, congenital deafness, and heterochromia iridis that are due to what defect in melanocytes?
A. Melanin production
B. Melanosome production
C. Epidermal precursors
D. Autoimmune destruction of melanocytes
E. Neural crest migration

73. This patient was born with colloidin membrane but no erythroderma or bullae. He now has thick platelike scaling. What is the normal function of the gene that is defective in this disorder?

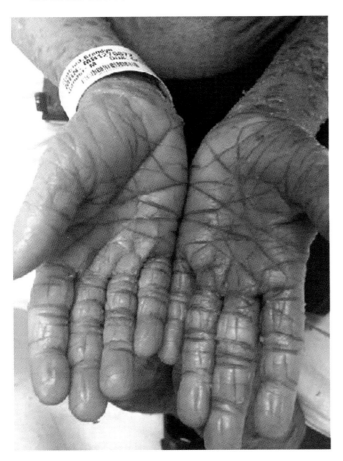

A. Development of lamellar bodies
B. Cross-linking proteins for cornified envelope formation
C. Keratin assembly
D. Cell adhesion between keratinocytes
E. Adhesion of keratinocytes to basement membrane

74. Which of the following does NOT explain differences in pigmentation between skin phototypes II and V?
A. Size of the melanosomes
B. Number of melanosomes
C. Number of melanocytes
D. Melanosome degradation
E. Distribution of melanosomes in keratinocytes

75. A patient presents with the rash shown. Which immune cell is primarily responsible for this disease process?

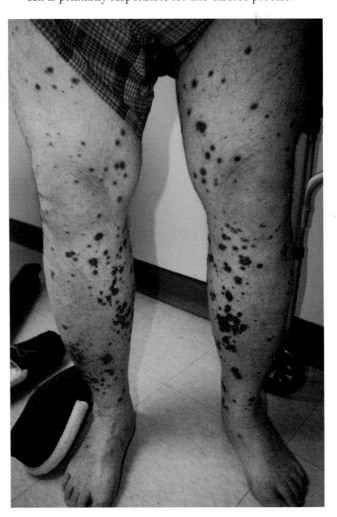

A. Plasma cells
B. Neutrophils
C. Histiocytes
D. Plasmacytoid dendritic cells
E. Th2 T cells

76. A 13-year-old girl presents for evaluation of this birthmark, which has recently become thicker and is getting irritated. The pathogenesis of this lesion is the same as which of the following conditions arising in a female patient?

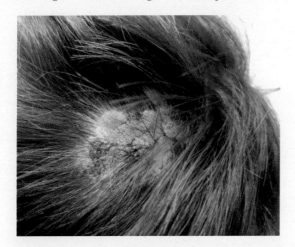

A. Ichthyosis with confetti
B. Incontinentia pigmenti
C. CHILD syndrome
D. Phylloid hypomelanosis
E. Wooly hair nevus

77. A 2-year-old boy presents for evaluation of very dry skin since early infancy. On examination he has fine brown scale that is most prominent on his lateral neck and anterior shins. He was born at term by cesarean section after failure to progress and has a history of an undescended testicle. His parents have no similar skin findings and are interested in having other children. What is the risk of having a second child with the same condition?
A. 25% risk, regardless of the sex of the child
B. 50% risk, regardless of the sex of the child
C. 25% risk for a male, 0% risk for a female
D. 50% risk for a male, 0% risk for a female
E. Negligible risk, as this most likely arose via sporadic mutation

78. Loss-of-function mutations in a specific epidermal gene causes this skin pathology. The gene, and its translated protein, was named because of its ability to interact with what other epidermal proteins?

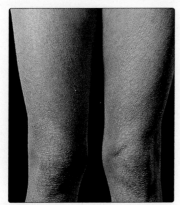

With permission from Gawkrodger DJ, et al., Keratinization and blistering syndromes, in Gawkrodger DJ, et al. (eds), *Dermatology: An Illustrated Colour Text*, 6th ed., 2017, Elsevier, 94–95 (fig. 47.1).

A. Loricrin
B. Keratins
C. Transglutaminases
D. Connexins
E. Aquaporins

79. The clinical and microscopic hair findings in this 2-year-old girl are most likely due to which of the following?

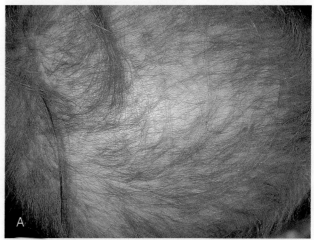

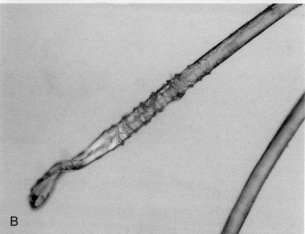

With permission from Bender AM, *Disorders of the Hair and Nails Pediatric Dermatology*, 2013, Elsevier, chapter 8, 211–239.

A. Defects of the inner root sheath
B. *SPINK5* mutation
C. Mutations in hair keratins
D. Chemical or thermal treatments
E. Fungal infection
F. *ATP7A* mutation

80. You are called to the neonatal intensive care unit to evaluate a 1-day-old infant with erosions and blistering of perioral, buttock, and acral skin. Bulla contents are sterile. Biopsy sample from an induced blister demonstrates cleavage within the lamina lucida. Which gene is most likely to be mutated in this condition?
A. Keratin 5
B. Keratin 10
C. Plectin
D. Laminin 332
E. Collagen VII

GENERAL DERMATOLOGY

1. A. Amoxicillin
The patient has developed SDRIFE, symmetrical drug-related intertriginous and flexural exanthema. Patients typically present with a localized exanthematous eruption of flexural zones. This drug-induced eruption most commonly occurs from beta-lactam antibiotics. It has also been associated with other antimicrobials, such as metronidazole, clindamycin, valacyclovir, and terbinafine.
Bolognia J, Schaffer J, Cerroni L, eds. *Dermatology*. [Philadelphia]: Elsevier, 2018 (ch. 21).

2. B. Oral contraceptive
The patient has a fixed drug eruption, which typically manifests with a round pink-dusky patch or plaque that may vesiculate and classically resolves with hyperpigmentation. The most common sites of involvement are the hands, feet, genitalia, lips, and face. The first presentation typically occurs within 1–2 weeks of starting a culprit drug; however, subsequent exposure may result in recurrent lesions within 24 hours. Common drug culprits include pseudoephedrine, NSAIDs, acetaminophen, antibiotics, barbiturates, aspirin, proton pump inhibitors, dapsone, and antifungals. Oral contraceptives are not classically associated with fixed drug eruptions. Pseudoephedrine can result in nonpigmenting fixed drug eruptions.
Bolognia J, Schaffer J, Cerroni L, eds. *Dermatology*. [Philadelphia]: Elsevier, 2018 (ch. 21).

3. B. Liver
This patient has drug reaction with eosinophilia and systemic symptoms (DRESS), also referred to as drug hypersensitivity syndrome. This drug eruption can affect multiple organ systems, including the thyroid, liver, heart, kidney, and lungs, with the liver being the most common extracutaneous site of involvement. It is important to stop the offending drug and start systemic corticosteroids with a slow taper to avoid rebound. It should also be noted that while peripheral hypereosinophilia is one of the criteria for diagnosis, it is not necessary and may rarely be absent. Myocarditis and thyroiditis can develop later in the course of the disease, thus close monitoring is necessary.
Bolognia J, Schaffer J, Cerroni L, eds. *Dermatology*. [Philadelphia]: Elsevier, 2018 (ch. 21).

4. D. No effect on the fetus
This patient has polymorphic eruption of pregnancy, formerly referred to as pruritic urticarial papules and plaques of pregnancy (PUPPP). It is characterized by urticarial papules and plaques that present in the third trimester of pregnancy with a predilection for striae and sparing of the umbilicus. There is no associated risk to the fetus. The rash does not usually recur in subsequent pregnancies.
Pemphigoid gestationis should be considered and ruled out, as there is increased fetal risk for small for gestational age and for prematurity. Clinical presentation includes urticarial papules and plaques with bulla, as seen in classical bullous pemphigoid, which develops later in pregnancy or postpartum. The umbilicus is usually involved, and recurrence in subsequent pregnancies may occur. Intrahepatic cholestasis of pregnancy presents with severe pruritus without primary cutaneous disease late in pregnancy. Bile acids are elevated and jaundice may occur. Diagnosis of this condition is important, as there is

increased risk of prematurity, fetal distress, and stillbirths. Recurrence is common.
Bolognia J, Schaffer J, Cerroni L, eds. *Dermatology*. [Philadelphia]: Elsevier, 2018 (ch. 27).

5. A. Chest x-ray
This patient has evidence of extramammary Paget disease (EMPD), manifesting with pink-red vegetative plaques with "strawberries and cream" appearance. Screening for internal malignancy with colonoscopy, cystoscopy, and prostate exam/prostate-specific antigen is indicated. EMPD can be primary or secondary. Primary disease results from an intraepithelial adenocarcinoma, while secondary EMPD results from contiguous spread of an adjacent or contiguous invasive cancer, most commonly gastrointestinal or genitourinary. Immunohistochemistry may show positivity for CK20 in the setting of secondary EMPD, while primary EMPD classically is positive for GCFDP-15.
Bolognia J, Schaffer J, Cerroni L, eds. *Dermatology*. [Philadelphia]: Elsevier, 2018 (ch. 73).

6. C. Primary systemic amyloidosis
This patient has primary systemic amyloidosis, which is associated with plasma cell dyscrasia. Cutaneous manifestations include a larger rubbery tongue (macroglossia); gingival papules or nodules; and periorbital waxy nodules, pinch purpura, and ecchymosis. Less commonly, sclerodermoid changes of the scalp may occur, as well as cutis vertices gyrate, hemorrhagic bullae, and nail dystrophy resembling lichen planus secondary to amyloid infiltration of the nail matrix or bed. Systemic involvement includes nephropathy, cardiomyopathy, neuropathy (carpal tunnel), and hepatomegaly.
Nodular amyloid is classified as a primary (localized) amyloidosis and presents as waxy papules or plaques on the trunk. The nodular variant may uncommonly be associated with a plasma cell dyscrasia and rarely progresses to systemic involvement. Sarcoidosis commonly manifests with red-brown periorificial papules without pinch purpura. Xanthelasma commonly presents on the eyelids with yellow-waxy papules and plaques.
Bolognia J, Schaffer J, Cerroni L, eds. *Dermatology*. [Philadelphia]: Elsevier, 2018 (ch. 47).

7. B. Sarcoidosis
This Kodachrome depicts sarcoidosis on the posterior neck and scalp. Note the red-brown granulomatous papules coalescing into annular plaques with central hypopigmentation on the scalp (discoid lupus erythematosus would be in the differential of these scalp lesions). Skin manifestations are present in one-third of patients with this systemic granulomatous disorder. Acne keloidalis nuchae occurs on the occipital scalp and posterior neck with pustules, papules, and keloidal scars. Elastosis perforans serpiginosa (EPS) also may involve the neck but presents with linear and serpiginously arranged pink-red papules. Down syndrome and various genodermatoses are associated with EPS. Granuloma annulare is another granulomatous disease that presents with annular plaques composed of smaller papules. Scalp involvement is unlikely to occur. Disseminate and recurrent infundibulofolliculitis (Hitch and Lund disease) presents in young adults with monomorphic follicular papules, often arranged linearly. Trunk and neck involvement are common.
Bolognia J, Schaffer J, Cerroni L, eds. *Dermatology*. [Philadelphia]: Elsevier, 2018 (ch. 93).

8. A. Morphea

The hypopigmented plaque on the trunk with a red-lilac rim is consistent with morphea. The inflammatory border indicates an active lesion. The sclerosis present in morphea can extend into the fat or underlying fascial structures and may cause joint contractures. Inflammatory morphea may present as an expanding red patch, and erythema chronicum migrans is the differential diagnosis but classically has a targetoid appearance with concentric rims without hypopigmentation centrally. Calciphylaxis can present as painful, firm indurated plaques in fatty areas that may ulcerate, in association with retiform purpura and/or livedo reticularis. Nephrogenic systemic fibrosis occurs with exposure to gadolinium-based contrast in the setting of renal disease. The disease presents as symmetric, indurated hyperpigmented plaques on the extremities with "ameboid" configuration.
Bolognia J, Schaffer J, Cerroni L, eds. *Dermatology*. [Philadelphia]: Elsevier, 2018 (ch. 44).

9. D. Pulmonary artery aneurysm

Mucocutaneous manifestations of Behçet disease include recurrent oral and genital ulcerations (classically aphthae), pathergy, erythema nodosum, papulopustular lesions, and pseudofolliculitis. Ocular involvement occurs in a majority of patients most commonly manifesting as uveitis. Other systemic manifestations include arthritis, GI ulcerations, cranial nerve palsy, glomerulonephritis, myocarditis, pulmonary artery aneurysms, deep venous thrombosis, and both occlusive and aneurysmal arterial disease. Pulmonary fibrosis may occur uncommonly with end-stage lung involvement and is associated with dermatomyositis, which does not present with pustular lesions. Hyperostosis may be found in patients with synovitis acne pustulosis hyperostosis (SAPHO) syndrome, but erythema nodosum and recurrent oral ulcerations are not part of this syndrome. Photosensitivity is seen in a variety of connective tissue diseases, including systemic lupus erythematosus.
Bolognia J, Schaffer J, Cerroni L, eds. *Dermatology*. [Philadelphia]: Elsevier, 2018 (ch. 36).

10. C. Pigment network

This is a pigmented basal cell carcinoma. Dermatoscopic features include arborizing vessels, leaflike structures, spoke-wheel areas, large blue-gray ovoid nests, multiple blue-gray globules, and ulceration. Pigment network would be absent and present in a melanocytic lesion.
Bolognia J, Schaffer J, Cerroni L, eds. *Dermatology*. [Philadelphia]: Elsevier, 2018 (ch. 108).

11. A. Oral cephalexin
   B. Bacterial culture

Impetigo is a common contagious superficial skin infection with a predominance for pediatric patients and may be bullous or nonbullous. The most common pathogen is *Staphylococcus aureus*. *Group A beta hemolytic streptococcus* is another important cause of nonbullous impetigo. Antibiotics (topical or oral depending on the severity) should be started while awaiting culture results. Therapy can be tailored pending results and clinical course. Eczema herpeticum is on the differential diagnosis but presents with monomorphic punched-out ulcers in a background of atopic dermatitis or other skin condition (e.g., Darier disease). Treatment is with an oral antiviral agent such as acyclovir or valacyclovir, while topical steroids should treat the underlying dermatitis.
Bolognia J, Schaffer J, Cerroni L, eds. *Dermatology*. [Philadelphia]: Elsevier, 2018 (ch. 74).

12. B. Bacterial infection

Pitted keratolysis is a noninflammatory bacterial infection of palmoplantar skin and most commonly affects the soles. Small 1–7 mm craterlike depressions are present. Hyperhidrosis, prolonged occlusion, and increased skin surface pH are predisposing factors. *Kytococcus sedentarius* is the most common cause. Other bacteria implicated include *Dermatophilus congolensis*, *corynebacterium*, and *actinomyces spp*. Malodor is often associated due to sulfur-containing compounds released by the bacteria. Topical antibiotics often lead to rapid resolution, including erythromycin, clindamycin, and mupirocin, as well as azole antifungals.
Tinea pedis is another infectious disease of the feet that presents with red scaly patches and plaques. Epidermolysis bullosa is an inherited blistering disorder that may affect palmoplantar skin with vesicles and bulla in areas of friction. Additionally, dyshidrotic dermatitis may occur on soles with deep-seated vesicles on the feet (usually along Wallace's lines). When associated with atopic dermatitis, a filaggrin mutation may be implicated. Tumor necrosis factor alpha inhibitors can cause a paradoxical psoriasiform dermatitis, which has a predilection for the palms and soles.
Bolognia J, Schaffer J, Cerroni L, eds. *Dermatology*. [Philadelphia]: Elsevier, 2018 (ch. 74).

13. A. Initiate oral corticosteroids
   B. Hold isotretinoin
   D. Discontinue anabolic steroid supplements
   E. Bacterial culture

The patient has acne fulminans triggered by isotretinoin. This can be a challenging condition to treat. Isotretinoin should be temporarily discontinued to get the skin under better control first with systemic steroids (0.5–1.0 mg/kg). Once there is improvement while on steroids (2–4 weeks), low-dose isotretinoin (0.1–0.25 mg/kg) can be initiated. As the condition improves, systemic steroids should be tapered as the isotretinoin dose is slowly increased. Refractory cases may be treated with the addition of dapsone or TNF-alpha inhibitors. A bacterial culture can be taken in case of superinfection. Anabolic steroids or whey protein should be inquired about and discontinued. Increasing the isotretinoin dose may worsen the acne fulminans. Radiation is not standard of care for acne fulminans and has been rarely used to treat keloids and dissecting cellulitis.
Bolognia J, Schaffer J, Cerroni L, eds. Dermatology. [Philadelphia]: Elsevier, 2018 (ch. 36).
Greywal T, et al. Evidence-based recommendations for the management of acne fulminans and its variants. *J Am Acad Dermatol*. 2017;77(1):109–117.

14. A. Adalimumab

Granuloma annulare is a benign cutaneous condition of unknown etiology. It commonly presents as annular plaques on the dorsal hands, arms, legs, and/or feet. Other clinical presentations include papular, subcutaneous, macular, and perforating lesions. Some studies have suggested a possible association with systemic disease, such as diabetes mellitus, hyperlipidemia, and thyroid disease, as well as HIV and hepatitis B and C infections. Drug-induced granuloma annulare has also been reported. Possible culprits include TNF-α inhibitors, amlodipine, allopurinol, diclofenac, gold, anti-programmed death 1 agents, and BRAF inhibitors. TNF-alpha blockers may also cause interstitial granulomatous drug reactions.
Bolognia J, Schaffer J, Cerroni L, eds. *Dermatology*. [Philadelphia]: Elsevier, 2018 (ch. 93).

15. C. Polyomavirus

Merkel cell carcinoma (MCC) is a cutaneous neuroendocrine tumor that is aggressive in nature. It typically occurs in older adults, most commonly presenting on the head and neck. Histopathologically, the tumor is comprised of uniform, small, round-to-oval blue cells with a sheetlike, trabecular, or nested growth pattern.

Immunohistochemistry can be used for both diagnostic and prognostic purposes. Characteristically, MCC has a CK-20 positive perinuclear dotlike pattern. In addition, neuroendocrine markers such as chromogranin, synaptophysin, somatostatin, calcitonin, and vasoactive intestinal peptide are positive. S100 is characteristically negative as is thyroid transcription factor (TTF-1), the latter of which helps distinguish MCC from cutaneous metastases of other small cell carcinomas (pulmonary and extrapulmonary). Polyomavirus has been identified in approximately 80% of MCCs, and its positivity can aid in diagnosis. In terms of prognosis, increased p63 expression is associated with clinically aggressive behavior. Likewise, MCCs negative for CK20 and for Merkel cell polyomavirus are more aggressive in nature.

Bolognia J, Schaffer J, Cerroni L, eds. *Dermatology.* [Philadelphia]: Elsevier, 2018 (ch. 115).

Moshiri AS, et al. Polyomavirus-negative Merkel cell carcinoma: a more aggressive subtype based on analysis of 282 cases using multimodal tumor virus detection. *J Invest Dermatol.* 2017;137:819–827.

16. D. Macrocephaly

Darier disease is an autosomal dominant disorder caused by a mutation in the calcium ATPase pump in the endoplasmic reticulum (SERCA2). The abnormal intracellular calcium signaling leads to impaired processing of junctional proteins. As a result, there is acantholysis due to disrupted epidermal adhesion and dyskeratosis due to an increase in apoptosis. The peak onset of the condition is during puberty.

Clinically, there are scattered keratotic red-brown papules, which are sometimes crusted, primarily concentrated in a "seborrheic" distribution—trunk, scalp, face, and lateral neck. Guttate hypopigmentation and hypomelanocytic macules admixed with the keratotic papules, as seen here, may be found in patients with darker skin types. On the hands, keratotic papules and keratin depressions are often seen. Less commonly, a thick and spiked focal keratoderma is found. The oral mucosa is involved in 15%–50% of patients with painless white papules or rugose plaques, and the hard palate is the most common site of involvement. In some patients there can be salivary gland obstruction, which can cause painful glandular swellings. Macrocephaly is not a feature of Darier disease but rather seen in tuberous sclerosis, which may present with guttate leukoderma in infancy.

Bolognia J, Schaffer J, Cerroni L, eds. *Dermatology.* [Philadelphia]: Elsevier, 2018 (ch. 59).

17. C. Ginkgo

Herbal supplements are increasingly utilized to treat a variety of conditions. Because the public largely perceives these "natural" therapies as harmless, patients often omit them from their medication lists. It is important to specifically ask patients about any herbal supplements they may be taking, as several are associated with an increased risk of bleeding and others may interact with medications commonly prescribed in dermatology.

Ginkgo (*ginkgo biloba*), garlic, and ginger supplements are all associated with spontaneous bleeding. Ginseng, on the other hand, can reduce the anticoagulant response to warfarin. Goldenseal (berberine) is associated with nervousness, confusion, nausea, and tremors. *Glycyrrhiza glabra* is found in licorice and has potential drug interactions with cyclosporine, digoxin, prednisone, and thiazides.

Bolognia J, Schaffer J, Cerroni L, eds. *Dermatology.* [Philadelphia]: Elsevier, 2018 (ch. 131).

18. A. Thrombotic thrombocytopenic purpura

Valacyclovir is an antiviral medication utilized in the treatment of herpes zoster infections. Systemic antiviral therapy needs to be dose adjusted for patients with renal impairment. An additional concern is with immunocompromised patients receiving valacyclovir, in whom thrombotic thrombocytopenic purpura and hemolytic uremic syndrome have been reported.

Any severely immunocompromised patient such as this is at risk of dissemination of his/her infection; however, that is not a result of the treatment with antiviral medication. Liver failure and acute respiratory distress syndrome are not known complications of treatment of zoster with valacyclovir.

Bolognia J, Schaffer J, Cerroni L, eds. *Dermatology.* [Philadelphia]: Elsevier, 2018 (ch. 127).

19. C. Lichen planus

Nail changes are observed in approximately 10% of patients with lichen planus; however, patients can also have isolated nail lichen planus. Multiple nails are typically affected, and the common clinical findings are longitudinal ridging and fissuring, nail thinning, and dorsal pterygium. Dorsal pterygium, as seen on the fourth digit here, is due to adhesion of the proximal nail fold to the nail bed due to matrix destruction and disappearance of the nail plate.

Systemic sclerosis is associated with ventral pterygium, which is characterized by the adhesion of the distal nail plate to the hyponychium, resulting in pain during nail trimming. Associated pitting and ulcers may be found. Common findings in nail psoriasis include irregular pitting, "oil drops," and onycholysis with an erythematous border. Onychomycosis can be difficult to differentiate from other causes of nail dystrophy, especially toenail psoriasis; however, typical clinical features include onycholysis, subungual hyperkeratosis with subungual debris, and yellow-orange nail plate discoloration.

Bolognia J, Schaffer J, Cerroni L, eds. *Dermatology.* [Philadelphia]: Elsevier, 2018 (ch. 71).

20. B. Cloves

Myroxylon pereirae (balsam of Peru) is a naturally occurring fragrance and commonly identified allergen. While allergy to balsam of Peru is most commonly observed in patients with fragrance allergy, it is also seen in those with allergies to spices, such as cloves, Jamaican pepper, and cinnamon.

Bolognia J, Schaffer J, Cerroni L, eds. *Dermatology.* [Philadelphia]: Elsevier, 2018 (ch. 14).

21. E. All of the above

Multiple eruptive dermatofibromas (MEDF) have been described in association with autoimmune disease, including systemic lupus, myasthenia gravis, dermatomyositis, Sjögren syndrome, and pemphigus vulgaris. Other associated conditions include HIV, pregnancy, hematologic malignancy, atopic dermatitis, Down syndrome, diabetes mellitus, ulcerative colitis, and mycosis fungoides. Initiation of several immunosuppressants including glucocorticoids, azathioprine, methotrexate, cyclophosphamide, and anti-TNF alpha therapy has also been described as a trigger of eruptive dermatofibromas.

Bolognia J, Schaffer J, Cerroni L, eds. *Dermatology.* [Philadelphia]: Elsevier, 2018 (ch. 116).

Callahan S, Matires K, Shvartsbeyn M, Brinster N. Multiple eruptive dermatofibromas. *Dermatol Online J.* 2015;21(12).

22. C. Tendon friction rubs are more commonly seen in patients with limited cutaneous systemic sclerosis than in patients with diffuse cutaneous systemic sclerosis.

There are two major clinical subtypes of systemic sclerosis differentiated by the degree of skin involvement. Limited cutaneous systemic sclerosis (lcSSc), formerly called CREST syndrome, involves the distal extremities and face, while diffuse cutaneous systemic sclerosis (dcSSc) involves the distal and proximal portions of the extremities, the trunk, and the face. Pulmonary arterial hypertension is more common in lcSSc while interstitial lung disease is more common in dsSSc. Anticentromere antibody occurs in 40% of patients with lcSSc but only in 5% of patients with dcSSc. Anti-RNA polymerase III antibody occurs in 1% of patients with lcSSc and in 10% of patients with dcSSc. Renal disease may be associated. Anti-topoisomerase I (Scl-70) antibody occurs in 5% of patients with lcSSc and in 20% of patients with dcSSc. Tendon friction rubs is described as a leathery feel to the tendons during active and passive motion and are seen in 5% of patients with lcSSc and in 70% of patients with dcSSc. Tendon friction rubs are caused by fibrous deposits on the surface of tendon sheaths and overlying the fascia. They may also be seen in eosinophilic fasciitis.

Bolognia J, Schaffer J, Cerroni L, eds. *Dermatology.* [Philadelphia]: Elsevier, 2018 (ch. 43).

23. D. Atenolol

Hydroxychloroquine may enhance the QTc-prolonging effects of ziprasidone, procainamide, amiodarone, sotalol, and quinidine. The combination of tamoxifen and hydroxychloroquine may increase the risk of retinal toxicity. The American Academy of Ophthalmology recommends regular annual screening (as opposed to screening every 5 years) for patients taking tamoxifen and hydroxychloroquine concomitantly. Hydroxychloroquine may also increase the serum concentration of digoxin. Hydroxychloroquine may decrease metabolism of beta-blockers that are metabolized via the CYP2D6-mediated pathway. Beta-blockers eliminated primarily by renal mechanisms, such as atenolol, nadolol, and sotalol, are not involved in this interaction (however, sotalol may interact with hydroxychloroquine via concomitant QTc prolongation as described previously).

Bolognia J, Schaffer J, Cerroni L, eds. *Dermatology.* [Philadelphia]: Elsevier, 2018 (ch. 43).

Leden I. Digoxin-hydroxychloroquine interaction? *Acta Med Scand* 1982;211:411–412.

24. B. Parapoxvirus

Orf, also known as contagious pustular dermatitis, is caused by a poxvirus of the genus *Parapoxvirus.* The infection typically resolves spontaneously within 6 to 8 weeks. Treatment for persistent lesions includes imiquimod and surgical excision. Cutaneous anthrax is on the differential but typically presents with a nonpainful papule that subsequently vesiculates and evolves into an ulcer with black eschar. Milker's nodules can look identical to Orf clinically but are transmitted by cows rather than sheep. Herpetic whitlow manifests as painful vesicles on the finger that may recur and is caused by herpesvirus.

Bolognia J, Schaffer J, Cerroni L, eds. *Dermatology.* [Philadelphia]: Elsevier, 2018 (ch. 81).

25. C. Penicillin

Acute generalized exanthematous pustulosis (AGEP) classically presents as numerous nonfollicular sterile pustules on a background of edematous erythema starting initially in the intertriginous areas and face. The eruption rapidly extends to the trunk and extremities. Fever and leukocytosis are often present. The most common triggers are antibiotics (aminopenicillins and macrolides), antifungals, the calcium channel blocker diltiazem, and antimalarials. Onset may be rapid with culprit medication starting days before the rash. Resolution occurs spontaneously after discontinuation of the offending agent within 1–2 weeks.

26. D. Trimethoprim/sulfamethoxazole

Livedo reticularis, a vascular reaction pattern characterized by a netlike discoloration on the extremities and trunk, is a manifestation of decreased blood flow to the skin. Livedo reticularis may be idiopathic/physiologic or secondary to an underlying vasculopathic or autoimmune connective tissue disease. Several medications have been associated with triggering livedo reticularis, including amantadine, quinidine, bismuth, catecholamines, minocycline, heparin, and interferon. Trimethoprim/sulfamethoxazole has not been reported to be associated with livedo reticularis.

Gibbs MB, English JC 3rd, Zirwas MJ. Livedo reticularis: an update. *J Am Acad Dermatol.* 2005;52(6):1009–1019.

27. B. *Corynebacterium tenuis*

Trichomycosis axillaris is a superficial bacterial infection of the hair (axillary or pubic) characterized by yellow, black, or red 1–2 mm granular nodules or concretions that stick to the hair shaft. Corynebacterium (mostly *Corynebacterium tenuis*) is the most common causative agent. *Piedraia hortae* is the causative agent of black piedra, which is characterized by pebble-sized masses irregularly distributed along the hair shafts in the beard, scalp, brows, or eyelashes. *Kytococcus sedentarius* is the most common causative agent of pitted keratolysis, which presents as depressed lesions on the plantar surface of the feet. *Trichosporon asahii* is the cause of white piedra. *Corynebacterium minutissimum* is the most common causative agent of erythrasma.

Bolognia J, Schaffer J, Cerroni L, eds. *Dermatology.* [Philadelphia]: Elsevier, 2018 (ch. 74).

28. E. *Tunga penetrans*

Tungiasis is caused by the chigger flea, *Tunga penetrans,* a sand flea found in Africa, India, and Central and South America. Female impregnated fleas burrow into the skin of the feet causing severe irritation, inflammation, and secondary bacterial infections. *Dermatobia hominis* is the human botfly found in the Americas and is one of the causative agents of myiasis. *Cordylobia anthropophaga* is the tumbu fly that causes myiasis in sub-Saharan Africa. *Cochliomyia hominivorax* is also known as the screw worm fly and is another cause of myiasis in the new world. *Ancylostoma Braziliense* is one of the causative agents of cutaneous larva migrans, which presents as a pruritic cordlike migratory plaque usually on the soles of the feet.

Bolognia J, Schaffer J, Cerroni L, eds. *Dermatology.* [Philadelphia]: Elsevier, 2018 (ch. 84).

29. A. Montelukast

Eosinophilic granulomatosis with polyangiitis is a multiorgan necrotizing vasculitis. Classic features include asthma,

neuropathy, migratory pulmonary infiltrates, paranasal sinus anomalies, tissue eosinophilic infiltrates, and peripheral blood eosinophilia. Cutaneous manifestations include leukocytoclastic vasculitis (palpable purpura), subcutaneous nodules on the scalp and extremities, urticaria, livedo racemosa, and papulonecrotic lesions, especially on the elbows. There are reports in the medical literature of eosinophilic granulomatosis with polyangiitis arising after initiation of Montelukast therapy.
Bolognia J, Schaffer J, Cerroni L, eds. *Dermatology.* [Philadelphia]: Elsevier, 2018 (ch. 24).

30. **D.** Lungs
Patients with cutaneous blastomycosis most likely have primary pulmonary infection with subsequent dissemination to the skin. This scenario is much more common than primary cutaneous inoculation. The classic presentation is multiple crusted, verrucous plaques; ulcers; and papulopustules.
Bolognia J, Schaffer J, Cerroni L, eds. *Dermatology.* [Philadelphia]: Elsevier, 2018 (ch. 77).

31. **E.** All of the above can occur in association with this condition
Cutaneous changes seen with hypothyroidism can include dry, rough, coarse skin that is cool and pale. Cutaneous myxedema can result in boggy and edematous skin. Yellow skin discoloration (carotenoderma) and capillary fragility may occur. Acquired ichthyosis, palmoplantar keratoderma, and eruptive and/or tuberous xanthomas are other associations. Hair changes associated with hypothyroidism can include coarse, brittle, slow-growing hair (increase in telogen hair phase); alopecia of the lateral third of the eyebrows (madarosis); and increased incidence of alopecia areata.
Bolognia J, Schaffer J, Cerroni L, eds. *Dermatology.* [Philadelphia]: Elsevier, 2018 (ch. 53).

32. **C.** Lung carcinoma
This photo represents paraneoplastic hypertrichosis lanuginosa acquisita, which has been most commonly associated with lung cancer. Less commonly it has been described with other adenocarcinomas arising in the large bowel, breast, uterus, genitourinary tract, and myeloma.
Bolognia J, Schaffer J, Cerroni L, eds. *Dermatology.* [Philadelphia]: Elsevier, 2018 (ch. 70).

33. **B.** Lung carcinoma
The photograph demonstrates velvety thickening of the palms with a ridged or corrugated appearance. This finding is tripe palms, also known as acanthosis palmaris, and is predominantly associated with gastric or lung cancer, although it is less frequently described in association with other malignancies or as an idiopathic condition. When tripe palms occurs concurrently with acanthosis nigricans, gastric cancer is more likely associated. However, when it occurs without acanthosis nigricans, lung cancer is the most common malignancy. Less commonly it may occur with tumors of the head and neck or genitourinary tract.
Bolognia J, Schaffer J, Cerroni L, eds. *Dermatology.* [Philadelphia]: Elsevier, 2018 (ch. 53).

34. **C.** *Aedes aegypti*
Dengue fever, also known as "break-bone," fever is characterized by sudden high fever, backache, retro-orbital pain, bone/joint pain, weakness, and malaise. It is caused by an arbovirus (RNA virus), which is transmitted by *Aedes aegypti* mosquito. The rash of Dengue may be

morbilliform with islands of white sparing; petechiae and conjunctival hemorrhage may occur. *Phlebotomus papatasi* is the vector for Old World cutaneous leishmaniasis. The Culex mosquito is the vector for several arboviruses, including the West Nile virus. *Lutzomyia verrucosum*, a sandfly, is a vector for New World leishmaniasis. *Xenopsylla cheopis*, the rat flea, is the vector for murine typhus (caused by *Rickettsia typhi*).
Bolognia J, Schaffer J, Cerroni L, eds. *Dermatology.* [Philadelphia]: Elsevier, 2018 (ch. 81).

35. **A.** Primary syphilis
A painless chancre with an indurated border is characteristic of primary syphilis. Associated painless lymphadenopathy ("buboes") is also a common feature. Unlike syphilitic chancres, chancroid (caused by *Haemophilus ducreyi*) presents with painful ulcerations. Primary syphilitic chancres usually heal spontaneously within 3 to 6 weeks even without treatment. In contrast, the primary lesions of lymphogranuloma venereum (LGV) (caused by the L1, L2, and L3 serovars of *Chlamydia trachomatis*) usually resolve within a few days. Inguinal lymphadenopathy in LGV is usually unilateral but may be bilateral in a minority of cases, and enlargement of inguinal and femoral nodes may result in a "groove sign," which is pathognomonic of LGV.
Bolognia J, Schaffer J, Cerroni L, eds. *Dermatology.* [Philadelphia]: Elsevier, 2018 (ch. 82).

36. **A.** Ophthalmic
The ophthalmic branch of the trigeminal branch is involved in ophthalmic zoster. This presentation accounts for 10%–15% of all cases of varicella zoster. It is important to consider ocular involvement with nasal tip lesions (Hutchinson's sign). The other nerve branches listed are not involved in ophthalmic zoster. Evaluation by ophthalmology is indicated.
Bolognia J, Schaffer J, Cerroni L, eds. *Dermatology.* [Philadelphia]: Elsevier, 2018 (ch. 80).

37. **E.** 13
Heck disease, characterized by numerous papules on the gingival, buccal, or labial mucosa, is associated with human papillomavirus 13 or 32 exclusively. This condition is more prevalent in natives of Greenland, South America, and South Africa and is rare among Caucasians. HPV 3 and 10 are detected in flat warts and can be found in lesions of epidermodysplasia verruciformis. HPV 4 may be detected in common warts as well as Butcher's wart. HPV 7 is frequently found in Butcher's warts.
Bolognia J, Schaffer J, Cerroni L, eds. *Dermatology.* [Philadelphia]: Elsevier, 2018 (ch. 79).

38. **C.** Primary effusion lymphoma
Human herpes virus 8 (HHV-8), a double-stranded DNA virus, is pathogenic in Kaposi sarcoma, primary effusion lymphoma, and Castleman disease. Primary effusion lymphoma, seen predominantly in patients with AIDS, is a rare type of B-cell lymphoma. HHV-6 and HHV-7 has been implicated in pityriasis rosea. HHV infections are not associated with angiosarcoma, pyogenic granuloma, or bacillary angiomatosis.
Bolognia J, Schaffer J, Cerroni L, eds. *Dermatology.* [Philadelphia]: Elsevier, 2018 (ch. 80).

39. **D.** Diabetes
Granuloma annulare is a benign, noninfectious, granulomatous condition of the skin disease that is usually

asymptomatic and self-limited. It typically presents with annular erythematous plaques that are most commonly found on the dorsal surfaces of the hands and feet. Generalized and perforating variants are most closely associated with diabetes.

Bolognia J, Schaffer J, Cerroni L, eds. *Dermatology.* [Philadelphia]: Elsevier, 2018 (ch. 93).

40. C. Artificially sweetened, low-calorie drinks

Aspartame, a frequently utilized synthetic sweetener that is transformed in the liver to formaldehyde, has been associated with systemic contact dermatitis. Aspartame can be found in chewable vitamins and low-calorie drinks and foods. Matiz et al. reported a case of a young boy with generalized erythema and eyelid dermatitis who improved with discontinuation of his montelukast chewable tablets, which contained aspartame.

Bolognia J, Schaffer J, Cerroni L, eds. *Dermatology.* [Philadelphia]: Elsevier, 2018 (ch. 14).

Matiz C, Jacob SE. Systemic contact dermatitis in children: how an avoidance diet can make a difference. *Pediatr Dermatol.* 2011;28(4):368–374.

Aquino M, Rosner G. Systemic contact dermatitis. *Clin Rev Allergy Immunol.* 2019;56(1):9–18.

PEDIATRIC DERMATOLOGY

41. C. Onychomadesis

Hand-foot-mouth disease (HFMD) is a viral illness that most frequently affects young children. Patients present with pink-red macules on the palms and soles that develop into vesicles, which are often oval-shaped with a gray center. The dorsal hands and feet, buttocks, and perineum are also commonly involved. The associated enanthem consists of red macules on the palate, buccal mucosa, and tongue that develop into vesicles and erosions. There is often preceding or concurrent fever and malaise, and onychomadesis may occur 1–2 months after the illness. HFMD can be caused by multiple enteroviruses, including coxsackievirus serotypes A16, A10, and A6. Coxsackie A6 has recently emerged as a cause of atypical and severe HFMD, which exhibits more widespread eruptions and more frequently affects adults than other serotypes.

Hypothyroidism is a delayed complication of drug reaction with eosinophilia and systemic symptoms; subacute sclerosing panencephalitis is a delayed complication of measles infection; herpes simplex encephalitis is a possible complication of herpes simplex infection; and aplastic anemia is a possible complication of parvovirus B19 infection.

Bolognia J, Schaffer J, Cerroni L, eds. *Dermatology.* [Philadelphia]: Elsevier, 2018 (ch. 81).

42. E. Reassurance

Nevus simplex (salmon patch) is a common congenital vascular lesion present in up to 80% of neonates in which blanchable, poorly defined pink macules and patches are found over the forehead, glabella, eyelids, philtrum, occipital scalp, and/or posterior neck. With the exception of lesions over the nape of the neck, nevus simplex usually fade in the first few years of life and most often do not require treatment. Nevus simplex should not be confused with port wine stains (PWSs), which are well-demarcated congenital red macules and patches that are caused by a somatic activating mutation in G Protein Subunit Alpha Q (GNAQ). In contrast to nevus simplex, PWSs do not fade

and may darken and develop nodules over time if left untreated.

MRI with gadolinium and ophthalmologic examination are appropriate in the workup of Sturge-Weber syndrome, which presents with a PWS involving the V1 segment of the face. Laryngoscopy would be indicated for the workup of a patient with a lower facial or "beard" hemangioma, which can be a marker of laryngeal hemangiomatosis. Pulsed dye laser would be appropriate for the treatment of facial PWS. Treatment is not needed for nevus simplex unless lesions persist.

Bolognia J, Schaffer J, Cerroni L, eds. *Dermatology.* [Philadelphia]: Elsevier, 2018 (ch. 104).

43. B. Gastrointestinal polyps

Peutz-Jeghers syndrome is an autosomal dominant disorder characterized by pigmented macules on the oral mucosa and digits that are present at birth or appear during childhood. The disorder is caused by mutations in *STK11*, and affected individuals have hamartomatous intestinal polyposis that may result in intussusception. They also have an increased risk of breast, ovarian, pancreatic, GI, and other cancers. Of note, Laugier-Hunziker syndrome is characterized by a similar distribution of lentigines as in Peutz-Jeghers syndrome; however, it does not have internal manifestations.

Pulmonic stenosis, electrocardiogram defects, and deafness are characteristic features of Noonan syndrome with multiple lentigines (formerly known as LEOPARD syndrome), an autosomal dominant disorder that features lentigines on the face, neck, and upper trunk but not specifically on the oral mucosa or digits. Multiple skin cancers are found in xeroderma pigmentosum, which is due to autosomal recessive defects in DNA-repair proteins and is characterized by lentigines predominantly in sun-exposed sites.

Bolognia J, Schaffer J, Cerroni L, eds. *Dermatology.* [Philadelphia]: Elsevier, 2018 (chs. 53 and 112).

44. A. Anti-DNase B

This patient has guttate psoriasis, which is often associated with a preceding streptococcal infection. In over half of patients, an elevated anti-streptolysin O, anti-DNase B, or Streptozyme titer is found. Atypical lymphocyte count is often elevated in drug reaction with eosinophilia and systemic symptoms (B); antihistone antibodies are elevated in most cases of drug-induced systemic lupus erythematosus; aldolase is elevated in dermatomyositis (D); anti-dsDNA is a marker of systemic lupus (E).

Bolognia J, Schaffer J, Cerroni L, eds. *Dermatology.* [Philadelphia]: Elsevier, 2018 (ch. 8).

45. A. Metastatic squamous cell carcinoma

Recessive dystrophic epidermolysis bullosa (RDEB) is characterized by blisters below the lamina densa due to autosomal recessive mutations in collagen VII. Patients experience fragile skin, erosions, blisters, and atrophic scarring with milia. Patients with RDEB-generalized/severe (previously Hallopeau-Siemens) commonly have pseudosyndactyly ("mitten deformities"), digital and limb contractures, corneal ulcerations and scarring, and microstomia. The leading cause of death in RDEB patients at or after mid-adolescence is cutaneous squamous cell carcinoma (SCC). The cutaneous SCCs in RDEB tend to be indistinct, difficult to fully excise, and are often recurrent locally with subsequent metastases that do not respond well to chemotherapy or radiation.

Patients with severe EB may develop chronic renal failure, and RDEB-generalized/severe is associated with an

approximately 10% risk of mortality from renal failure by 35 years of age. Lethal bacterial sepsis is now comparatively rare in EB patients, and when it does occur, it typically affects infants with generalized-severe disease. Finally, some patients with RDEB-generalized/severe may develop fatal dilated cardiomyopathy; however, this is not the leading cause of death.
Bolognia J, Schaffer J, Cerroni L, eds. *Dermatology*. [Philadelphia]: Elsevier, 2018 (ch. 32).

46. **D.** Congenital hypertrophy of the retinal pigment epithelium (CHRPE)
Gardner syndrome (GS) is an autosomal dominant disorder caused by mutations in the tumor suppressor gene *APC*, which encodes a protein responsible for downregulating the *Wnt/β-catenin* pathway. GS patients develop premalignant colonic polyps, with colorectal carcinoma occurring in nearly 100% of affected patients in the absence of surgical intervention.
Up to 50% of GS patients develop multiple epidermoid cysts during the first and second decade of life, some of which may have pilomatricoma-like changes. Up to 80% of GS patients exhibit osteomas, most commonly in the jaw. Affected individuals may also have desmoid tumors, fibromas, dental anomalies, and other tumors. Approximately 75% of GS patients exhibit CHRPE, which is present at birth and may be an early sign of the disorder. Early diagnosis of GS is critical to allow for screening, and prophylactic colectomy is indicated when polyp formation begins.
Sebaceous adenomas are characteristic of Muir-Torre syndrome. Multiple trichilemmomas and oral papillomas may be found in Cowden syndrome (multiple hamartoma syndrome). Bifid ribs may be found in Gorlin syndrome (basal cell nevus syndrome).
Bolognia J, Schaffer J, Cerroni L, eds. *Dermatology*. [Philadelphia]: Elsevier, 2018 (ch. 63).

47. **B.** Reassurance
F. Discussion of pulsed dye laser therapy
A spider angioma (nevus araneus) is a common telangiectasia composed of a central vascular papule (arteriole) with radiating capillaries. While multiple lesions in adults may be associated with liver disease, pregnancy, or estrogen therapy, these lesions are usually idiopathic in children and are found in up to 15% of healthy children and young adults. Spider angiomas may regress spontaneously but many persist, and such lesions may be treated with pulsed dye laser or electrocoagulation.
Transthoracic contrast echocardiography, MRI of the brain, and Doppler ultrasonography of the liver may be performed in patients with hereditary hemorrhagic telangiectasia (HHT) to screen for arteriovenous malformations (AVMs) in the lung, brain, and liver, respectively. Annual testing for hemoglobin and hematocrit is recommended for HHT patients over age 35 to detect substantial bleeding due to gastrointestinal AVMs.
Bolognia J, Schaffer J, Cerroni L, eds. *Dermatology*. [Philadelphia]: Elsevier, 2018 (ch. 104 and 106).

48. **C.** Recurrent fevers during infancy
Hypohidrotic ectodermal dysplasia (HED) is a disorder characterized by decreased sweating, hypotrichosis, and abnormal dentition. HED is most commonly caused by a mutation in ectodysplasin (ED1), which results in an X-linked recessive inheritance pattern. However, autosomal dominant and autosomal recessive variants exist due to mutations in genes that affect the same pathway. HED patients exhibit sparse light hair, darkening of the skin under

the eyes, peg-shaped or missing teeth, and characteristic facial features including frontal bossing. Nails are typically unaffected. HED patients have an increased risk for hyperthermia due to impaired sweating, and infants may have multiple febrile episodes before a diagnosis of HED is made. Premature atherosclerosis is found in Hutchinson-Gilford progeria syndrome and Werner syndrome. Short, thickened fingernails are characteristic of hidrotic ectodermal dysplasia (Clouston syndrome) in which patients have affected hair and nails with normal teeth and sweating. Angiokeratoma corporis diffusum is characteristic of Fabry disease as well as other lysosomal storage disorders.
Bolognia J, Schaffer J, Cerroni L, eds. *Dermatology*. [Philadelphia]: Elsevier, 2018 (ch. 63).

49. **E.** Perifollicular erythema and follicular hyperkeratosis
Monilethrix is an inherited disorder of the hair shaft characterized by ellipse-shaped nodes of normal hair thickness separated by abnormal constrictions throughout the hair shaft. Affected individuals have normal-appearing hair at birth, which is then replaced by fragile, short, brittle hair. Affected areas often exhibit perifollicular erythema and follicular hyperkeratosis. Monilethrix is most commonly inherited in an autosomal dominant manner due to mutations in the hair cortex–specific keratin genes *KRT86* and *KRT81*, though an autosomal recessive form has been identified due to mutations in *Dsg4*.
Traumatic heat styling causes bubble hair and can also contribute to acquired trichorrhexis nodosa. Both Bazex-Dupre-Christol and Rombo syndrome patients exhibit pili torti. In both syndromes affected individuals are at increased risk of basal cell carcinomas. Menkes kinky hair disease is characterized by pili torti and trichorrhexis nodosa as well as mental retardation and diffuse hypopigmentation. Netherton syndrome patients exhibit trichorrhexis invaginata, trichorrhexis nodosa, ichthyosis linearis circumflexa, and severe atopy.
Bolognia J, Schaffer J, Cerroni L, eds. *Dermatology*. [Philadelphia]: Elsevier, 2018 (ch. 69).

50. **D.** Start low-potency topical steroid plus barrier cream
This patient has irritant contact dermatitis, which is the most common cause of diaper dermatitis. It classically presents as glazed erythema with punched-out erosions most prominent on the buttocks, genitalia, and inner thighs with sparing of skin folds. It occurs as the result of dampness and exposure to urine and feces. Treatment with mild corticosteroids is helpful acutely, and barrier creams containing zinc oxide along with frequent diaper changes can help prevent recurrences. This is a common occurrence in children and is very unlikely to indicate parental neglect or abuse (A). Skin biopsy is not necessary given the classic clinical presentation (B). Checking zinc levels is important when acrodermatitis enteropathica is suspected; however, this typically also involves perioral skin and acral areas and presents with more sharply demarcated scaly patches and/or erosions (C). This is not a bacterial infection, so amoxicillin would not be appropriate (E).
Bolognia J, Schaffer J, Cerroni L, eds. *Dermatology*. [Philadelphia]: Elsevier, 2018 (ch. 13).

DERMATOPATHOLOGY

51. **C.** Interleukin-23
The diagnosis is psoriasis. Histologic features of psoriasis that can be seen in the photomicrograph include: regular

acanthosis, parakeratosis, thin suprapapillary plates, neutrophils in the stratum corneum, and minimal spongiosis. Based on this diagnosis, the correct choice is IL-23. IL-27 is not a current therapeutic target in psoriasis, nor is it being actively pursued as one. IL-17, however, is a target in psoriasis. IL-23 promotes TH17 cell activity, which in turn secretes IL-17, so these two cytokines are closely related. Guselkumab was recently approved for psoriasis and targets IL-23. Ustekinumab targets both IL-12 and IL-23.

Therapies that target IL-4, IL-13, and/or IL-31 are either already FDA approved or undergoing clinical development for atopic dermatitis and related disorders. These histologic features in this case are not typical of atopic dermatitis, even that with overlying lichen simplex chronicus (LSC). Dupilumab targets IL-4/IL-13 and is FDA approved for atopic dermatitis. Agents targeting IL-31 are also being targeted for atopic dermatitis. The histologic features of atopic dermatitis are nonspecific but include more prominent spongiosis. Compact hyperkeratosis and irregular acanthosis can be seen; however, the acanthosis would not be expected to be so regular and "test-tube-like" as in this case.

Bolognia J, Schaffer J, Cerroni L, eds. *Dermatology*. [Philadelphia]: Elsevier, 2018 (ch. 8).

52. C. Serum ferritin level

The diagnosis in this case is porphyria cutanea tarda (PCT). The most prominent histologic feature (besides the subepidermal split) is "festooning" of the dermal papillae with minimal inflammatory infiltrate. Other histologic features of PCT include "caterpillar bodies" (intraepidermal amorphous basement membrane material) and hyaline perivascular PAS+ material associated with superficial dermal vessels. DIF is typically negative; however, it can be positive on occasion when IgM and C3 staining is found in the superficial dermal vessels.

Serum ferritin levels can be used to screen for hemochromatosis, which is associated with PCT, particularly when there is a positive family history. Patients should also be screened for alcohol use, HIV, and hepatitis C, and renal function should also be evaluated. Collagen VII antibodies can be seen in bullous lupus or epidermolysis bullosa acquisita; BP180 and BP230 antibodies are found in bullous pemphigoid; and ceruloplasmin is helpful in evaluating for Wilson disease, which is not associated with PCT. Serum protein electrophoresis (SPEP) with IFE (immunofixation) are used to detect plasma cell dyscrasias, which are not associated with PCT.

Bolognia J, Schaffer J, Cerroni L, eds. *Dermatology*. [Philadelphia]: Elsevier, 2018 (ch. 49).

53. D. *CARD14*

The patient presents with typical features of pityriasis rubra pilaris (PRP); however, presentation at a very young age combined with prominent involvement of the face are clues for the ultimate underlying diagnosis of CAPE—*CARD14*-associated papulosquamous eruption—which is due to heterozygous mutations in the *CARD14* gene. Histologic features of PRP shown in the photomicrograph include acanthosis and so-called checkerboard alteration between orthokeratosis and parakeratosis. Suprapapillary plates are often thicker than in typical psoriasis. Although not show here, parakeratosis around follicles (corresponding to the follicular prominence seen clinically) would also support the diagnosis. Ustekinumab has been reported as an effective treatment for CAPE.

Keratin 10 (greater than keratin 1) mutations are seen in ichthyosis with confetti (IWC) (as well as epidermolytic ichthyosis). Although IWC has confetti-like islands of normal skin, this condition is present at birth and would not be expected to have other features of PRP or the histologic findings described in the vignette. The normal islands of skin in IWC are due to revertant mosaicism over time. *ABCA12* mutation is seen in harlequin ichthyosis. STS (steroid sulfatase) gene mutations are seen in X-linked ichthyosis. HLA-B27 polymorphism is seen in reactive arthritis.

Craiglow BG, et al. CARD14-associated papulosquamous eruption: a spectrum including features of psoriasis and pityriasis rubra pilaris. *J Am Acad Dermatol*. 2018 Sep;79(3):487–494.

54. B. Trametinib

Vemurafenib inhibits the mutant BRAF protein, which is found in 50% of cutaneous melanomas. Patients taking BRAF inhibitors can develop SCCs, keratoacanthomas, and benign squamous proliferations (squamous papillomas, as shown here) due to paradoxical activation of the MAP kinase (MAPK) pathway in keratinocytes with wild-type BRAF and/or RAS mutations. Squamous papillomas from BRAF inhibitors can have verrucous features as shown here.

BRAF is part of the MAPK pathway. Trametinib inhibits the MEK protein, which is also part of the MAPK pathway (further downstream). Combining BRAF and MEK inhibitors in BRAF mutant melanoma has been shown to have the dual benefit of increasing efficacy against the melanoma and reducing adverse effects, including the development of SCCs, keratoacanthomas, and papillomas, as seen here. Acitretin and nicotinamide can be used for chemoprophylaxis but are not the correct choice in this setting given the dual benefit of adding an MEK inhibitor.

Bolognia J, Schaffer J, Cerroni L, eds. *Dermatology*. [Philadelphia]: Elsevier, 2018 (ch. 128).

55. A. BAP1 syndrome—ophthalmology

The biopsy shows a lesion composed of epithelioid/Spitzoid melanocytes, features that can be seen in "*BAP1* nevi." Intranuclear inclusions are another clue to this diagnosis. BAP1 is a tumor-suppressor gene; a defective copy of BAP1 is inherited in patients with familial BAP1 syndrome.

When a BAP1 nevus is suspected, as in this case based on the histologic features of the nevus and the presence of multiple dome-shaped pink nevus-like papules clinically, loss of nuclear BAP1 staining can be used to confirm the diagnosis. BAP1 nevi can occur sporadically, but as discussed later, several features in this case suggest it is syndromic. In BAP1 syndrome, loss of BAP1 staining is the result of inactivation of the second "good" copy of BAP1, which is thought to lead to formation of the lesion. For sporadic BAP1 nevi to form, both copies of BAP1 must undergo somatic mutation/inactivation.

Clinically, BAP1 tumors present similarly to Spitz nevi with flesh-colored to pink-red dome-shaped papules. BAP1 cancer syndrome is characterized by atypical nevi/tumors composed of epithelioid melanocytes (as shown here), uveal melanomas, and mesothelioma (as seen in the patient's father). Given the risk of uveal melanomas in this patient with suspected BAP1 syndrome, referral to ophthalmology in addition to genetic testing is appropriate.

None of the other diagnoses fit as well with the presentation and histologic findings. Familial atypical multiple mole melanoma syndrome presents with atypical pigmented nevi and melanoma and has an increased risk of pancreatic cancer due to germline *CDKN2A* mutations.

Carney (NAME/LAMB) presents with lentigines, blue nevi (including epithelioid), psammomatous melanotic Schwannomas, and can be associated with the development of atrial myxomas. Peutz-Jeghers presents with perioral and mucosal lentigines and has an increased risk of several cancers, including gastrointestinal tumors. This is not a cutaneous mosaic disorder.

Haugh AM, Njauw CN, Bubley JA, et al. Genotypic and phenotypic features of BAP1 cancer syndrome: a report of 8 new families and review of cases in the literature. *JAMA Dermatol.* 2017 Oct 1;153(10):999–1006.

56. B. CK 20

The staining pattern shown demonstrates a perinuclear dot pattern, characteristic of CK20 (cytokeratin 20) staining in Merkel cell carcinoma. CK20 can also be used to differentiate desmoplastic trichoepithelioma (positive) from basal cell carcinoma (negative). INSM21 (insulinoma-associated protein 1), a sensitive nuclear marker of neuroendocrine differentiation, is positive in Merkel cell carcinoma but shows nuclear staining, not cytoplasmic staining accentuated near the nucleus in a glob or "dot" pattern. Merkel cell polyomavirus (MCPyV) can be detected in many but not all Merkel cell carcinomas (highly UV-mutated tumors are often negative for MCPyV), and MCPyV staining is predominantly nuclear. CD20 marks B cells and would not be expected to be positive here. CD30 is positive in anaplastic large-cell lymphoma, cutaneous T-cell lymphoma with large-cell transformation, and lymphomatoid papulosis.

Bolognia J, Schaffer J, Cerroni L, eds. *Dermatology.* [Philadelphia]: Elsevier, 2018 (ch. 115).

57. E. Paraffinoma

Paraffinomas (aka sclerosing lipogranulomas) result from subcutaneous or intradermal injection of oil-based substances such as paraffin, silicone, or wax, often for cosmetic indications. Location on the penis is common, as in this case. Histologically, as pictured in the photomicrograph, numerous vacuolated spaces of varying sizes in the dermis are typically seen, sometimes referred to as "Swiss cheese" appearance. In paraffinoma, a sclerotic stroma is also typically present. Foreign body giant cells may also be noted.

The other diagnoses would not be expected to show "Swiss cheese" vacuolation of the dermis on biopsy. Chancroid would be expected to show three zones of change on biopsy: a superficial zone of necrosis, fibrin, and neutrophils; granulation tissue; and lymphocytes and plasma cells. The diagnosis of chancroid, caused by *Haemophilus ducreyi*, is confirmed clinically by gram stain showing gram-negative bacilli in a "school of fish" pattern. Primary syphilis shows a very similar histologic pattern to chancroid; spirochetes may be identified on special stains, and syphilitic serologies confirm the diagnosis (e.g., Venereal Disease Research Laboratory [VDRL] test, rapid plasma reagin [RPR], fluorescent treponemal antibody absorption [FTA-ABS]). Herpes simplex virus shows ballooning degeneration of keratinocytes with multinucleate giants cells. Invasive squamous cell carcinoma would demonstrate atypical keratinocytes.

Bolognia J, Schaffer J, Cerroni L, eds. *Dermatology.* [Philadelphia]: Elsevier, 2018 (ch. 100).

58. D. Large dendritic-shaped cells around a hair follicle

A common feature of lentigo maligna is extension of atypical melanocytes down adnexal structures. The confocal image shown in this case displays large dendritic/elongate cells (white in color; marked by blue arrow) in association with a hair follicle (marked by red arrow). Extension of melanocytes down adnexal structures can be seen clinically with dermoscopy (perifollicular hyperpigmentation), histologically, and with confocal as discussed here. Even if one were not trained in confocal, given this cardinal feature of lentigo maligna, one should be able to be deduce the correct answer.

Loss of adnexal structures is not seen in lentigo maligna, where prominent hair follicles are found clinically and histologically. The hair follicle in the field has a honeycomb pattern of keratinocytes and is not consistent with a nerve. Pagetoid spread is not shown here; given the presence of a hair follicle, we know we are in the lower (not upper) epidermis and most likely in the basal layer. Of note, Langerhans cell can appear similar to melanocytes on confocal (white cells with dendritic extensions in the epidermis) but would be expected to extend down hair follicles.

59. A. Urinalysis and stool guaiac

The biopsy shows leukocytoclastic vasculitis (LCV) characterized by neutrophilic infiltrate and karyorrhexis centered on blood vessels in the superficial dermis. Fibrin deposition in the vessels (as nicely illustrated here) is a key feature. Erythrocyte extravasation is also commonly noted. A DIF can also be performed when suspecting LCV and/or Henoch-Schönlein purpura (HSP) to rule out IgA positivity in dermal blood vessels. It was not performed in this case; however, given the presence of LCV in a child and distribution of lesions on buttocks and lower extremities, there should be concern for HSP. The most common extracutaneous manifestations of HSP include: arthritis (75%), GI involvement (50%–75% of patients) including GI bleeding in 30% of patients, and renal involvement (in 40% of patients) with accompanying hematuria (40%) and proteinuria (25%).

Given the frequency of GI and renal involvement, the presence of blood in the stool and the urine should be evaluated with urinalysis (including microscopic examination) and stool guaiac. If GI involvement is suspected (based on clinical symptoms and/or a positive stool guaiac), a gastroenterologist may be consulted due to the risk of intussusception. Creatinine is important to check as well, but hepatic and lung involvement are atypical and so should not be a priority. Basic labs including a CBC and complete metabolic panel would be indicated as well, but urinalysis and guaiac are most essential.

Bolognia J, Schaffer J, Cerroni L, eds. *Dermatology.* [Philadelphia]: Elsevier, 2018 (ch. 24).

60. D. SPEP and IFE

The diagnosis is erythema elevatum diutinum (EED). EED is hypothesized to be a chronic form of leukocytoclastic vasculitis (LCV) that leads to or is associated with fibrosis. Pictured in the photomicrograph is the characteristic onion skin or lamellar fibrosis that is described in EED. Neutrophilic infiltrate and karyorrhectic debris can also be seen in the photomicrograph and are characteristic of EED histologically.

EED is associated with HIV, IgA gammopathy, beta-hemolytic strep, and less commonly other infectious, inflammatory and neoplastic (hematopoietic malignancies) disorders. Once a diagnosis of EED is made, potential underlying etiologies should be ruled out.

This is not a sclerotic fibroma; however, there is a resemblance between EED and this diagnosis histologically. Sclerotic fibromas have a plywood-like collagen that can appear vaguely similar to the fibrosis in EED; however, sclerotic fibromas are less cellular and should not have prominent neutrophilic infiltration with karyorrhexis.

Sclerotic fibromas can be a maker of Cowden. EED can be associated with hematopoietic malignancies but most commonly myelodysplasia, myeloproliferative disorders, and Hairy cell leukemia, not CTCL (TCR v-beta testing) and other T-cell malignancies. EED is not associated with tuberous sclerosus (TSC1/2 genes).
Bolognia J, Schaffer J, Cerroni L, eds. *Dermatology.* [Philadelphia]: Elsevier, 2018 (ch. 24).

PROCEDURAL DERMATOLOGY

61. D. Glycolic acid
Glycolic acid is not a component of a Jessner's peel, a superficial depth peel. Jessner's peel penetrates to the superficial papillary dermis and is considered a superficial peel, which can be used to treat dyspigmentation and fine wrinkles. Other superficial peels include glycolic acid, 30% salicylic acid, and 10%–20% trichloroacetic acid (TCA).
Bolognia J, Schaffer J, Cerroni L, eds. *Dermatology.* [Philadelphia]: Elsevier, 2018 (ch. 154).

62. C. Deep subcutaneous adipose superficial to the fascia
Undermining on most areas of the forehead, cheeks, chin, neck, trunk, and extremities should be performed within the subcutaneous adipose, as there is minimal resistance to tissue movement, and there are rarely critical anatomic structures in this plane. Undermining in the deep subcutis will avoid the subdermal vascular plexus at junction of dermis and subcutis and preserve this plexus with the advancing skin. On the temple, where the temporal branch of the facial nerve travels on the superficial surface of the fascia in an area with minimal subcutaneous adipose, undermining should be performed within the mid-subcutaneous adipose to avoid damage to the nerve. Undermining in general cannot be performed within the dermis. On the nose, undermining is generally performed in the submuscular/fascial plane. On the scalp and superior forehead, undermining may be performed deep to the fascia (galea) overlying the periosteum, but on many areas of the cheek there is no underlying bone. Incising until one encounters periosteum is not recommended in this area.
Bolognia J, Schaffer J, Cerroni L, eds. *Dermatology.* [Philadelphia]: Elsevier, 2018 (ch. 142).

63. B. Supraorbital nerve tracking to ophthalmic nerve and trigeminal ganglion
The supraorbital nerve is a branch of cranial nerve V_1 that supplies sensation to the lateral forehead and frontal scalp. The nerve emerges from the supraorbital foramen at superior orbital rim near the site of the SCC in the image. The supraorbital nerve and supratrochlear nerve join proximally in the ophthalmic nerve (CN V_1), which can be tracked proximally to the trigeminal ganglion in the skull base. Perineural SCC tracking this far proximally is nearly inoperable, although skull-base resection may be considered. The temporal nerve is a branch of the facial nerve (CN VII) that supplies motor innervation to the frontalis muscle of the forehead. From these muscles it tracks proximally to the parotid gland, where it joins with the other branches of the facial nerve, enters the skull via the stylomastoid foramen, and traverses the bony facial canal to the geniculate ganglion.
Bolognia J, Schaffer J, Cerroni L, eds. *Dermatology.* [Philadelphia]: Elsevier, 2018 (ch. 142).

64. E. Nothing, proceed directly to wide local excision
With an adequate biopsy confirming melanoma in situ and no evidence of dermal invasion, the risk of metastatic disease is less than 1%. Thus no additional workup is necessary prior to definitive surgical excision. Genetic testing is not indicated for sporadic melanoma in situ unless there is a strong family history suggestive of an inherited cancer predisposition syndrome.
Bolognia J, Schaffer J, Cerroni L, eds. *Dermatology.* [Philadelphia]: Elsevier, 2018 (ch. 113).

65. E. No antibiotics are indicated
Structural disease of native heart valves such as mitral or aortic regurgitation are not indications for antibiotic prophylaxis. According to guidelines of the American Heart Association and the American College of Cardiology, only the following patients require perioperative antibiotic prophylaxis: patients with prosthetic cardiac valves, patients with a history of prior infective endocarditis, cardiac transplant recipients with valve regurgitation due a structurally abnormal valve, or patients with unrepaired or prosthetically repaired congenital heart disease. Moreover, antibiotic prophylaxis is only indicated for procedures on inflamed skin or procedures that breach the oral or nasal mucosa. For cutaneous surgery on normal skin, antibiotic prophylaxis is not recommended.
Bolognia J, Schaffer J, Cerroni L, eds. *Dermatology.* [Philadelphia]: Elsevier, 2018 (ch. 151).

66. D. This is exclusively a result of hemosiderin deposition
Postinflammatory hyperpigmentation is the most frequent complication of sclerotherapy, occurring in up to 30% of patients. It results from a combination of hemosiderin deposition and postinflammatory hyperpigmentation after vessel destruction. Hypercoagulability syndromes, use of nonsteroidal antiinflammatory drugs or minocycline, high total body iron stores, or vessel fragility (e.g., as seen in elderly patients) may predispose to this adverse sequela. Hyperpigmentation is more commonly seen after treatment with hypertonic saline but can also develop with detergent sclerosants.
Bolognia J, Schaffer J, Cerroni L, eds. *Dermatology.* [Philadelphia]: Elsevier, 2018 (ch. 155).

67. D. 95%
For primary basal cell carcinoma without infiltrative or high-risk histologic features that is less than 2 centimeters in diameter on low-risk locations such as the trunk and proximal extremities, electrodesiccation and curettage (ED&C) is a highly effective procedure. With an appropriately performed ED&C, ensuring adequate depth and breadth of treatment, the cure rate is comparable to standard surgical excision, approximately 95%. Mohs surgery may achieve greater cure rates of 98%–99% but is generally not indicated for these lesions when simpler methods of treatment (ED&C or standard excision) are effective.
Bolognia J, Schaffer J, Cerroni L, eds. *Dermatology.* [Philadelphia]: Elsevier, 2018 (ch. 150).

68. B. Staged interpolation flap placed over cartilage graft
This defect includes full-thickness loss of the alar rim as well as loss of epidermis, dermis, and musculature on the nasal tip and alar body. To prevent collapse of the alar rim, cartilage grafting is required. Only a staged interpolation flap such as a paramedian forehead flap will provide a robust vascular supply to support optimal healing of the

flap and cartilage graft. Given the size of the defect, single-stage local nasal flaps would not be able to provide adequate coverage without unacceptable distortion of the nose. Full-thickness and split-thickness skin grafts may be used over cartilage grafts on the nose, but the vascular supply is tenuous and there is increased risk of graft necrosis.
Bolognia J, Schaffer J, Cerroni L, eds. *Dermatology*. [Philadelphia]: Elsevier, 2018 (chs. 147 and 148).

69. B. Benzyl alcohol
Benzyl alcohol is the preservative agent in bacteriostatic saline. When botulinum toxin is reconstituted in saline with this preservative, patients report less pain with injection and the shelf life after reconstitution is longer. According to a study, 90% of patients reported that injections that included the preservative to be less painful than the preservative-free injections and that average reduction in pain was approximately 55%.
Murad M, Dover JS, Arndt KA. Pain associated with injection of botulinum A exotoxin reconstituted using isotonic sodium chloride with and without preservative: a double-blind, randomized controlled trial. *Arch Dermatol*. 2002; 138(4):510–514.

70. B. Multiple sclerosis
Patients with a history of myasthenia gravis, Eaton-lambert syndrome, or amyotrophic lateral sclerosis should not be treated with botulinum toxin injections. This is because botulinum toxin prevents release of acetylcholine from presynaptic motor neurons and can potentially worsen these conditions. On the contrary, botulinum toxin has been used to treat certain symptoms and complications of multiple sclerosis.
Bolognia J, Schaffer J, Cerroni L, eds. *Dermatology*. [Philadelphia]: Elsevier, 2018 (ch. 159).

BASIC SCIENCE

71. B. Postzygotic mutation
Postzygotic mutation present in a subset of somatic cells from a developing embryo, which creates somatic mosaicism that follows lines of Blaschko. Importantly not all somatic mosaicism lesions follow lines of Blaschko, but mutations in epidermal cells as those seen in epidermal nevi classically do. Thus the pattern of lesions caused by somatic mosaicism is often due to what cell type harbors the mutation.
Bolognia J, Schaffer J, Cerroni L, eds. *Dermatology*. [Philadelphia]: Elsevier, 2018 (ch. 62 and 109).

72. E. Neural crest migration
Waardenburg syndrome is due to a defect in melanosome migration from neural crest precursors. Defects in melanin production cause oculocutaneous albinism and defects in melanosome production can cause Hermansky-Pudlack syndrome. Defects in melanosome transfer cause Chédiak-Higashi syndrome and Griscelli syndrome. Autoimmune destruction of melanocytes cause vitiligo.
Bolognia J, Schaffer J, Cerroni L, eds. *Dermatology*. [Philadelphia]: Elsevier, 2018 (ch. 65 and 66).

73. B. Cross-linking proteins for cornified envelope formation
Lamellar ichthyosis presents with collodion membrane and subsequent thick platelike scale and hyperlinearity of palms and is most often caused by defect in transglutaminase 1 (TGM1). The normal function of TGM1 is to cross-link proteins for cornified envelope formation on corneocytes. Defect in lamellar body's formation causes harlequin ichthyosis. Defects in keratin assembly are often due to defects in specific keratins contributing to distinct ichthyoses, erythrokeratodermas, epidermolysis bullosa simplex, and palmoplantar keratodermas. Defects in cell adhesion between keratinocytes cause Hailey-Hailey and Darier disease. Defects in the adhesion of keratinocytes to the basement membrane causes the various subtypes of epidermolysis bullosa.
Bolognia J, Schaffer J, Cerroni L, eds. *Dermatology*. [Philadelphia]: Elsevier, 2018 (ch. 56 and 67).

74. C. Number of melanocytes
Human pigmentation has many contributing genetic factors. In terms of melanocyte biology, differences in the size of melanosome, number of melanosomes, distribution of melanosomes in keratinocytes, and degradation of melanosomes all contribute to pigmentary skin phototypes. For instance, darker skin generally has larger melanosomes, decreased melanosome degradation, and melanosomes transferred as individual organelles rather than membrane-bound clusters. The number of melanocytes is not significantly different between the skin phototypes.
Bolognia J, Schaffer J, Cerroni L, eds. *Dermatology*. [Philadelphia]: Elsevier, 2018 (ch. 65 and 66).

75. B. Neutrophils
Cutaneous small-vessel vasculitis presents with histological evidence of leukocytoclastic vasculitis, including neutrophil attack of the blood vessels and leukocytoclasia. Plasma cells are predominant in zoon's balanitis and may be found in biopsies of syphilis; histiocytes are predominant in histiocytic disorders such as Langerhans cell histiocytosis; plasmacytoid dendritic cells are important in the pathogenesis of autoimmune disorders, such as lupus or psoriasis; Th2 T-cell response is associated with conditions such as atopic dermatitis.
Bolognia J, Schaffer J, Cerroni L, eds. *Dermatology*. [Philadelphia]: Elsevier, 2018 (ch. 24).

76. E. Wooly hair nevus
This patient has a nevus sebaceous, which is caused by somatic (postzygotic) mutations in *HRAS* or *KRAS*. Wooly hair nevus also arises as the result of somatic mosaicism (in *HRAS* or *BRAF*). Ichthyosis with confetti is an example of a disorder that exhibits revertant mosaicism (A); incontinentia pigmenti and CHILD syndrome are X-linked dominant disorders that produce lesions in lines of Blaschko in females as a result of functional mosaicism (lyonization) (B, C); phylloid hypomelanosis usually results from mosaic trisomy 13 (D).
Bolognia J, Schaffer J, Cerroni L, eds. *Dermatology*. [Philadelphia]: Elsevier, 2018 (ch. 55 and 62).

77. D. 50% risk for a male, 0% risk for a female
The vignette describes a patient with X-linked recessive ichthysis. As the name implies, this is an X-linked recessive disorder. Because the patient's mother is a carrier, there is a 50% chance that a male child will inherit the disorder. While there is a 50% chance that a female child will be a carrier of the disease, because of the inheritance pattern there is no risk for an affected female child.
Bolognia J, Schaffer J, Cerroni L, eds. *Dermatology*. [Philadelphia]: Elsevier, 2018 (ch. 57).

78. B. Keratins

The disease pictured is ichthyosis vulgaris, which is associated with mutations in the gene *FLG*, which encodes the protein filaggrin. Filaggrin is short for "filament aggregating protein" because of its ability to aggregate keratin intermediate filaments in the upper granular layer and stratum corneum during skin barrier formation.

Bolognia J, Schaffer J, Cerroni L, eds. *Dermatology.* [Philadelphia]: Elsevier, 2018 (ch. 57).

79. A. Defects of the inner root sheath

Loose anagen syndrome most commonly occurs in young, fair-haired girls; boys and dark-haired children are less commonly affected. These patients have defects of the inner root sheath that result in easily and painlessly plucked hair. Trichoscopy reveals ruffled cuticles and misshapen bulbs. This condition typically improved with age and does not require intervention. A diagnostic clue is the "painless pluck," where a clump of hair is easily pulled from the child's head without any associated pain.

Netherton syndrome is caused by mutations in *SPINK 5*, resulting in hair abnormalities, including trichorrhexis invaginata and trichorrhexis nodosa. Mutations in hair cortex–specific keratin genes *KRT86* and *KRT81* cause monilethrix. Chemical or thermal treatments can result in acquired trichorrhexis nodosa. Tinea capitis is caused by fungal infection of the hair shaft. Mutations in *ATP7A* result in defective copper transport and cause Menkes kinky hair disease, which is characterized by the hair abnormalities pili torti and trichorrhexis nodosa.

Bolognia J, Schaffer J, Cerroni L, eds. *Dermatology.* [Philadelphia]: Elsevier, 2018 (ch. 69).

80. D. Laminin 332

The clinical and pathological descriptions support a diagnosis of junctional epidermolysis bullosa, most commonly resulting from mutations in laminin 332. The resulting cleavage plane occurs at the hemidesmosome. Keratin 5 is mutated in epidermolysis bullosa simplex, whereas collagen VII is mutated in dystrophic epidermolysis bullosa. Plectin is mutated in a subtype of epidermolysis bullosa simplex, which also presents with muscular dystrophy. Keratin 10 mutation is seen in epidermolytic ichthyosis.

Bolognia J, Schaffer J, Cerroni L, eds. *Dermatology.* [Philadelphia]: Elsevier, 2018 (ch. 27; table 32.1 and fig. 32.1).

GENERAL DERMATOLOGY

1. The patient is exposed to surfactants at work and develops a pruritic hand eruption. Patch testing is strongly positive to ethylenediamine. Which of the following medications may cause a systemic contact dermatitis in this patient?

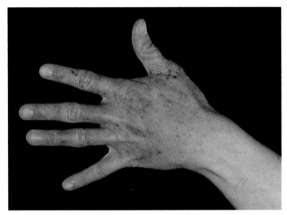

Courtesy Rosemary Nixon, MD. With permission from Nixon RL, Mowad CM, and Marks JG, in Bolognia, *Dermatology*, 2018, Elsevier, 242–261 (fig. 14.3).

  A. Erythromycin
  B. Hydroxyzine
  C. Amoxicillin
  D. Deflazacort
  E. Hydralazine

2. What is the diagnosis?

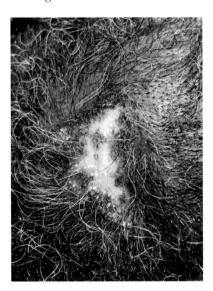

  A. Lichen planopilaris
  B. Discoid lupus erythematosus
  C. Tinea capitis
  D. Folliculitis decalvans

3. This 28-year-old female has a history of worsening alopecia, oral ulcers, fatigue, and joint pains for which she takes intermittent acetaminophen and ibuprofen for the past 5 years. She recently returned from vacation in Mexico with the following eruption. She has not been given any prescription medications in the past several months. The most likely diagnosis is:

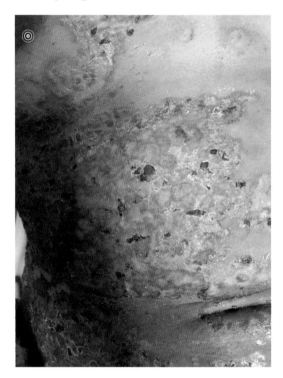

  A. Cutaneous herpes simplex virus
  B. Pemphigus vulgaris
  C. Acute lupus erythematosus
  D. Bullous pemphigoid

4. This 54-year-old athletic patient reports an asymptomatic eruption in his bilateral axillae for the past two decades. What is the diagnosis?

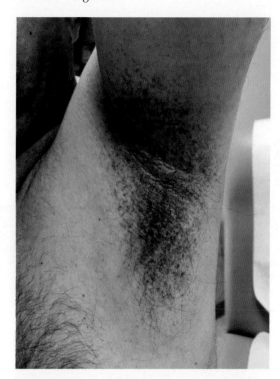

A. Erythrasma
B. Dowling-Degos disease
C. Allergic contact dermatitis
D. Acanthosis nigricans

5. The patient has a history of untreated Crohn disease. Biopsy was performed of the lesions in the figure and did not reveal viral changes of human papillomavirus infection but did show:

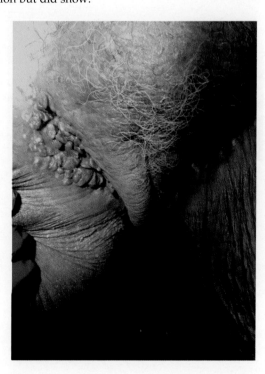

A. Granulomatous infiltrate in the dermis
B. Donovan bodies
C. Koilocytosis
D. Spirochetes

6. What is the next best step?

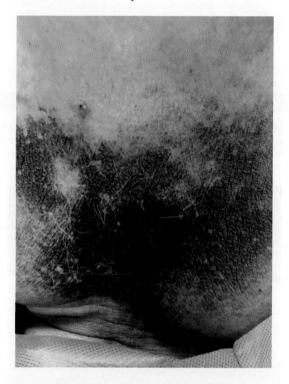

A. Check HbA1c
B. Alcohol swab to the area
C. Minocycline
D. Prescription for urea

7. The diagnosis is:

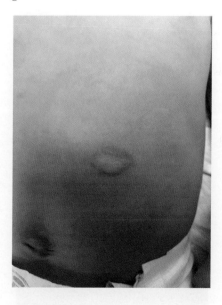

A. Arthropod bite
B. Urticaria
C. Mastocytoma
D. Langerhans histiocytosis

8. An oily substance is extruded upon palpation of these nontender cystic lesions. The patient also has lesions on the chest. What other finding may be present?

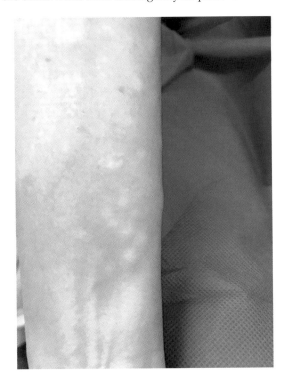

A. Nail dystrophy
B. Colon cancer
C. Renal cell carcinoma
D. Myotonic dystrophy

9. Which of following is most likely associated with this mucosal finding?

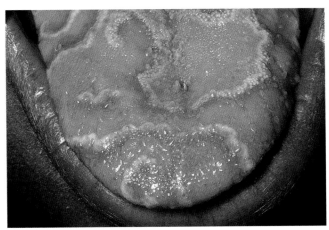

With permission from Allen CM, et al., Oral disease, in Bolognia JL, Schaffer JV, and Cerroni L (eds.), *Dermatology*, 2018, Elsevier, 1220–1242 (fig. 72.3).

A. Vitamin deficiency
B. Candidiasis
C. Smoking
D. Psoriasis
E. Ulcerative colitis

10. A 66-year-old male with a history of drug abuse is seen as an inpatient for the following cutaneous findings. What laboratory abnormality is expected?

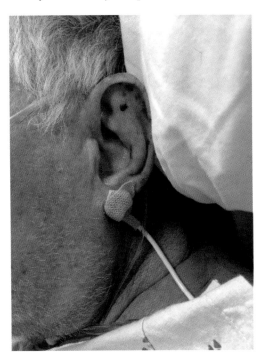

A. Eosinophilia
B. Elevated protein C
C. Elevated antineutrophil cytoplasmic antibodies
D. Elevated antistreptolysin O

11. Which of the following medications may be associated with this patient's skin findings?

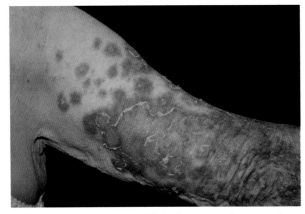

With permission from Jeffrey PC, in Cutaneous lupus erythematosus: Reflecting on practice-changing observations over the past 50 years, *Clinics in Dermatology*, 2018, 36(4):442–449.

A. Terbinafine
B. Hydrochlorothiazide
C. Omeprazole
D. Adalimumab
E. All of the above

12. A 75-year-old man presents with these clinical findings. He is also noted to have longitudinal and horizontal ridging of multiple nails. Which of the following malignancies is most likely to be associated?

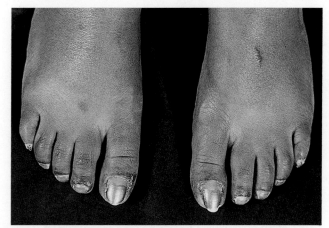

With permission from James WD, Dermal and Subcutaneous Tumors, in *Andrews' Diseases of the Skin Clinical Atlas*, 2018, Elsevier, chapter 28, 405–435.

    A. Laryngeal
    B. Lung
    C. Bladder
    D. Gastrointestinal
    E. Prostate

13. Which of the following is NOT part of the diagnostic criteria for the following condition?

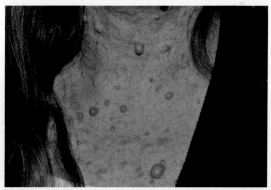

With permission from Hernández MA, Duat Rodríguez A, Part I. Dermatological clinical criteria diagnostic of the disease, *Dermatology* (Actas DermoSifiliográficas, English edition), 2016, volume 107, issue 6, pages 454–464 (fig. 7).

    A. Axillary freckling
    B. First-degree relative with the syndrome
    C. Ash leaf spots
    D. Optic gliomas

14. What is the most common anatomic location for sebaceous carcinoma?
    A. Axilla
    B. Forehead
    C. Eyelid
    D. Lip

15. What type of hyperlipoproteinemia is characterized by eruptive xanthomas without associated systemic metabolic disease?
    A. Type I
    B. Type II
    C. Type III
    D. Type IV
    E. Type V

16. This patient was found to have high titers of desmoglein 3. On review of his medication list, you suggest discontinuing which of the following medications?

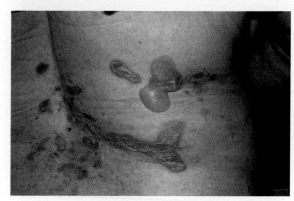

Courtesy Dr Lawrence Lieblich.

    A. Fluconazole
    B. Captopril
    C. Furosemide
    D. Spironolactone

17. The patient who is 30 weeks pregnant presents with a diffusely pruritic eruption. Mineral oil preparation from the skin scrapings reveals the following finding. What is the treatment of choice for this patient?

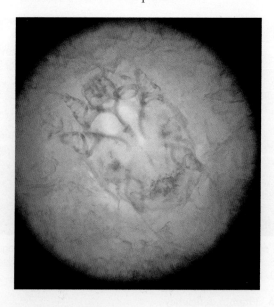

    A. Permethrin cream
    B. Lindane lotion
    C. Crotamiton lotion

D. Oral ivermectin pills
E. Malathion lotion

18. A 2-year-old boy presents to the emergency department with seizures, history of hoarse cry since birth, and CT scan of the head showing bilateral sickle-shaped calcification in the temporal lobes. You are consulted for vesicles on the face but also notice few skin-colored papules on the eyelid margins and ice-pick scars on the face. What gene is mutated?
A. *Col V*
B. *ABCC6*
C. *LMX-1B*
D. *ECM1*

19. An otherwise healthy 25-year-old woman presents with the following after exposure to water. Which test is indicated?

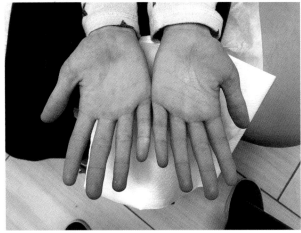

Courtesy Roman Bronfenbrener, MD, Philadelphia, PA.

A. Filaggrin sequencing
B. Cystic fibrosis transmembrane conductance regulator (CFTR) mutation screen
C. Starch-iodine test
D. RPR

20. This healthy 45-year-old female with no systemic symptoms presents with the following eruption. Diagnosis is:

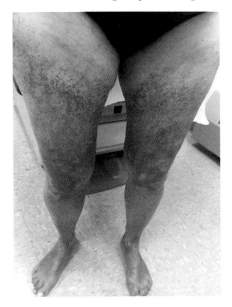

A. Generalized essential telangiectasia
B. Angioma serpiginosum
C. Systemic lupus erythematosus
D. Rothmund-Thomson syndrome

21. What drug is NOT associated with these lesions?

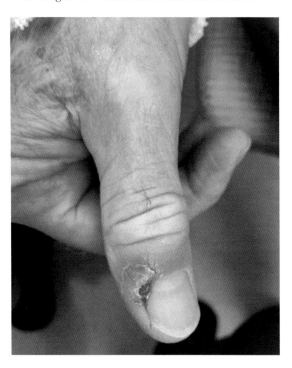

A. Indinavir
B. Isotretinoin
C. Tetracycline
D. Cetuximab

22. What is the diagnosis?

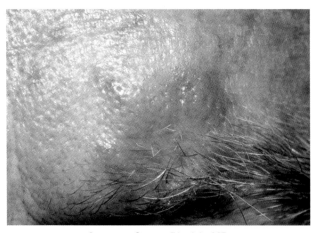

Courtesy Steven Binnick, MD.

A. Granuloma faciale
B. Angiolymphoid hyperplasia with eosinophilia
C. Leprosy
D. B-cell lymphoma

23. A 16-year-old male presents to your office for evaluation after his sibling was just diagnosed with NAME syndrome

(Carney complex). Which of the findings below would NOT be a pertinent finding in regards to this diagnosis? (may have more than one correct answer)
- **A.** Blue macules on his extremities
- **B.** Brown macules of the right eye medial canthus and nasal sidewall
- **C.** History of atrial myxoma
- **D.** Pulmonary stenosis
- **E.** Vertical striae on the abdomen
- **F.** Enlarged facial bone structure
- **G.** Patchy scalp hair loss
- **H.** Testicular nodule

24. A healthy middle-aged male presented with this eruption after spending the weekend on his snowmobile in frigid temperatures. This was caused by:

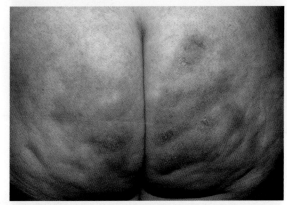

With permission James WD, *Andrews' Diseases of the Skin Clinical Atlas*, Elsevier, 2018, chapter 23, 331–338.

- **A.** Reaction to a medication
- **B.** Autoimmune disease
- **C.** Foreign body reaction
- **D.** Environmental exposure
- **E.** Malignancy

25. An 84-year-old man has been treated for rosacea for many years. He has similar pigmentary changes on cheeks, shins, forearms, and dorsal hands. What are the histologic findings of the following hyperpigmented condition?

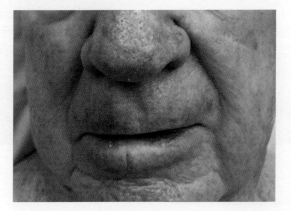

- **A.** Increased basal epidermal melanin
- **B.** Brown-black granules in dermal macrophages, positive Perls, and Fontana-Masson stains
- **C.** Brown-black granules in dermal macrophages, positive for Perls' stain only

- **D.** Yellow-brown, large, banana-shaped aggregates in the dermis

26. A patient with HIV presents with this asymptomatic lesion for the past week. He has no medication allergies. What is the recommended treatment?

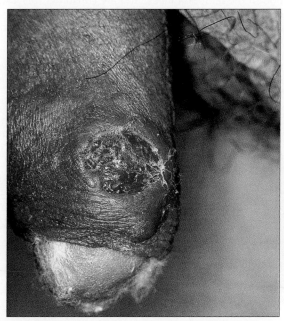

With permission from Lupi O, *Tropical Dermatology*, 2017, Elsevier, chapter 26, 313–345.

- **A.** IM benzathine penicillin
- **B.** Doxycycline
- **C.** IM ceftriaxone
- **D.** Acyclovir
- **E.** Azithromycin

27. What is the most likely allergen?

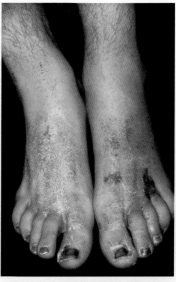

Courtesy of Steven Binnick, MD.

- **A.** Tocopheryl acetate
- **B.** Methylchloroisothiazolinone

  C. Potassium dichromate
  D. Glyceryl thioglycolate

28. Which choice is NOT a criterion for systemic mastocytosis?
  A. Atypical mast-cell morphology
  B. Aberrant mast-cell surface phenotype
  C. Serum/plasma serotonin levels
  D. Serum/plasma tryptase levels
  E. c-*Kit* mutation

29. A protester presents urgently from a demonstration after being sprayed with pepper spray. What do you tell her to do?
  A. Rinse off with water only
  B. Apply a class 1 topical steroid
  C. Rinse with water and soap followed by vegetable oil soak
  D. Do not rinse, apply talcum powder

30. You are consulted to see a 24-year-old graduate student in the ICU with cardiogenic shock, hemolysis, and acute kidney injury with a solitary necrotic eschar on the inner arm. She reports it originally was exquisitely painful, had a marblelike appearance with blood blisters, and developed within a few hours after noticing a mild burning sensation in the area while she was camping in the Ozarks while home in Arkansas last week. What is the toxin responsible for this reaction?
  A. Alpha-latrotoxin
  B. Sphingomyelinase-D
  C. Agatoxin
  D. Hyaluronidase
  E. A & B
  F. B & D
  G. B & C

31. What is the best treatment for this tender and fluctuant lesion in an otherwise healthy 25-year-old man who works in the hospital and presents with leg pain and fever?

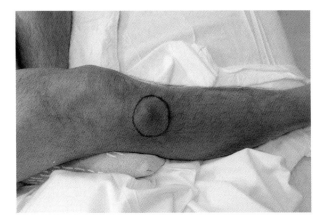

  A. Incision and drainage
  B. Trimethoprim-sulfamethoxazole
  C. High-potency topical steroids
  D. Cephalexin
  E. Itraconazole
  F. A & B

32. A 29-year-old woman who is 12 weeks pregnant presents with these expanding lesions on her popliteal fossae, buttocks, and legs over the past week. She also reports associated low-grade fevers and generalized malaise for which she has been taking acetaminophen. What is the best next step?

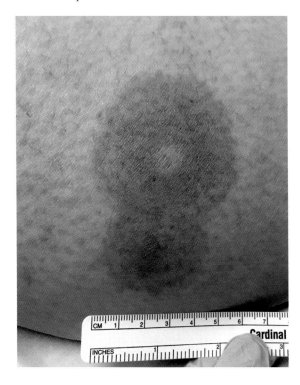

  A. Start amoxicillin
  B. Check RPR
  C. Discontinue acetaminophen
  D. Biopsy for H&E and direct immunofluorescence
  E. Doxycycline

33. A 4-year-old boy presents with his mother to the pediatric emergency department with acute onset fever, rhinorrhea, and severe irritability upon examination. What is the best management?

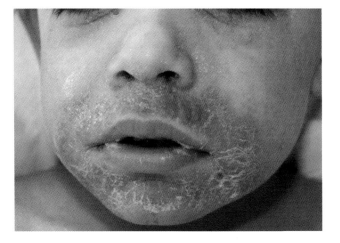

  A. Bleach baths and topical steroids
  B. Intravenous immunoglobulin and aspirin
  C. Hospitalize and intravenous antistaphylococcal antibiotics
  D. Detailed drug history and cyclosporine

34. What is the most appropriate test for this 50-year-old man with a history of intravenous drug use presenting with fevers and these painless lesions?

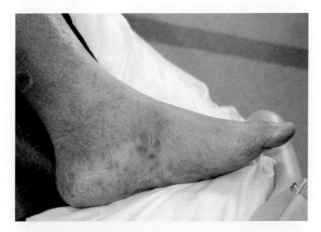

   A. KOH and fungal culture
   B. Urine toxicology screen and Anti-neutrophil cytoplasmic antibodies
   C. HIV screen
   D. Blood cultures and echocardiography

35. A 7-year-old boy presents with fevers, severe headache, and abdominal pain for the past 3 days and a new rash that appeared today. He denies any sick close contacts or recent travel. What is the treatment of choice?

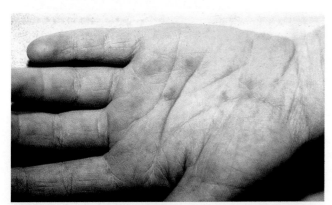

With permission Rickettsia rickettsii and other spotted fever group rickettsiae (rocky mountain spotted fever and other spotted fevers), in Mandell GL, et al. (eds.), *Principles and Practice of Infectious Diseases,* 8th edition, 2015, Churchill Livingstone: New York.

   A. Oral doxycycline
   B. Supportive care only
   C. Stop acetaminophen and change to NSAIDs
   D. IV ceftriaxone
   E. Oral ivermectin

36. This 11-year-old healthy boy presents with the following skin lesions on the face and thigh. He also complains of fever and headache. What is the most likely mode of transmission?

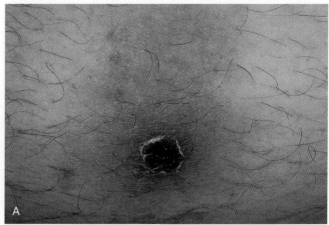

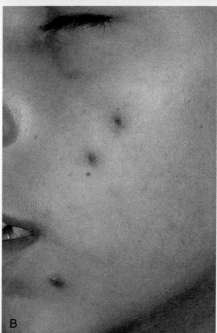

With permission from Walker DH, Blanton LS, *Dermatology,* 2018, Elsevier, 1319–1328 (fig. 76.8).

   A. Cat flea
   B. House mouse mite
   C. Brown dog tick
   D. Human body louse

37. A 38-year-old man complains of asymptomatic hair loss over the past 3 months. He denies scalp pruritus. What is the most appropriate test for this condition?

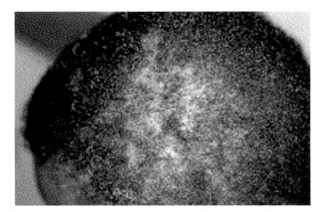

With permission from Zeltser R, et al., *Clin Dermatol* 2004, volume 22, issue 6, 461–468 (fig. 8).

    A. Fungal culture
    B. Antinuclear antibody
    C. VDRL
    D. TSH

38. A 37-year-old man presents with the following painful lesions. He reports unprotected sexual activity and multiple partners. What is the most likely causal agent?

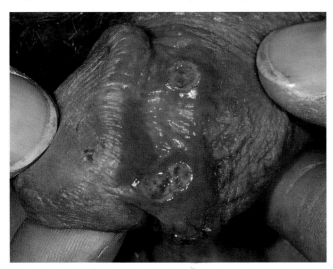

With permission from Habif TB, *Clinical Dermatology*, 6th edition, 2016, Elsevier, 1–74.

    A. *Neisseria gonorrhoeae*
    B. *Chlamydia trachomatis L1-3*
    C. *Klebsiella granulomatis*
    D. *Hemophilus ducreyi*
    E. *Treponema pallidum*

39. The patient presented with new onset lesions on the face and oral mucosa. What is the best diagnostic test for these lesions?

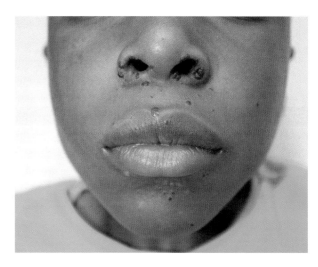

    A. Enterovirus PCR from nasopharyngeal swab
    B. Histopathological identification of noncaseating granulomas
    C. History checking for topical corticosteroid use
    D. Patch testing

40. What is the best treatment for this condition?

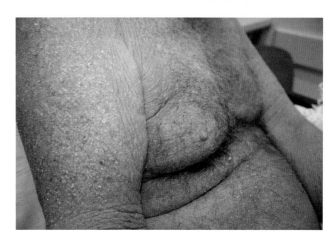

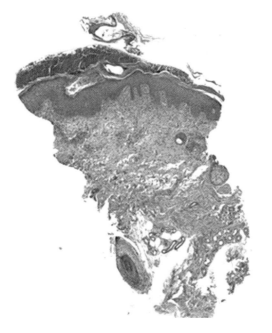

A. Open-wet dressings and topical steroids
B. Topical permethrin and oral ivermectin
C. Cyclosporine
D. Supportive care only

PEDIATRIC DERMATOLOGY

41. Which of the following is the most likely diagnosis for this boy, who also exhibits hypertrichosis and coarse facies?

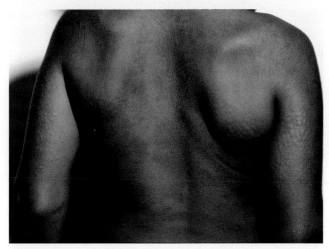

Courtesy Paul Honig, MD.

A. Phakomatosis pigmentovascularis type II
B. Trisomy 21
C. Giant congenital nevus
D. Hunter syndrome
E. McCune-Albright syndrome

42. This otherwise healthy teenage girl presents with a several-month history of the below eruption. She is at increased risk of developing all of the following EXCEPT:

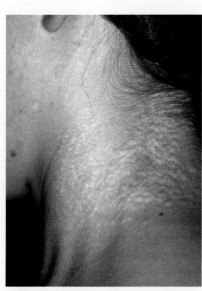

With permission from James WD, *Andrews' Diseases of the Skin Clinical Atlas*, 2018, Elsevier, chapter 25, 351–359.

A. Angioid streaks
B. Myocardial infarction
C. Cerebral hemorrhage
D. Atherosclerosis
E. Gastric artery hemorrhage
F. Restrictive lung disease
G. Mitral valve prolapse
H. Blindness

43. A 7-year-old boy presents with recurrent episodes of the pictured rash over the face, trunk, and extremities, accompanied by fever, abdominal pain, pain in his limbs, and conjunctivitis. The rash is transient and self-resolves after 1–2 days. Biopsy of the rash shows a sparse perivascular and interstitial neutrophilic infiltrate within the dermis, and the rash has been nonresponsive to oral diphenhydramine. Which of the following is a long-term treatment for this patient?

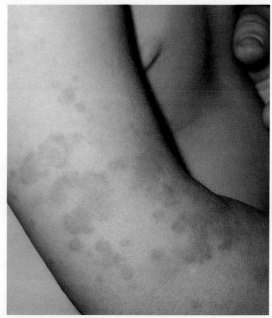

With permission from Nguyen TV, *Journal of the American Academy of Dermatology*, volume 68, issue 5, 834–853.

A. Cetirizine
B. Adalimumab
C. Prednisone
D. Rituximab
E. Anakinra

44. A 7-month-old boy is referred for severe atopic dermatitis. His mother reports that he also bruises easily, has had recurrent ear infections, and has been hospitalized for pneumonia. On exam, in addition to findings consistent with severe atopic dermatitis, there are petechiae and ecchymoses of the hard palate and skin. Which of the following lab abnormalities is most likely to be found in this patient?
A. Elevated IgM
B. Giant granules in platelets
C. Thrombocytopenia
D. Low IgE
E. Low IgA
F. Neutrophilia
G. Prolonged PTT

45. This 19-year-old patient has had the pictured skin condition since infancy. He was born via cesarean section because of failure of labor to progress, and he has a similarly affected uncle. Based on his likely diagnosis, he should be counseled that he has an increased risk of which of the following?

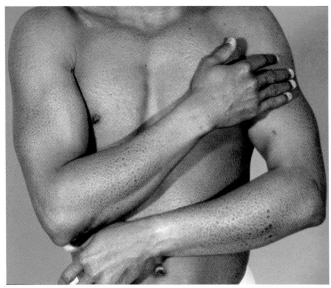

With permission from James WD, *Andrews' Diseases of the Skin Clinical Atlas*, 2018, Elsevier, chapter 27, 379–404.

A. Blindness due to corneal opacities
B. Progressive spastic di- and tetraplegia
C. Collodion membrane in an affected offspring
D. Testicular cancer
E. Sensorineural hearing impairment

46. A 7-year-old girl presents with a 6-month history of a pink-red plaque on the leg that has recently ulcerated. Biopsy shows collections of histiocytes, and a sterile culture for bacterial, fungal, and mycobacterial growth is negative. She also has the below ocular findings, which first developed 4 years ago. Her mother reports progressive impairment in her ability to walk. Based on her likely diagnosis, she has an increased risk of developing which of the following?

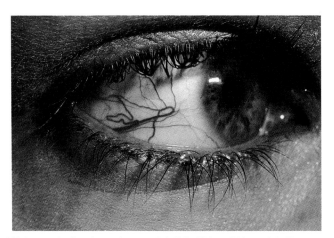

With permission from Antonovich DD, Thiers BH, and Jeffrey PC, in Dermatologic manifestations of internal malignancy, *Cancer of the Skin*, 2nd edition, 2011, 367–378 (fig. 34.9).

A. Pulmonary arteriovenous malformation
B. Glaucoma
C. Cold abscesses
D. Myelokathexis
E. Lymphoma

47. This 2-week-old otherwise healthy infant presents with this skin lesion, and a biopsy was performed as shown. What is the most appropriate next step?

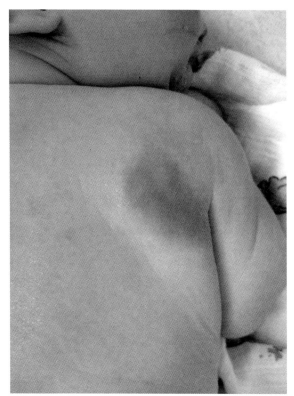

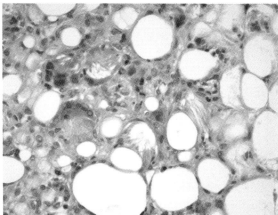

With permission from James WD, *Andrews' Diseases of the Skin Clinical Atlas*, 2018, Elsevier, chapter 23, 331–338 (*top figure*) and Darling MD, *Dermatology Secrets Plus*, 2016, Elsevier, chapter 19, 170–178 (*lower figure*).

A. Report suspected nonaccidental trauma
B. Systemic antibiotics
C. Serial monitoring of calcium
D. MRI of the chest/abdomen/pelvis
E. Admission to the neonatal ICU
F. Reassurance

48. Wright stain of a pustule from this otherwise healthy 12-hour-old infant would most likely reveal which of the following?

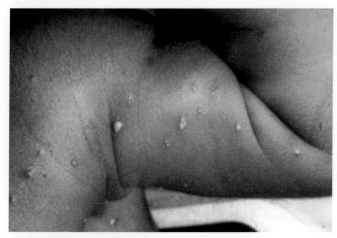

With permission from Gleason, in *Avery's Diseases of the Newborn*, Tenth edition, 2018, Elsevier (fig. 106.2).

A. Eosinophils
B. Neutrophils
C. Yeast
D. Multinucleated giant cells
E. Lymphocytes
F. Mast cells

49. A teenage patient with the pictured dental findings may also exhibit any of the following EXCEPT:

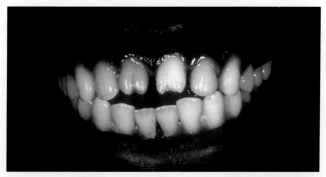

With permission from James WD, *Andrews' Diseases of the Skin Clinical Atlas*, 2018, Elsevier, chapter 18, 251–261.

A. Parrot pseudoparalysis
B. Saddle nose
C. Symmetric knee swelling
D. Deafness
E. Enlargement of the medial third of the clavicle
F. Interstitial keratitis
G. Radial periorificial scars

50. Skin biopsy of this lesion is most likely to show which of the following?

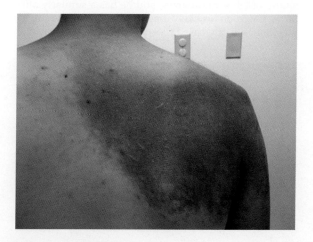

A. Tightly packed capillaries in discrete lobules
B. Tracking of melanocytes around and within appendages, vessels, or nerves
C. Proliferation of smooth muscle bundles in the dermis
D. Large hypertrophied nerves
E. Increased dermal collagen bundles

DERMATOPATHOLOGY

51. A 1-year-old boy presents with papules. A biopsy is performed. Bedside examination of one of the lesions would demonstrate which of the following findings?

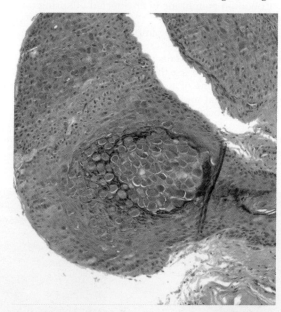

Reprinted with permission from Chen et al., in Molluscum contagiosum virus infection, *The Lancet Infectious Diseases*, 2013, 13:877–888. (© Elsevier)

A. Hemophagocytosis
B. Donovan bodies
C. Owl's eye inclusions
D. Multinucleate giant cells
E. Henderson-Paterson bodies

52. A 50-year-old man presents with numerous papules, some linearly arrayed on a background of shiny, indurated plaques on his back and neck. A skin biopsy is performed. Alcian blue staining (as shown) is ordered in addition to normal H&E evaluation. Which of the following is the correct diagnosis?

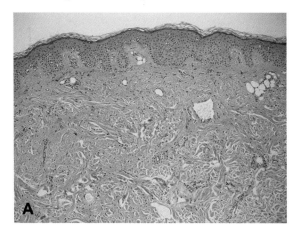

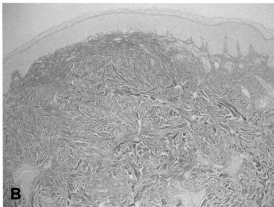

With permission from Rey and Luria, *J Am Acad Dermatol*, 2008, volume 60, 1038 (fig. 2).

    A. Scleromyxedema
    B. Scleredema
    C. Granuloma annulare
    D. Actinic granuloma
    E. Lupus erythematosus

53. You receive teledermatology consult with no associated information except for patient demographics (70-year-old female), one clinical photograph, and one histologic image from a skin biopsy. Medical records and a history from the referring clinician will be solicited. However, given the likely diagnosis, what is the single most important piece of medical information to specifically request?

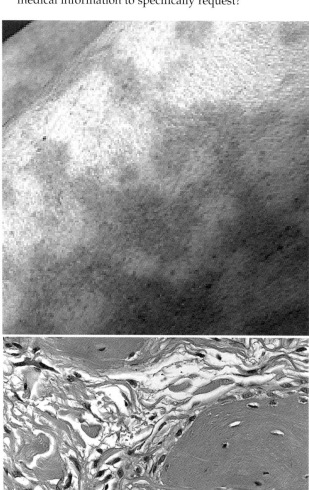

With permission from Girardi, et al., *J Am Acad Dermatol*, 2011, volume 65, 1101–1103 (figs. 1 and 38).

    A. History of Albright hereditary osteodystrophy
    B. History of radiation
    C. Prior treatment with bleomycin
    D. History of CREST/scleroderma
    E. Exposure to gadolinium contrast

54. The tumor shown may be associated with which one of the following viruses?

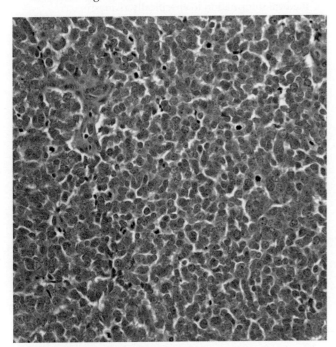

   A. Epstein-Barr virus (EBV)
   B. Human T-lymphotropic virus (HTLV)
   C. Human papilloma virus (HPV)
   D. Polyoma virus

55. What is the best diagnosis?

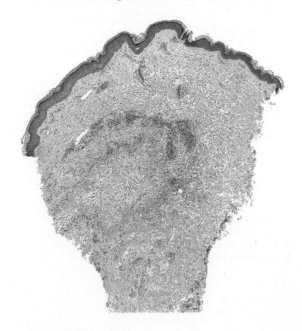

   A. Dermatofibroma
   B. Granuloma annulare
   C. Necrobiosis lipoidica
   D. Sarcoidosis

56. What is the best diagnosis for this solitary lesion?

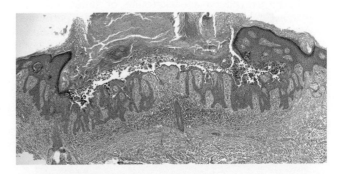

   A. Acantholytic actinic keratosis
   B. Acantholytic dyskeratotic acanthoma
   C. Epidermolytic dyskeratotic acanthoma
   D. Herpesvirus infection

57. What is the best diagnosis?

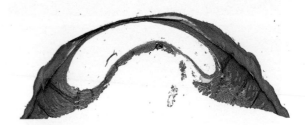

   A. Hidrocystoma
   B. Digital mucous cyst
   C. Pilar cyst
   D. Branchial cyst

58. Which of the following is the most likely genetic aberration associated with this lesion?

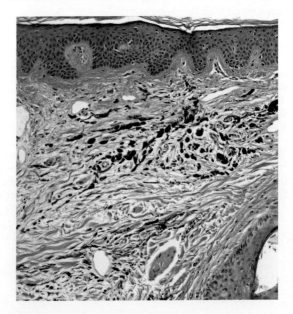

   A. *BRAF* mutation
   B. *GNAQ* mutation
   C. *C-KIT* mutation
   D. *PDGFB* translocation

59. What is the best diagnosis?

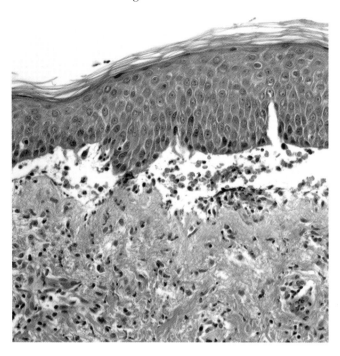

A. Bullous pemphigoid
B. Bullous lupus erythematosus
C. Pemphigus vulgaris
D. Dermatitis herpetiformis

60. What is the best diagnosis?

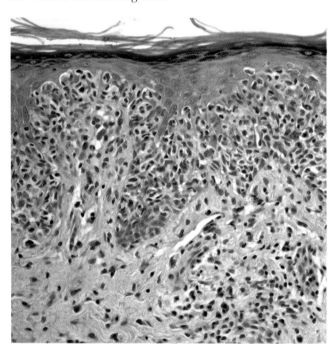

A. Squamous cell carcinoma in situ/Bowen disease
B. Extramammary Paget disease
C. Mycosis fungoides/cutaneous T-cell lymphoma (CTCL)
D. Intraepidermal Merkel cell carcinoma

PROCEDURAL DERMATOLOGY

61. A 69-year-old male presents to your office 1 week after Mohs surgery for treatment of a basal cell carcinoma on the upper nasal sidewall. The site was repaired with a flap closure. He complains of excessive tearing following the surgery. Which structure was likely injured?
A. Lacrimal gland
B. Tarsus
C. Nasolacrimal duct
D. Anterior ethmoid artery

62. A 20-year-old male presents to your office for evaluation of lesions within the radiation field for treatment of medulloblastoma as a child. On exam he is noted to have an eroded papulonodule on the right neck and numerous acrochordons on his left neck, as shown. What gene mutation should this patient be tested for?

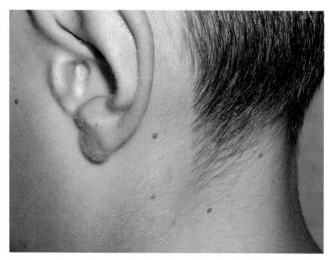

With permission from Feito-Rodriguez M, et al., *J Amer Acad Dermatol*, 2009, Volume 60, Issue 5, 857–961.

A. *PTCH*
B. *PTEN*
C. *Notch1*
D. *P53*
E. *TSC1*

63. Appropriate antibiotic regimens for patients that require prophylaxis prior to dermatologic surgery for a lesion on the leg include all of the following EXCEPT:
A. Cephalexin 2g PO x 1
B. TMP-SMX DS 1 tablet PO x 1
C. Clindamycin 300 mg PO x 1
D. Levofloxacin 500 mg PO x 1

64. What is the porphyrin responsible for the efficacy of photodynamic therapy?
A. Aminolevulinic acid
B. Protoporphyrin IX
C. Coproporphyrinogen II
D. Uroporphyrinogen II

65. A 51-year-old female has Mohs surgery performed for a basal cell carcinoma in the right external auditory meatus. The lesions are removed with three Mohs stages and the 1.5 x 2.0 cm circumferential wound is allowed to heal by second intention. One week after surgery, the patient returns to your office complaining of severe pain and fullness with muffled hearing in the right ear. Appropriate management would include which of the following:
- **A.** Ibuprofen 600 mg PO q6–8h and instructions for vinegar soaks
- **B.** Ciprofloxacin PO x 7 days
- **C.** Referral to otolaryngology for evaluation of a wick placement in the external auditory meatus
- **D.** A and B
- **E.** B and C

66. A 34-year-old female presents for treatment with pulsed-dye laser for erythrotelangiectatic rosacea and photo-damage-associated telangiectasias. She is a saleswoman and needs to return to work tomorrow for a meeting and is concerned about bruising. Which would be the most appropriate pulse duration for her?
- **A.** 1.5 ms
- **B.** 3 ms
- **C.** 10 ms
- **D.** 40 ms

67. A 58-year-old renal transplant recipient has been surgically treated for seven invasive SCCs and three SCC in-situs in the last 2 years. She also has more than 30 actinic keratoses on the face, scalp, and upper extremities. Her renal transplant was performed 5 years ago and is functioning well. She is maintained on tacrolimus and mycophenolate mofetil immunosuppression. Which of the following interventions will have the greatest impact in reduction of future skin cancer for this patient?
- **A.** Oral acitretin
- **B.** Oral niacinamide
- **C.** Topical 5-fluorouracil
- **D.** Topical imiquimod
- **E.** Change immunosuppression to sirolimus-based regimen

68. A patient presents to your office for consideration of soft tissue filler. After review of the possible adverse reactions, she states that she wants to avoid treatment of areas most prone to injection into a vessel. Which of the following treatment areas have the highest risk of vascular occlusion?
- **A.** Nasolabial folds and tear troughs
- **B.** Upper lip and lateral temples
- **C.** Glabella and perinasal area
- **D.** Nasal dorsum and lateral cheeks

69. A patient underwent treatment with hyaluronic acid filler in the nasolabial folds 1 day ago. She calls the office complaining of severe pain and redness of the upper lip area. She is instructed to come into the office for evaluation and management. Management options of this condition include all of the following EXCEPT:
- **A.** Cold compresses
- **B.** Application of nitropaste
- **C.** Initiation of oral aspirin therapy
- **D.** Hyperbaric oxygen
- **E.** Flushing the area with serial injections of hyaluronidase

70. A patient underwent treatment with a deep chemical peel, which resulted in the following complications seen in the photo. Which of the ingredients of the

Baker-Gordon peel is responsible for causing the complications pictured?

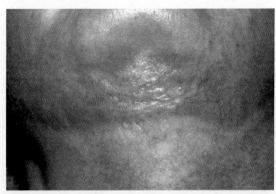

With permission Monheit GD, Chastain M, Chemical and mechanical skin resurfacing, In *Dermatology*. 2018, 2593–2609, Elsevier (fig. 154.11).

- **A.** Phenol
- **B.** Croton oil
- **C.** Septisol
- **D.** Resorcinol

BASIC SCIENCE

71. The patient shown most likely has a mutation in a protein with which of the following functions?

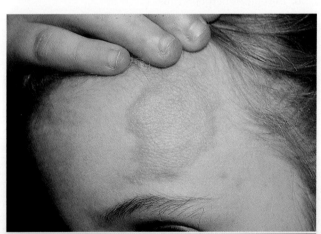

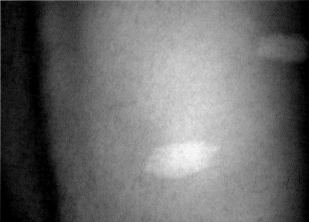

Courtesy Steven Binnick, MD.

A. Negatively regulate Ras signaling
B. DNA mismatch repair
C. Downregulated the Wnt/β-catenin signaling pathway
D. Negatively regulate mTOR signaling
E. Glycosphingolipid metabolism

72. An 11-year-old girl with a history of squamous cell carcinoma is brought to your office for total body skin examination. Her cutaneous examination is notable for poikiloderma as shown in the figure. She has no known developmental anomalies. Which of the following is most likely responsible for these manifestations?

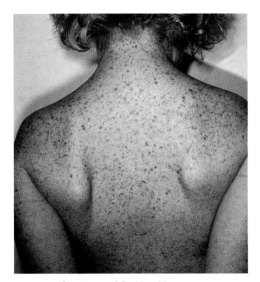

Courtesy of Dr Ken Kraemer.

A. Increased rates of sister chromatid exchange and chromosomal instability
B. Defective transcription-coupled nucleotide excision repair
C. Defective DNA replication
D. Defective formation of the nuclear envelope
E. Defective nucleotide excision repair

73. Distraught parents bring their teenage son to you for further evaluation of recurrent episodes of thrush, chronic paronychia, and dental anomalies. He was recently diagnosed with hypoparathyroidism. He was adopted from overseas, and his family history is unknown. You suspect an underlying syndrome due to a defect in which gene?
A. *STAT1*
B. *STAT3*
C. *DOCK8*
D. *AIRE*
E. *CARD14*

74. An 8-year-old girl and her similarly affected father present with the skin findings shown. What is the most likely cause?

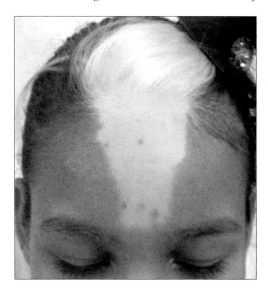

A. Autoimmune destruction of melanocytes
B. Defective melanin synthesis
C. Defective migration of melanoblasts
D. Overgrowth of *Malassezia furfur*
E. Chemical depigmentation

75. An 8-year-old boy is referred to your office for evaluation of nodular lesions on his lower extremities. Examination is notable for yellow-red papulonodules with central punctum. You also note several atrophic scars and the findings shown. What is the most common etiologic mutation in this condition?

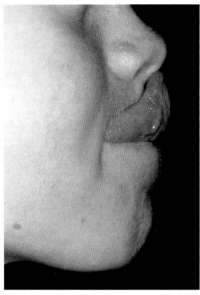

With permission from James WD, Elston DM, McMahon PJ, Abnormalities of dermal fibrous and elastic tissue, in *Andrews' Diseases of the Skin Clinical Atlas*, 2017, Elsevier, 351–359 (fig. 25–32).

A. Type V collagen
B. Tenascin X
C. Type III collagen
D. Fibrillin 1
E. ABCC6

76. A 14-month-old boy is brought to your office for evaluation of a rash, which has waxed and waned over the past several months. Which of the following cell types is responsible for these findings?

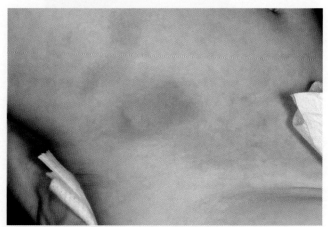

With permission from Paller AS, Mancini AJ (eds), Cutaneous tumors and tumor syndromes, in *Hurwitz Clinical Pediatric Dermatology*, 5th edition, 2016, Elsevier, 193–229 (fig. 9-52).

- **A.** Neutrophils
- **B.** Mast cells
- **C.** Eosinophils
- **D.** Lymphocytes
- **E.** Langerhans cells

77. A 40-year-old man presents with numerous yellow papules on the face, chest, back, and abdomen. Biopsy reveals lobules of sebaceous glands within the dermis. He reports a strong family history of colon cancer. What is the function of the mutated genes in the associated condition?
- **A.** Mismatch repair
- **B.** Activation of smoothened
- **C.** ATPase/calcium signaling
- **D.** Connexin gap junction signaling
- **E.** Lysosomal transport

78. Keratinopathies represent genetic disorders of the keratin genes. For example, epidermolytic ichthyosis is caused by mutations in keratin 1 or keratin 10. Keratins are intermediate filament proteins that share a common domain organization as shown in the image, where a central coiled-coil helical rod domain is flanked by head and tail regions. The rod domain itself has four regions denoted helix 1A, 1B, 2A, and 2B. Which two regions of keratins are "mutational hot spots" for the majority of missense mutations associated with keratinopathies?

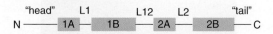

- **A.** Head and tail domains
- **B.** 1A and 2A domains
- **C.** 1B and 2B domains
- **D.** 1A and 1B domains
- **E.** 1A and 2B domains

79. The syndrome responsible for this clinical presentation is associated with mutations in which intercellular junction protein?

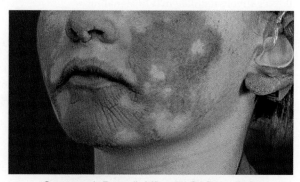

Courtesy, L Russell, MD, and SJ Bale, PhD.

- **A.** Cadherin
- **B.** Desmoplakin
- **C.** Keratin
- **D.** Occludin
- **E.** Connexin 26
- **F.** Connexin 43

80. You are treating a patient with this eruption using first-line adult therapy. What is the primary molecular target of the drug you prescribe?

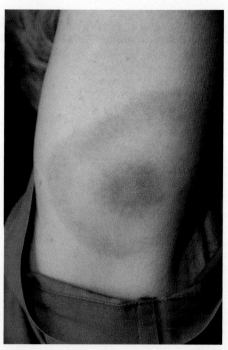

With permission from CDC Public Health Image Library, image identification number 9875. Photo credit James Gathany, accessed November 3, 2016, http://phil.cdc.gov/.

- **A.** DNA gyrase
- **B.** RNA Polymerase
- **C.** 30S ribosomal subunit
- **D.** 50S ribosomal subunit
- **E.** Folic acid metabolism
- **F.** Cell wall synthesis

GENERAL DERMATOLOGY

1. B. Hydroxyzine
Ethylenediamine is used in various medications and industrial mixtures as a preservative, emulsifier, and stabilizer. Patients sensitized to ethylenediamine may have a systemic contact dermatitis with ingestion of hydroxyzine, cetirizine, piperazine, and aminophylline.
Bolognia J, Schaffer J, Cerroni L, eds. *Dermatology.* [Philadelphia]: Elsevier, 2018 (ch. 14).
Aquino M, Rosner G. Systemic contact dermatitis. *Clin Rev Allergy Immunol.* 2019;56(1):9–18.

2. B. Discoid lupus erythematosus
This patient has discoid lupus erythematosus. Discoid lesions may result in scarring alopecia, as seen in this case, along with classic follicular plugging, central hypopigmentation, and peripheral hyperpigmentation. Antinuclear antibody may be positive in a small subset of cutaneous discoid lupus patients, although most do not go on to develop systemic lupus. Treatment includes intralesional steroids, antimalarial drugs, oral retinoids, or immunomodulatory agents such as methotrexate or mycophenolate mofetil in severe cases. Lichen planopilaris is another type of cicatricial alopecia, which presents with perifollicular scale and erythema. Loss of follicular ostia occurs as the disease progresses. Patients may have burning, itching, and tingling of the scalp. Kerion presents as boggy plaques with overlying alopecia as a complication of tinea capitis. Pustules, scale, and broken hairs are key clinical features of tinea capitis. Folliculitis decalvans, another cicatricial alopecia, presents as follicular papulopustules, which results in destruction of the hair follicle. *Staphylococcal aureus* may be cultured.
Bolognia J, Schaffer J, Cerroni L, eds. *Dermatology.* [Philadelphia]: Elsevier, 2018 (ch. 69).

3. C. Acute lupus erythematosus
The patient has diffuse erosions and skin necrosis in the setting of systemic lupus (history of fevers, photosensitivity, joint pain, alopecia, and oral ulcers), possibly triggered by excessive ultraviolet exposure and consistent with a toxic epidermal necrolysis (TEN)-like presentation of acute cutaneous lupus erythematosus. This falls within the spectrum of acute syndrome of apoptotic pan-epidermolysis (ASAP), a clinical syndrome manifesting with necrosis and cleavage of the epidermis with significant apoptosis. The differential diagnosis includes Stevens-Johnson Syndrome (SJS)/TEN, immunobullous disease, TEN-like acute graft-versus-host disease, and TEN-like lupus erythematosus. In addition to history and review of systems, other physical signs of cutaneous lupus (e.g., discoid lesions or Subacute cutaneous lupus erythematosus) and serological tests (ANA, dsDNA, Sm, SSA, SSB) may help establish the diagnosis. Workup should include a biopsy and DIF. Histology of TEN-like lupus demonstrates epidermal necrosis with inflammatory perivascular infiltrate with neutrophils. DIF may reveal deposition of immunoglobulins in the basement membrane as well as complement in dermal vessels. Treatment for TEN-like conditions is similar to that of classical drug-induced TEN, including supportive skin care and immunosuppression. Other bullous presentations of lupus include bullous systemic lupus and Rowell syndrome (EM-like lesions associated with lupus).
Bolognia J, Schaffer J, Cerroni L, eds. *Dermatology.* [Philadelphia]: Elsevier, 2018 (ch. 41).

4. B. Dowling-Degos disease
Dowling-Degos disease is an uncommon autosomal dominant condition with variable penetrance caused by loss-of-function mutations in the keratin 5 gene (*KRT5*). Patients present with reticulated hyperpigmentation in flexural areas. Additional features include comedone-like lesions on the back or neck, pitted perioral scars, epidermoid cysts, and hidradenitis suppurativa. Treatments are variable and limited, including hydroquinone, topical retinoids, topical steroids, and laser therapy. Erythrasma is a bacterial infection caused by *Corynebacterium minutissimum* and presents with brown scaly patches in intertriginous areas. Allergic contact dermatitis of the axillae typically presents with pruritus or burning, erythema, and scale. Acanthosis nigricans is in the differential diagnosis of Dowling-Degos disease and presents with velvety thickened plaques in the axilla and neck associated with impaired insulin regulation.
Bolognia J, Schaffer J, Cerroni L, eds. *Dermatology.* [Philadelphia]: Elsevier, 2018 (ch. 67).

5. A. Granulomatous infiltrate in the dermis
The patient has vulvar swelling and infiltrative lesions in the inguinal folds in the setting of known Crohn disease. This Kodachrome represents cutaneous Crohn disease, which can present as a manifestation of known Crohn disease or present prior to bowel disease. A key clinical clue is vulvar swelling. Other manifestations of cutaneous Crohn include ulcers (knifelike), fissures, sinus tracts, or vegetating plaques. Pyostomatitis vegetans of the oral mucosa is associated with inflammatory bowel disease (classically ulcerative colitis) and manifests as snail-like pustules on an inflamed base. Hidradenitis suppurativa is also in the differential for cutaneous Crohn. Colonoscopy with biopsy should be performed if there is a high suspicion for inflammatory bowel disease. There is no consistent correlation between the appearance of skin lesions and intestinal Crohn disease activity. Donovan bodies (rod-shaped organisms in the cytoplasm of histiocytes) are found in granuloma inguinale, a sexually transmitted disease caused by *Klebsiella granulomatis*. Clinical presentation includes beefy red nodules that later erode and form ulcers in the perianal area and genitals. Primary syphilis presents with a painless ulcer (chancre) on the mucosa, not with vulvar swelling and infiltrative lesions. It is important to recognize the cutaneous manifestations of Crohn disease.
Bolognia J, Schaffer J, Cerroni L, eds. *Dermatology.* [Philadelphia]: Elsevier, 2018 (ch. 93).

6. B. Alcohol swab to the area
Terra firma–forme dermatosis results from extensive retention hyperkeratosis. The mid-back location is common. It is easily diagnosed by rubbing an alcohol swab on the lesions, with immediate removal of the discoloration revealing normal underlying skin. While lesions can respond to keratolytics such as urea and ammonium lactate, the best next step would be using an alcohol swab to diagnose the condition. Treatment includes washing the area thoroughly and keratolytics. HbA1c should be checked in patients with acanthosis nigricans (AN), which is associated with hyperinsulinemia. Minocycline is the treatment of choice for confluent and reticulated papillomatosis (CARP), which presents as reticulated keratotic and pigmented papules on the chest and back and sometimes intertriginous areas. While important to consider AN and CARP in the differential diagnosis of this eruption, the use of an alcohol swab will avoid further unnecessary diagnostic tests and inappropriate treatments.
Bolognia J, Schaffer J, Cerroni L, eds. *Dermatology.* [Philadelphia]: Elsevier, 2018 (ch. 109).

7. C. Mastocytoma

Mastocytomas are localized presentations of cutaneous mastocytosis, which usually present in infancy. Clinically, they are red-brown cobblestoned plaques or nodules, which become accentuated with rubbing on the skin, known as Darier sign. Urticaria pigmentosa is another presentation of cutaneous mastocytosis in childhood with diffuse red-brown papules that become accentuated with skin rubbing. Telangiectasia macularis eruptiva perstans (TMEP) is a form of cutaneous mastocytosis in adults that presents with red-brown macules and papules with overlying telangiectasia. Arthropod reactions and urticaria may also form wheals but without the presence of an underlying cobblestoned plaque. Cutaneous manifestations of Langerhans cell histiocytosis vary and may present like seborrheic dermatitis with more discrete papules (often purpuric) and crusting to eroded nodular plaques in the case of congenital self-healing reticulohistiocytosis (Hashimoto-Pritzker disease), which presents early in infancy.
Bolognia J, Schaffer J, Cerroni L, eds. *Dermatology*. [Philadelphia]: Elsevier, 2018 (ch. 118).

8. A. Nail dystrophy

The Kodachrome and clinical description is that of steatocystoma multiplex, which are asymptomatic cysts that contain a yellow oily fluid. They are commonly found on the chest, axilla, and groin but can present in other areas (as seen here). They may be inherited in an autosomal dominant fashion due to mutation in the *KRT17* gene. They also may occur in the setting of pachyonychia congenita type 2, which can present with palmoplantar keratoderma and nail dystrophy. Colon cancer occurs in Gardner syndrome, which may present with multiple cutaneous epidermoid cysts. The yellowish color seen in these lesions should help distinguish steatocystomas from the epidermal cysts seen in Gardner. Cutaneous leiomyomas are smooth muscle tumors that present as painful red-brown papules or plaques. They may be seen in hereditary leiomyomatosis and renal cell cancer (HLRCC) syndrome or Reed syndrome. Renal cell carcinoma and uterine fibromas are also part of the syndrome. Pilomatrixomas are adnexal tumors usually found on the head and neck. They present as firm (rock-hard) nodules that may have a bluish hue. Multiple lesions may be seen in Gardner syndrome, myotonic dystrophy, and Rubinstein-Taybi syndrome.
Bolognia J, Schaffer J, Cerroni L, eds. *Dermatology*. [Philadelphia]: Elsevier, 2018 (ch. 110).

9. D. Psoriasis

The Kodachrome depicts geographic tongue, which is associated with psoriasis and atopy. This condition histologically resembles psoriasis. Median rhomboid glossitis presents with redness, and loss of lingual papillae in the midline of the tongue may be caused by oral candidiasis. Vitamin deficiencies (especially B12) may lead to atrophic glossitis. Smoking is a risk factor for oral black hairy tongue. Ulcerative colitis may be associated with pyostomatitis vegetans and recurrent aphthous stomatitis.
Bolognia J, Schaffer J, Cerroni L, eds. *Dermatology*. [Philadelphia]: Elsevier, 2018 (ch. 72).

10. C. Elevated antineutrophil cytoplasmic antibodies

There are subtle retiform purpuric patches on the ear helices in the setting of drug abuse history. This should raise concern for levamisole-associated vasculitis. The differential for retiform purpura in acral areas also includes antiphospholipid syndrome and type I cryoglobulinemia. Other diseases that cause retiform purpura include cholesterol emboli (which presents with extensive livedo reticularis and retiform purpura and ulcers in the distal extremities), septic emboli from endocarditis, warfarin blue toe syndrome, and hypercoagulable states (e.g., postsepsis protein C/S deficiency, essential thrombocytosis, heparin-induced thrombocytopenia). The patient most likely has levamisole-induced vasculitis, which is a contaminant found in cocaine. Levamisole is an antihelminthic agent, which increases the stimulant effects. Patients with this condition present with purpura and necrosis of the ears, nose, cheeks, and extremities; leukocytoclastic vasculitis-like lesions; ecchymoses; and systemic vasculitis. Pyoderma gangrenosum-like lesions have also been reported. Greater than 80% of patients will have antibodies to p-antineutrophil cytoplasmic antibody (ANCA). Approximately 50% may have elevated antibodies to c-ANCA. Eosinophilia may be seen with cholesterol emboli. Elevated antiphospholipid antibodies are found in antiphospholipid syndrome and Sneddon syndrome. Elevated cryoglobulins are found in cryoglobulinemia. It is important to consider the entire differential diagnosis and workup in evaluating a patient with retiform purpura.
Bolognia J, Schaffer J, Cerroni L, eds. *Dermatology*. [Philadelphia]: Elsevier, 2018 (ch. 89).

11. E. All of the above.

Subacute cutaneous lupus erythematosus (SCLE) presents with annular and polycyclic plaques with scale in photopredominant distribution. SCLE may be associated with systemic lupus or can be drug-induced. Common medications, including terbinafine, hydrochlorothiazide, proton pump inhibitors (such as omeprazole), and TNF-alpha inhibitors have been associated with drug-induced SCLE. Other culprits include calcium channel blockers, antiepileptics, taxanes, and thrombocyte inhibitors. A thorough drug history is important in the evaluation of SCLE.
Bolognia J, Schaffer J, Cerroni L, eds. *Dermatology*. [Philadelphia]: Elsevier, 2018 (ch. 41).

12. A. Laryngeal

The clinical findings described above are consistent with Bazex syndrome, also known as acrokeratosis paraneoplastica. Patients present with acral, violaceous, and psoriasiform plaques, which typically involve the fingers, toes, nose, and helices. Longitudinal and horizontal ridging of the nails occurs in 75% of patients. This syndrome is most commonly linked to malignancies of the upper aerodigestive tract.
Bolognia J, Schaffer J, Cerroni L, eds. *Dermatology*. [Philadelphia]: Elsevier, 2018 (ch. 53).

13. C. Ash leaf spots

Neurofibromatosis type 1 (NF1) is an autosomal dominant syndrome due to mutations in the *neurofibromin* gene. Diagnostic criteria for NF1 require at least two of the following: six or more café au lait macules, at least two neurofibromas or one plexiform neurofibroma, axillary and inguinal "freckling," at least two Lisch nodules (iris hamartomas), characteristic osseous lesions (sphenoid wing dysplasia, thinning of long bone cortex, pseudoarthrosis), or a first-degree family member with NF1. Patients with NF1 have a predilection toward tumor development, both benign and malignant (e.g., malignant peripheral nerve sheath tumor). Other reported tumors include optic gliomas, pheochromocytoma, carcinoid, CNS tumors, and juvenile myelomonocytic leukemia. Ash leaf spots are found in tuberous sclerosis not neurofibromatosis.
Bolognia J, Schaffer J, Cerroni L, eds. *Dermatology*. [Philadelphia]: Elsevier, 2018 (ch. 61).

14. C. Eyelid
Sebaceous carcinoma is an uncommon malignant adenocarcinoma of sebaceous differentiation. They can be sporadic or associated with Muir-Torre syndrome (MTS). The most common location for sebaceous carcinoma is periocular, followed by the head and neck region and less commonly the trunk. The development of sebaceous carcinoma or other sebaceous neoplasms outside of the head and neck region should raise suspicion for MTS—other features include keratoacanthomas and associated tumors, including gastrointestinal and genitourinary. Treatment of sebaceous carcinoma is primarily surgical.
Bolognia J, Schaffer J, Cerroni L, eds. *Dermatology*. [Philadelphia]: Elsevier, 2018 (ch. 111).

15. A. Type I
Eruptive xanthomas may occur in several types of familial hyperlipoproteinemia, but the presence of eruptive xanthomas without other metabolic systemic disease is only seen in type I (familial LPL deficiency, familial hyperchylomicronemia). Type II (familial defective apo B 100, familial hypercholesterolemia) and type III (familial dysbetalipoproteinemia) both exhibit tuberoeruptive xanthomas, plane xanthomas, and tendinous xanthomas and are associated with atherosclerosis. Type IV (endogenous familial hypertriglyceridemia) exhibits eruptive xanthomas, non-insulin-dependent diabetes mellitus, and obesity. Type V is associated with eruptive xanthomas and diabetes mellitus.
Bolognia J, Schaffer J, Cerroni L, eds. *Dermatology*. [Philadelphia]: Elsevier, 2018 (ch. 92).

16. B. Captopril
Drug-induced pemphigus is more commonly seen in pemphigus foliaceus and occurs less commonly in pemphigus vulgaris. Patients with drug-induced pemphigus exhibit similar autoantibody types to sporadic pemphigus (Desmoglein 1, 3). The most commonly implicated drugs are penicillamine and captopril. Other drugs that have been reported include other Angiotensin-converting enzyme inhibitors, penicillin, nifedipine, and piroxicam. Discontinuation of the medication is important, as many patients achieve remission with removal of the culprit medication. Furosemide is commonly implicated in drug-induced bullous pemphigoid. While patients typically manifest with flaccid bullae, tense bullae may also be occasionally seen in pemphigus.
Bolognia J, Schaffer J, Cerroni L, eds. *Dermatology*. [Philadelphia]: Elsevier, 2018 (ch. 29).

17. A. Permethrin cream
Permethrin cream is considered safe in pregnancy and is the treatment of choice in this population. Sulfur ointment is another treatment modality considered safe during pregnancy. Lindane should not be used in pregnant women as its use has been associated with neural tube defects and mental retardation. There is lack of safety data for the use of crotamiton lotion or oral ivermectin pills in the pregnant population. Malathion is not used to treat scabies but is a treatment option for pediculosis capitis (head lice).
Bolognia J, Schaffer J, Cerroni L, eds. *Dermatology*. [Philadelphia]: Elsevier, 2018 (ch. 84).

18. D. *ECM1*
Lipoid proteinosis is a rare autosomal recessive disorder due to mutations in extracellular matrix protein 1 (*ECM1*) gene. It is a deposition disorder, in which hyaline material is deposited in various organs. Initial presentation is early in life with a hoarse or weak cry. Early stages of lipoid proteinosis are characterized by erosions; vesicles; and scarring on the face, extremities, and mouth. Later stages are characterized by thickening of the skin with waxy papules and nodules forming on the face, axillae, and scrotum. String of beadlike papules on the eyelid margins is characteristic. These patients can have neurologic manifestations, including seizures, and have a characteristic radiographic finding of sickle-shaped calcifications in the temporal lobes of the brain. *Col V* mutations are seen in Ehlers-Danlos; *ABCC6* mutations are seen in pseudoxanthoma elasticum; and *LMX-1B* mutations are seen in Nail-Patella syndrome.
Bolognia J, Schaffer J, Cerroni L, eds. *Dermatology*. [Philadelphia]: Elsevier, 2018 (ch. 48).

19. B. Cystic fibrosis transmembrane conductance regulator mutation screen
Aquagenic keratoderma or aquagenic wrinkling of the palms and soles is an acquired keratoderma characterized by development of thickened white pebbly papules or plaques on the palms after immersion in water. Symptoms include burning and pain, which resolve after drying the skin. Aquagenic keratoderma is found in approximately 25% of cystic fibrosis (CF) carriers and is very common in CF patients. Genetic screening for CFTR mutations is recommended, as this condition typically develops in women in their second decade and is important for family planning decisions.
Bolognia J, Schaffer J, Cerroni L, eds. *Dermatology*. [Philadelphia]: Elsevier, 2018 (ch. 58).

20. A. Generalized essential telangiectasia
Generalized essential telangiectasia (GET) is an idiopathic progressive disorder characterized by development of widespread innumerable telangiectasias. Telangiectasias often start symmetrically on the bilateral lower extremities and may progress to generalized involvement.
GET is not associated with underlying systemic disease. The main entity in the differential diagnosis is a cutaneous collagenous vasculopathy. Clinically these entities are very similar, but in cutaneous collagenous vasculopathy, there is typically a female predominance, lesions may be limited to the trunk, and on pathology there is hyalinized concretions surrounding the basement membrane of the affected vessels. Both of these conditions are benign but may progress. Treatment includes vascular lasers. Systemic lupus erythematosus and other connective tissue diseases (e.g., CREST) may present with discrete telangiectasias. Angioma serpiginosum is a vascular disorder that presents as small red to purple macules in a serpiginous arrangement usually unilaterally on an extremity; however, the condition may become more widespread. Rothmund-Thomson syndrome is an inherited disorder with mutations in *RECQL4* gene. Patients present in infancy with erythema and edema of the face and extremities with significant poikiloderma that affects the dorsal arms, hands, and the buttocks. Osteosarcoma occurs in 10%–30% of patients with this syndrome.
Bolognia J, Schaffer J, Cerroni L, eds. *Dermatology*. [Philadelphia]: Elsevier, 2018 (ch. 106).

21. C. Tetracycline
Pyogenic granulomas (PGs) are rapidly growing reactive vascular benign neoplasms. They are common in children and young adults and often occur at a site of local trauma, although many are spontaneous. PGs commonly develop in the gingiva of pregnant women or may be medication related. Common medications include indinavir, systemic

retinoids, and epidermal growth factor receptor inhibitors; however, PG-like lesions in this setting are often periungual and thought to be a reaction to ingrown nails causing a foreign body reaction and hypergranulation tissue. Tetracyclines are not a reported cause of pyogenic granulomas but rather cause photo-onycholysis.
Bolognia J, Schaffer J, Cerroni L, eds. *Dermatology.* [Philadelphia]: Elsevier, 2018 (ch. 114).

22. **A.** Granuloma faciale
Granuloma faciale is an idiopathic eosinophilic dermatosis characterized by a pauci-lesional (typically solitary) red-brown plaque on the face, although it can affect extrafacial sites. A clinical clue is prominent follicular openings in the plaque as depicted in the figure. Biopsy characteristically shows a grenz zone, with a dense mixed infiltrate of lymphocytes, neutrophils, plasma cells, and numerous eosinophils. Leukocytoclastic vasculitis with neutrophilic dust may be present. There is no association with systemic disease. While often recalcitrant to treatment, topical and intralesional steroids, oral or topical dapsone, tetracycline antibiotics, topical calcineurin inhibitors, topical psoralen and ultraviolet A (PUVA), excision, cryosurgery, and pulsed dye laser or CO_2 laser have all been reported as treatment options.
Angiolymphoid hyperplasia with eosinophilia presents with pink to violaceous papules and nodules that favor the ear and scalp, and other areas of the head and neck. Leprosy may present with infiltrative nodules on the face, especially the ear. B-cell lymphoma or pseudolymphoma may present with violaceous shiny papules or nodules on the head and neck.
Bolognia J, Schaffer J, Cerroni L, eds. *Dermatology.* [Philadelphia]: Elsevier, 2018 (ch. 25).

23. **D.** Pulmonary stenosis
G. Patchy scalp hair loss
NAME/LAMB or Carney complex is an autosomal dominantly inherited disorder due to mutations in the *PRKAR1A* gene. It is characterized by a constellation of findings, including lentigines, blue nevi (including epithelioid), myxomas (mucocutaneous and atrial), endocrine neoplasia (adrenocortical, pituitary, thyroid, testes), psammomatous melanotic schwannomas, and myxoid mammary fibroadenomas. Striae may occur in the setting of Cushing syndrome, which may result from primary pigmented nodular adrenocortical disease. With pituitary adenomas, acromegaly may occur secondary to increased growth hormone production. Pulmonary stenosis is seen in LEOPARD syndrome. Patchy scalp hair loss is not characteristic of NAME.
Bolognia J, Schaffer J, Cerroni L, eds. *Dermatology.* [Philadelphia]: Elsevier, 2018 (ch. 53 and 112).

24. **D.** Environmental exposure
The patient has a panniculitis with firm red subcutaneous plaques in a fat-bearing area. Given distribution and clinical history, cold panniculitis is the diagnosis. Equestrian cold panniculitis is a specific type of cold panniculitis that appears on the thighs as red tender plaques following cold exposure in the setting of tight-fitting clothing. Vitamin K injection may cause Texier disease, which is a form of traumatic panniculitis due to phytonadione injections (vitamin K). This disorder involves development of painful sclerotic inflamed nodules on the buttocks and thighs ("cowboy holster pattern"), often sclerotic and with lilac-colored borders. It has been termed pseudoscleroderma and can persist for years. Lupus panniculitis presents as tender subcutaneous plaques on the arms, thighs, and face. Cutaneous T-cell lymphoma may present as a panniculitis (subcutaneous panniculitis-like

T-cell lymphoma), which favors the lower extremities. Silicone or other foreign body injections may cause a traumatic panniculitis.
Bolognia J, Schaffer J, Cerroni L, eds. *Dermatology.* [Philadelphia]: Elsevier, 2018 (ch. 100).

25. **B.** Brown-black granules in dermal macrophages, positive Perls, and Fontana-Masson stains
Minocycline hyperpigmentation can present in several forms. Type I: blue-black pigmentation in sites of inflammation or trauma/scars; type II: blue-gray macules and patches on normal skin, particularly shins and arms but can be seen in other sites; type III: muddy brown diffuse pigmentation in a photodistribution. Blue-black discoloration may also involve nails, bones, mucosa, teeth, and sclerae. Biopsy of type I minocycline hyperpigmentation shows pigment aggregates in the dermis that contain iron (positive for Perls stain). Biopsy of type II minocycline hyperpigmentation shows dermal macrophages with pigment granules that are positive for iron stains and Fontana-Masson (melanin)—the correct answer choice B. Type III minocycline hyperpigmentation shows increased melanin in the basal epidermis and dermal macrophages, where iron stains are negative. Increased basal epidermal melanin may occur in lentigines. The histology of ochronosis (choice D) is quite characteristic with yellow-brown, large, banana-shaped aggregates in the dermis.
Bolognia J, Schaffer J, Cerroni L, eds. *Dermatology.* [Philadelphia]: Elsevier, 2018 (ch. 67 and 127).

26. **A.** IM benzathine penicillin
The patient has primary syphilis (a painless chancre) in the setting of HIV. It is important to consider the other causes of genital ulcerations and STIs, including lymphogranuloma venereum (LGV), herpes simplex virus, granuloma inguinale, and chancroid. Recommended treatment for primary early syphilis is benzathine penicillin 2.5 million units IM in a single dose. Although patients with HIV are at higher risk for treatment failure and neurologic complications, these have not been shown to be prevented by more intense treatment regimens. It is recommended that patients with HIV be monitored more frequently and for a longer duration. IV aqueous penicillin is the treatment for neurosyphilis. Benzathine penicillin 2.4 million units IM for two doses is recommended for pregnant patients. Benzathine penicillin 2.4 million units IM weekly for three doses is recommended for late latent, cardiovascular, and gummatous syphilis, or retreatment of any stage syphilis. In penicillin-allergic patients, doxycycline, tetracycline, or ceftriaxone may be used. Acyclovir is used to treat genital herpes. Ceftriaxone can be used to treat gonorrhea or chancroid. Azithromycin may be used to treat chancroid. Doxycycline is the recommended treatment for LGV.
Bolognia J, Schaffer J, Cerroni L, eds. *Dermatology.* [Philadelphia]: Elsevier, 2018 (ch. 82).

27. **C.** Potassium dichromate
The Kodachrome depicts well-demarcated lichenified plaques indicative of a shoe contact dermatitis. Potassium dichromate is used for the leather tanning process and is a common allergen for leather shoe dermatitis. Other causes of shoe dermatitis include mercaptobenzothiazole, thiuram, and carbamix. If the shoe is dyed, then Paraphenylenediamine (PPD) may also be an allergen. Potassium dichromate is also found in wet cement and green pigment (e.g., paint, dyes, tattoo pigment). Tocopheryl acetate (vitamin E) may be found in creams and makeup.

Methylchloroisothiazolinone is found in personal care products as a preservative and baby/sanitary wipes. Glyceryl thioglycolate is the chemical that disrupts disulfide bonds in hair and is used for permanent or semipermanent waves.
Bolognia J, Schaffer J, Cerroni L, eds. *Dermatology.* [Philadelphia]: Elsevier, 2018 (ch. 14).

28. C. Serum/plasma serotonin levels
The WHO classification for the diagnosis of systemic mastocytosis requires either one major criterion plus one minor criterion or three minor criteria. The major criterion is multifocal dense infiltrates of mast cells in bone marrow or extracutaneous tissues. Minor criteria are: (1) >25% of mast cells in bone marrow or extracutaneous tissues are spindle or atypically shaped; (2) extracutaneous mast cells express CD2, CD25 or both; (3) presence of c-*KIT* codon 816 mutation in blood, bone marrow, or extracutaneous tissues; and (4) serum tryptase level is persistently >20 ng/ml. Serum serotonin measurement is not a criterion.
Bolognia J, Schaffer J, Cerroni L, eds. *Dermatology.* [Philadelphia]: Elsevier, 2018 (ch. 118).

29. C. Rinse with water and soap followed by vegetable oil soak
Capsaicin is the active ingredient in pepper spray, which causes a severe irritant contact reaction (erythema, burning, and edema but no dermatitis). It depolarizes nerves causing dose-related neuropathic pain and erythema due to vasodilation. Capsaicin is derived from the Solanaceae family, *Capsicum annuum* (hot pepper) plant. It is fat soluble and therefore insoluble in water. Rinsing with water or with soap alone will just spread the fat soluble substance more extensively. The best treatment is washing with soap and water followed by immersion in vegetable oil for at least one hour to help remove the fat soluble capsaicin. Antiseptic solutions and antidotes are also available.
Bolognia J, Schaffer J, Cerroni L, eds. *Dermatology.* [Philadelphia]: Elsevier, 2018 (ch. 17).

30. F. B & D
Loxosceles reclusa (brown recluse spider) bites cause dermonecrotic reactions and acute systemic disease, including shock, renal insufficiency, disseminated intravascular coagulation, and hemolysis. Most commonly found in south-central United States, they are found in attics, wood piles, and under radiators. Brown recluse spiders have a characteristic "fiddle-shaped" pattern on the cephalothorax, small body, and long legs. They only bite in self-defense. The bite initially can be painless or cause a burning sensation, followed by an exquisitely painful ischemic "marble"-patterned plaque within approximately 6 hours. Within a week this plaque can evolve to necrosis. Systemic reactions can occur as above. Treatment includes ice, elevation, and supportive care. Intradermal injection of anti-*Loxosceles* Fab antibody fragments (antivenin) can attenuate symptoms. Prednisone can be used for systemic symptoms. The primary toxin in loxoscelism is sphingomyelinase B with hyaluronidase also playing a less important role. Alpha-latrotoxin is involved in black widow spider bites (*Latrodectus*). Agatoxin is elaborated from American funnel web spider (hobo spider) bites.
Bolognia J, Schaffer J, Cerroni L, eds. *Dermatology.* [Philadelphia]: Elsevier, 2018 (ch. 85).

31. F. A & B
The figure shows an abscess, which is a walled-off purulent collection often found on hair-bearing areas, with surrounding erythema suggesting cellulitis. Simple abscesses

and furuncles can be treated with warm compresses and incision and drainage, or I&D (A). In complicated cases, such as those with associated cellulitis, systemic symptoms, or in immunocompromised hosts, oral antibiotics should be added. Furuncles are most commonly caused by *S. aureus* and are often methicillin-resistant (MRSA), thus antibiotic coverage for MRSA should include doxycycline, trimethoprim-sulfamethoxazole (B), or clindamycin. Bacterial culture should always be performed to monitor for antibiotic resistance. This patient has a risk factor for MRSA as he works in a hospital setting.
High-potency topical steroids (C) may be used for arthropod bites, which often present with pruritus and a central punctum at the puncture site. Arthropod reactions may be exaggerated (e.g., in Chronic lymphocytic leukemia patients) and present with vesicular or bullous lesions or multiple lesions. Cephalexin (D) is commonly used in the treatment of bacterial skin infections such as impetigo, cellulitis, and folliculitis but does not cover MRSA. Itraconazole (E) is an antifungal agent.
Bolognia J, Schaffer J, Cerroni L, eds. *Dermatology.* [Philadelphia]: Elsevier, 2018 (ch. 74).

32. A. Start amoxicillin
Disseminated erythema migrans may present several days to weeks after the development of a single primary lesion. These tend to be multiple smaller annular lesions and may be associated with flulike symptoms and regional lymphadenopathy. Classically lesions of erythema migrans present as expanding targetoid patches and may have edema or vesiculate centrally. Diagnosis of Lyme disease can be made clinically, and serologic studies are often negative in the first 2 weeks. Treatment of choice for pregnant women and children under 8 years of age is amoxicillin. All other patients with early Lyme disease should be treated with doxycycline (E).
While RPR (B) may be falsely positive during pregnancy and with Lyme disease, it is one of the screening tests for syphilis, another spirochete infection. Secondary syphilis may present with disseminated annular lesions but are often papulosquamous with involvement of the palms and soles. Fixed drug eruption (FDE) is a cutaneous drug reaction that appears as a round patch and recurs in the same area with re-exposure to the culprit drug, resolving with hyperpigmentation. Acetaminophen (C) has been associated with FDE, however, based on the vignette, her symptoms started prior to taking the medication. More common causes of FDE include sulfonamides, NSAIDs, tetracyclines, and pseudoephedrine (nonpigmenting).
Bolognia J, Schaffer J, Cerroni L, eds. *Dermatology.* [Philadelphia]: Elsevier, 2018 (ch. 74).

33. C. Hospitalize and intravenous antistaphylococcal antibiotics
Staphylococcal scalded skin syndrome (SSSS) is caused by systemically disseminated *S. aureus* exfoliative toxins that bind to desmoglein 1 and lead to skin pain and acantholysis of the epidermis. It is common in infants, children, and occasionally adults with chronic renal insufficiency. Clinically, SSSS initially presents with fever, malaise, purulent rhinorrhea, and/or conjunctivitis. This progresses to tender erythema on the face and intertriginous areas followed by generalized superficial epidermal desquamation. Radial fissuring with crust around the mouth and eyes, giving the appearance of a "sad clown," is classic. For severe SSSS, treatment of choice is hospitalization and IV antistaphylococcal antibiotics (C).
Bleach baths and topical steroids (A) would be indicated for an atopic dermatitis flare and reduction of *S. Aureus*

load on the skin. Intravenous Immune Globulin and aspirin (B) are the treatment of choice for Kawasaki disease, a form of multisystem vasculitis affecting infants and children. Classic Kawasaki disease requires high-grade fevers for greater than 5 days plus at least four of the following clinical criteria: (1) conjunctival injection without exudate; (2) oral mucosa changes; (3) extremity erythema, edema, or peeling, (4) polymorphous exanthema, (5) and cervical lymphadenopathy. Detailed drug history and treatment with cyclosporine (D) is one of the strategies for managing Stevens-Johnson syndrome (SJS), along with stopping all potential drug culprits, wound care, and multidisciplinary management. In SJS, dusky and tender skin with moist desquamation and mucosal involvement is typical.
Bolognia J, Schaffer J, Cerroni L, eds. *Dermatology.* [Philadelphia]: Elsevier, 2018 (ch. 74).

34. D. Blood cultures and echocardiography
This Kodachrome depicts Janeway lesions. These are painless hemorrhagic macules and papules on the palms and soles characteristic of infectious endocarditis. Other clinical findings include Osler nodes (tender, erythematous papules and nodules that favor finger pads), conjunctival and splinter hemorrhages, and retiform purpura. Symptoms include cough, dyspnea, fever, and chest pain. Endocarditis should always be excluded in IV drug users who present with these symptoms with blood cultures and an echocardiogram (D).
Tinea pedis and onychomycosis are common fungal infections of the feet and nails, respectively, and would not typically manifest with purpuric macules and papules. KOH and fungal culture would be the appropriate test to rule this out (A). Urine toxicology screen and ANCAs (B) are useful in the diagnosis of levamisole-induced vasculitis, a common contaminant in cocaine. This clinically presents with retiform purpura (classically with helical involvement), combined vasculopathy and vasculitis on histology, and patients may demonstrate positive ANCA serology (especially p-ANCA). HIV testing (C) should be performed in high-risk patients, including those with a history of IV drug use. This test, however, will not aid in the diagnosis associated with the clinical findings presented previously.
Bolognia J, Schaffer J, Cerroni L, eds. *Dermatology.* [Philadelphia]: Elsevier, 2018 (ch. 74 and 89).

35. A. Oral doxycycline
Rocky Mountain spotted fever (RMSF) is caused by *Rickettsia rickettsia* and spread by the dog ticks *Dermacenter variabilis* (Eastern Coast of the United States) and *D. andersoni* (Rocky Mountains and Western Coast of the United States). Patients typically develop fever, severe headaches, myalgias, and GI symptoms 1–2 weeks post-tick exposure. Three to 5 days later, 90% of patient's will develop a pink macular and/or petechial rash on the wrists and ankles with centripetal spread to the trunk. The rash is due to endothelial cell infection and damage, which, if left untreated, can lead to mortality in 25% of patients. All patients with suspected RMSF should be treated with oral doxycycline (A), regardless of age.
Supportive care (B) is the treatment of choice for many childhood viral illnesses, including hand, foot, and mouth disease (HFMD). HFMD typically presents with macular, papular, or vesicular lesions favoring the hands, feet, mouth, buttocks, genitalia, and thighs. Patients with atopic dermatitis may present with eczema coxsackium, which is in the differential diagnosis of eczema herpeticum. It typically follows an upper respiratory infection or GI viral illness and is highly contagious. This patient's associated

headaches and purpuric rather than vesicular lesions are more concerning for RMSF. NSAIDs (C) are used in the treatment of Kawasaki disease, a childhood multisystem vasculitis. IV ceftriaxone (D) is the treatment of choice for acute meningococcemia. While this may also present with headaches, fevers, and a petechial/purpuric eruption, these symptoms typically evolve more rapidly within 24 hours of onset. Oral ivermectin (E) is the treatment of choice for strongyloidiasis as well as crusted scabies.
Bolognia J, Schaffer J, Cerroni L, eds. *Dermatology.* [Philadelphia]: Elsevier, 2018 (ch. 76).

36. B. House mouse mite
Rickettsialpox is a vector-borne bacterial infection caused by *Rickettsia akari* and transmitted by *Liponyssoides sanguineus* (house mouse mite). Thus it occurs primarily in urban settings where mice live in close proximity to humans. Rickettsialpox presents as a papulovesicle at the bite site, then progressing to an eschar. Constitutional symptoms including fever, headache, and myalgias, as well as a disseminated eruption favoring the face, trunk, and extremities, may occur up to 1 to 2 weeks later. While infection is self-limited, treatment with doxycycline or other tetracyclines may shorten the duration of symptoms. *Ctenocephalides felis*, or cat fleas (A), transmit endemic typhus, cat flea–borne spotted fever, bacillary angiomatosis, and cat-scratch disease. *Rhipicephalus sanguineus*, or brown dog ticks (C), transmit Mediterranean spotted fever. This rickettsial infection is caused by *Rickettsia conorii*. Although it may present similar to rickettsialpox, the cutaneous eruption of Mediterranean spotted fever is generally said to favor the legs. *Pediculus humanus* var. *corporis*, or human body louse (D), transmit epidemic typhus.
Bolognia J, Schaffer J, Cerroni L, eds. *Dermatology.* [Philadelphia]: Elsevier, 2018 (ch. 76).

37. C. VDRL
Nonscarring alopecia can be classified by clinical distribution. This type of patchy, "moth-eaten" pattern can be seen in patients with secondary syphilis. Thus a VDRL nontreponemal screening test would be appropriate for this patient. Other clinical manifestations of secondary syphilis include a generalized maculopapular or papulosquamous (pityriasis rosea-like) eruption, copper-colored lesions on the palms and soles, condylomata lata on the genitals or oral mucosa, split papules at the oral commissures, sore throat, low-grade fevers, and lymphadenopathy.
A fungal culture (A) is an appropriate test to rule out tinea capitis. While this condition typically affects young, school-aged children, adults can also be affected. Tinea capitis classically presents with scaly patches of circumscribed alopecia with broken hairs and variable amounts of inflammation. It may also be associated with cervical and preauricular lymphadenopathy. ANA (B) is an appropriate test for a patient presenting with chronic cutaneous lupus. Discoid lupus may present on the scalp with circumscribed round to oval patches or plaques with alopecia with loss of hair follicles (scarring) and variable amounts of inflammation, atrophy, telangiectasias, and dyschromia. Systemic lupus may rarely present with a diffuse pattern of nonscarring alopecia. TSH (D) may be used to screen for thyroid disease, which may be associated with hair changes (brittle) and alopecia in hyperthyroidism or hypothyroidism, or alopecia areata (autoimmune thyroid disease).
Bolognia J, Schaffer J, Cerroni L, eds. *Dermatology.* [Philadelphia]: Elsevier, 2018 (ch. 82).

38. D. *Hemophilus ducreyi*

Chancroid is a sexually transmitted infection caused by *Hemophilus ducreyi* (D). It causes painful ulcers with ragged or undermined borders and a fibrinous base unlike syphilitic chancres (E), which are typically painless. The incidence of chancroid is higher in males, often affecting the prepuce, coronal sulcus, and frenulum. Giemsa stain will reveal the classic "school of fish" pattern of coccobacilli. Treatment of choice is azithromycin 1 gram given once.

Neisseria gonorrhoeae (A) causes gonorrhea. Patients present with urethritis and purulent discharge. Hemorrhagic and necrotic lesions are only seen with hematologic spread. Treatment of choice is a dual treatment with ceftriaxone and azithromycin. *Chlamydia trachomatis* serotypes L1-3 (B) causes lymphogranuloma venereum. Clinical presentation evolves over time: stage 1 disease presents in the first 1–2 weeks of infection with painless ulcers; stage 2 occurs up to 1 month later with painful buboes and inguinal lymphadenopathy above and below the Poupart ligament giving the classic "groove sign;" and stage 3 presents months to years later with proctocolitis, perirectal fissures, abscesses, and lymphadenopathy. Treatment of choice is doxycycline 100 mg twice daily for 3 weeks. *Klebsiella granulomatis* (C) causes granuloma inguinale, which classically presents as beefy red, chronic ulcers with friable granulation tissue. Giemsa stain will reveal "safety pin" Donovan bodies. Treatment of choice is azithromycin 1 gram weekly for at least 3 weeks.

Bolognia J, Schaffer J, Cerroni L, eds. *Dermatology*. [Philadelphia]: Elsevier, 2018 (ch. 82).

39. A. Enterovirus PCR from nasopharyngeal swab

Hand-foot-mouth disease (HFMD) is a common childhood infection caused by Coxsackie A16 virus. Less commonly, it can also be caused by Coxsackie A6 and other enteroviruses, with more atypical severe and widespread infection presenting in adults. HFMD can be diagnosed by enterovirus PCR from cutaneous vesicles or nasopharyngeal swab (A). Treatment is supportive. Eczema coxsackium may present with more widespread vesicular lesions, which appear similarly to eczema herpeticum in patients with atopic dermatitis.

Noncaseating granulomas (B) are classically seen in sarcoidosis, which classically presents with red-brown papules at periorificial sites. Periorificial dermatitis is an inflammatory condition presenting with pink papules and pustules around the mouth, nares, and eye, sparing the vermilion lip border. It is often triggered by topical or inhaled steroid use on the face (C). Patch testing (D) is used to diagnose allergic contact dermatitis.

Bolognia J, Schaffer J, Cerroni L, eds. *Dermatology*. [Philadelphia]: Elsevier, 2018 (ch. 81).

40. B. Topical permethrin and oral ivermectin

This patient is presenting with generalized dermatitis with crusting and histopathology demonstrating a scabies mite, consistent with crusted scabies. Given the high mite burden associated with this type of scabies, the CDC recommends combined topical and oral treatment (B).

Open-wet dressings with topical steroids (A) are useful for erythrodermic atopic dermatitis and other widespread eczematous conditions. Given its rapid response, cyclosporine (C) is one of the treatments of choice for erythrodermic psoriasis and other severe dermatitides.

Bolognia J, Schaffer J, Cerroni L, eds. *Dermatology*. [Philadelphia]: Elsevier, 2018 (ch. 84).

PEDIATRIC DERMATOLOGY

41. D. Hunter syndrome

The mucopolysaccharidoses are a family of diseases characterized by mutations in enzymes that break down glycosaminoglycans (GAGs). The resulting storage of excessive amounts of GAGs in various tissues causes intellectual disability, hepatosplenomegaly, skeletal abnormalities, and corneal clouding. Skin manifestations are generally nonspecific and include hypertrichosis, thickening of the skin, and coarse facies. Hunter syndrome is an X-linked recessive type of mucopolysaccharidosis caused by a mutation in *IDS* which encodes for the enzyme iduronate-2-sulfatase. Hunter syndrome patients exhibit specific characteristic skin-colored to white papules "pebbled" over the scapulae more frequently than the arms, lateral upper chest, and buttocks. Patients affected by Hunter syndrome or Hurler syndrome, another type of mucopolysaccharidosis, can present with extensive dermal melanocytosis.

Bolognia J, Schaffer J, Cerroni L, eds. *Dermatology*. [Philadelphia]: Elsevier, 2018 (ch. 48).

42. F. Restrictive lung disease

Pseudoxanthoma elasticum (PXE) is an autosomal recessive disorder due to loss-of-function mutations in the ATP-binding cassette transporter *ABCC6*. Affected individuals develop yellowish papules on flexural surfaces, often first appearing on the lateral neck, that coalesce into a cobblestoned plaque that is often described as "plucked chicken skin." Patients also develop ocular manifestations, including asymptomatic angioid streaks (rupture of Bruch's membrane) and choroidal neovascularization, which may lead to hemorrhage, scarring, and ultimately blindness. Patients may also develop calcification of elastic fibers in arterial walls, leading to atherosclerosis and complications including claudication, angina, and myocardial infarction. These calcified vessels are more likely to rupture, most frequently resulting in gastrointestinal or cerebral hemorrhage. PXE patients also have an increased risk of mitral valve prolapse. Further, those with PXE, PXE-like cutis laxa, and particularly autosomal recessive cutis laxa type I are at significantly increased risk of lung involvement, including emphysema and hypoplastic lungs, which may be fatal. These patients do not develop restrictive lung disease.

Bolognia J, Schaffer J, Cerroni L, eds. *Dermatology*. [Philadelphia]: Elsevier, 2018 (ch. 97).

43. E. Anakinra

Muckle-Wells syndrome (MWS) belongs to the family of autosomal-dominant autoinflammatory disorders called the cryopyrin-associated periodic syndromes (CAPS). These disorders are due to mutations in *NLRP3* and also include familial cold autoinflammatory syndrome and neonatal-onset multisystem inflammatory disease (NOMID). MWS may present at any age and typically presents with episodes of fever, widespread urticarial papules and plaques, abdominal pain, myalgias, and arthralgias, which may be accompanied by conjunctivitis and the development of sensorineural hearing loss. Secondary AA amyloidosis may complicate MWS in up to 25% of patients. Treatment of choice is an IL-1 antagonist such as anakinra.

Prednisone may mitigate symptoms of acute flares but is not a long-term treatment. TNF-inhibitors such as adalimumab may be appropriate for other autoinflammatory disorders such as familial Mediterranean fever; hyper-IgD syndrome; TNF-receptor-associated periodic syndrome;

Blau syndrome; or pyogenic arthritis, pyoderma gangrenosum, acne (PAPA) syndrome.
Bolognia J, Schaffer J, Cerroni L, eds. *Dermatology.* [Philadelphia]: Elsevier, 2018 (ch. 45).

44. C. Thrombocytopenia
Wiskott-Aldrich syndrome is an X-linked immunodeficiency due to mutations in the WAS protein (*WASP*), which results in abnormal T-cell function, small platelets with a reduced half-life, and reduced B-cell and NK-cell function. Patients may present initially with petechiae and ecchymoses of the oral mucosa and skin due to thrombocytopenia and platelet dysfunction, which are present at birth. Atopic dermatitis develops in the first few months of life and has a predilection for the face, scalp, and flexural areas, though more widespread involvement is common. Recurrent bacterial infections begin during early infancy and are most commonly due to encapsulated bacteria, resulting in otitis media, pneumonia, and meningitis. WAS patients are also more susceptible to herpes simplex virus, human papillomavirus, and *P. jiroveci*. In addition, there is increased risk for development of autoimmune diseases and non-Hodgkin's lymphoma. Treatment for WAS is with hematopoietic stem cell transplantation.
Laboratory evaluation in WAS patients reveals thrombocytopenia with small platelets, low IgM and elevated IgA, and IgE. Platelets and neutrophils that contain giant granules are found in Chédiak-Higashi syndrome. Neutrophilia is identified in leukocyte adhesion deficiency. Low IgA may be found in patients with selective IgA deficiency, common variable immunodeficiency (along with decreased IgG), or ataxia-telangiectasia syndrome (along with decreased IgE and $IgG_{2,4}$). Elevated IgM is found in hyper-IgM syndrome and may also be seen in hypohidrotic ectodermal dysplasia with immunodeficiency.
Bolognia J, Schaffer J, Cerroni L, eds. *Dermatology.* [Philadelphia]: Elsevier, 2018 (ch. 60).

45. D. Testicular cancer
Steroid sulfatase deficiency is an X-linked recessive disorder that presents in the neonatal period with mild erythroderma and peeling, followed by the development of dark-brown adherent scales over the trunk, extremities, and neck later in infancy or childhood. During birth, labor is often delayed. Asymptomatic comma-shaped corneal opacities occur in up to 50% of affected patients and do not affect visual acuity. There is an increased risk of cryptorchidism, and patients may also have an increased risk for developing testicular cancer and hypogonadism even if the testes have appropriately descended.
Progressive spastic di- and tetraplegia is characteristic of Sjögren-Larsson syndrome. Collodion membrane at birth is a common presenting feature in patients with autosomal recessive congenital ichthyosis (lamellar ichthyosis and congenital ichthyosiform erythroderma) and self-improving collodion ichthyosis. A collodion membrane may also be present in trichothiodystrophy and is rarely present in Sjögren-Larsson syndrome and infantile Gaucher disease. Congenital sensorineural hearing impairment is characteristic of keratitis-ichthyosis-deafness (KID) syndrome.
Bolognia J, Schaffer J, Cerroni L, eds. *Dermatology.* [Philadelphia]: Elsevier, 2018 (ch. 57).

46. E. Lymphoma
Ataxia telangiectasia (AT) is an autosomal recessive primary immunodeficiency disorder in which patients develop oculocutaneous telangiectasias and progressive cerebellar ataxia. The immunodeficiency results in particular susceptibility to sinus and respiratory tract infections. Bronchiectasis with respiratory failure is the most common cause of death. Serum levels of IgM are elevated, and levels of IgA, IgG, and IgE are decreased. Affected individuals also have increased sensitivity to ionizing radiation and a 70-fold to 200-fold increased risk of leukemia and lymphoma as well as increased risk of other malignancies. Carriers of AT are also at increased risk for malignancies, including breast cancer.
Patients present with truncal ataxia when learning to walk; however, the diagnosis of AT may not be recognized until the oculocutaneous telangiectasias develop. Telangiectasias first appear on the lateral and medial bulbar conjunctivae between 3–6 years of age and subsequently develop on the skin and hard and soft palate. Patients may also develop noninfectious granulomas.
Pulmonary arteriovenous malformations may occur in hereditary hemorrhagic telangiectasia. Glaucoma may occur in patients with Sturge-Weber syndrome. Cold abscesses may be found in autosomal dominant hyper-IgE (Job) syndrome. Myelokathexis (peripheral neutropenia with retention of neutrophils in the bone marrow) is found in WHIM syndrome (warts, hypogammaglobulinemia, infections, and myelokathexis).
Bolognia J, Schaffer J, Cerroni L, eds. *Dermatology.* [Philadelphia]: Elsevier, 2018 (ch. 60).

47. C. Serial monitoring of calcium
Subcutaneous fat necrosis of the newborn is a panniculitis that presents in the first few weeks of life in full-term neonates. Infants present with one to several red/violaceous indurated plaques, typically in fat-rich areas such as the back, cheeks, buttocks, or thighs. Possible precipitating factors include hypothermia, hypoglycemia, and perinatal hypoxemia. Biopsy shows a lobular panniculitis with a mixed infiltrate and needle-shaped clefts in adipocytes and giant cells. Subcutaneous fat necrosis may be complicated by hypercalcemia, and patients should undergo serial monitoring of calcium for at least 4 months. Treatment is supportive care and management of hypercalcemia if indicated.
Admission to the neonatal ICU may be appropriate for infants diagnosed with sclerema neonatorum, which occurs in severely ill premature neonates and is not a localized panniculitis. Reassurance alone is not appropriate as infants with subcutaneous fat necrosis may develop hypercalcemia and require monitoring.
Bolognia J, Schaffer J, Cerroni L, eds. *Dermatology.* [Philadelphia]: Elsevier, 2018 (ch. 100).

48. B. Neutrophils
Transient neonatal pustular melanosis is a benign, self-limited condition that develops in up to 5% of newborns with darkly pigmented skin and less commonly occurs in Caucasians. Infants are born with fragile superficial pustules without surrounding erythema. These pustules subsequently rupture and leave behind hyperpigmented macules with collarettes of scale. The hyperpigmented macules may persist for months. Wright stain of the pustule contents demonstrates neutrophils.
Erythema toxicum neonatorum rarely presents at birth and instead usually begins 24 to 48 hours after delivery with possible onset as late as 1–2 weeks of age. Affected infants present with pink-red macules, wheals, pustules and vesicles, and Wright stain of these pustules demonstrates eosinophils. Congenital candidiasis presents at birth or within the first few days of life with a widespread

eruption of pink-red papules, vesiculopustules, diffuse erythema and/or scaling, and yeast may be visible on smear of these pustules. Multinucleated giant cells would be seen in a Wright stain of a vesicle due to herpes simplex virus or varicella zoster virus.
Bologna J, Schaffer J, Cerroni L, eds. *Dermatology.* [Philadelphia]: Elsevier, 2018 (ch. 34).

49. A. Parrot pseudoparalysis
The stigmata of late congenital syphilis becomes apparent at some point after age 2 and may include characteristic dental findings such as Hutchinson teeth (pictured) and mulberry molars as well as interstitial keratitis, nerve deafness, saber shins, enlargement of the medial third of the clavicle (Higoumenakis sign), saddle nose, radial periorificial scars (periorificial rhagades), and symmetric painless knee swelling (Clutton joints). In contrast, manifestations of early congenital syphilis occur before age 2 and include Parrot pseudoparalysis (due to painful osteochondritis), snuffles, secondary syphilis-like papulosquamous eruption, bullae or erosions favoring acral sites, perioral and perianal fissures, lymphadenopathy, hepatosplenomegaly, and cachexia.
Bologna J, Schaffer J, Cerroni L, eds. *Dermatology.* [Philadelphia]: Elsevier, 2018 (ch. 82).

50. C. Proliferation of smooth muscle bundles in the dermis
This is a Becker nevus. These lesions are often associated with an underlying smooth muscle hamartoma. Tightly packed capillaries in discrete lobules are suggestive of a tufted angioma (A); tracking of melanocytes around appendages, vessels, and nerves is seen in congenital melanocytic nevi; large hypertrophied nerves are seen in neurofibromas (D); and increased dermal collagen bundles are suggestive of a collagenoma (E).
Bologna J, Schaffer J, Cerroni L, eds. *Dermatology.* [Philadelphia]: Elsevier, 2018 (ch. 70 and 112).

DERMATOPATHOLOGY

51. E. Henderson-Paterson bodies
The diagnosis is molluscum contagiosum. A crush preparation of molluscum lesion can be stained with Giemsa allowing the clinician to visualize Henderson-Paterson bodies, which are discrete purple ovals filling the majority of the cytoplasm of affected cells in molluscum. Henderson-Paterson bodies reflect viral cytoplasmic inclusions characteristic of molluscum and have a somewhat similar appearance to the affected cells histologically.
Multinucleate giant cells would be present in HSV or VZV. Donovan bodies are present in granuloma inguinale. Owls' eye inclusions can be seen on Giemsa stain in CMV, which is not the diagnosis. Hemophagocytosis is characteristic of hemophagocytic lymphohistiocytosis (HLH), a rare rapidly progressive and often fatal disorder of activated histiocytes that often presents with fevers, hepatosplenomegaly, and pancytopenia. It may be familial or secondary to infection. Skin findings are nonspecific and may include erythroderma, generalized purpuric macules and papules, and morbilliform rash.
Bologna J, Schaffer J, Cerroni L, eds. *Dermatology.* [Philadelphia]: Elsevier, 2018 (ch. 81).

52. A. Scleromyxedema
The diagnosis is scleromyxedema. Scleromyxedema presents as 2–3 mm waxy papules in a generalized distribution. Sclerodermoid changes are often present in surrounding skin, as in this case. Leonine facies and a "donut" sign over the proximal interphalangeal joints are classically seen and may be present clinically. Scleromyxedema is almost always associated with an IgG lambda monoclonal gammopathy. Histologically, scleromyxedema is characterized by increase in fibroblasts and collagen fibers in the dermis plus the presence of interstitial mucin (as demonstrated here on H&E and confirmed with Alcian blue staining). Scleredema most commonly presents as a woody induration of the upper back. Histologically a thickened dermis is noted with more variable interstitial mucin (typically most prominent in the deep dermis); however, there is no inflammatory infiltrate or increase in fibroblast cellularity in scleredema; in fact, the histologic changes are often so subtle, scleredema is considered in the "normal skin" histologic differential diagnosis. It is associated with diabetes, streptococcal infection, and IgG monoclonal gammopathy. While granuloma annulare and lupus can have mucin in the biopsy, the clinical and histologic features in this case are not suggestive of these diagnoses. Actinic granuloma typically does not have mucin and instead shows solar elastosis and central elastolysis (loss of elastic tissue).
Bologna J, Schaffer J, Cerroni L, eds. *Dermatology.* [Philadelphia]: Elsevier, 2018 (ch. 46).

53. E. Exposure to gadolinium contrast
Pictured in the clinical Kodachrome are so-called "patterned plaques" or "ameboid plaques," which are fairly characteristic of nephrogenic systemic fibrosis (NSF) due to gadolinium contrast exposure in patients receiving MRI with impaired renal function. Histologically, osseous metaplasia (also known as lollipop bodies) may be seen as illustrated in the figure, which are also characteristic of NSF. Albright hereditary osteodystrophy is associated with primary bone formation in the skin. However, patterned plaques are not typical of Albright, and Albright's patients typically die at a young age. Dystrophic calcinosis cutis can be seen in CREST/scleroderma; however, calcinosis cutis is not pictured histologically and typically appears as very basophilic, amorphous material on H&E stain. Radiation can lead to fibrosis and morphea; however, given the lollipop bodies histologically, a history of gadolinium exposure is most critical to make the diagnosis.
Bologna J, Schaffer J, Cerroni L, eds. *Dermatology.* [Philadelphia]: Elsevier, 2018 (ch. 43).

54. D. Polyoma virus
The figure illustrates sheets of small blue cells with a high nuclear to cytoplasmic ration, nuclear molding, and stippled nuclear chromatin. The differential diagnosis for a small, blue, round cell tumor in skin includes Merkel cell carcinoma, metastatic small cell lung carcinoma, and lymphoma cutis, among others. Cytokeratin 20 positivity (perinuclear dotlike or membranous pattern) is present in the vast majority of Merkel cell carcinomas (MCC) and distinguishes this tumor from the other entities in the differential diagnosis. MCC is associated with Merkel cell polyomavirus in approximately 80% of cases.
Polyomavirus is also associated with trichodysplasia spinulosa in immunosuppressed individuals. Epstein-Barr virus is linked to multiple lymphoproliferative disorders, such as extranodal NK/T-cell lymphoma, and post-transplant lymphoproliferative disorders, while HTLV-1 is seen with adult T-leukemia/lymphoma. High-risk HPV may be associated with cervical and oropharyngeal squamous cell carcinoma.
Bologna J, Schaffer J, Cerroni L, eds. *Dermatology.* [Philadelphia]: Elsevier, 2018 (ch. 115).

55. **B.** Granuloma annulare

Within the reticular dermis, there is a palisaded granuloma with mucinous degeneration at the center, surrounded by a rim of histiocytes with perivascular lymphocytes. The findings seen here are typical of granuloma annulare. Dermatofibroma demonstrates a proliferation of spindle and stellate fibrohistiocytes with collagen trapping at the periphery and does not have a palisaded appearance. Necrobiosis lipoidica typically involves the deep dermis and shows a tiered pattern with alternating collagen degeneration and inflammatory infiltrate. Sarcoidosis will demonstrate well-formed, "naked" granulomas composed of epithelioid histiocytes without significant lymphocytic infiltrate.

Bolognia J, Schaffer J, Cerroni L, eds. *Dermatology.* [Philadelphia]: Elsevier, 2018 (ch. 93).

56. **B.** Acantholytic dyskeratotic acanthoma

The figure illustrates a variant of benign keratosis with acantholysis and dyskeratosis, also known as acantholytic dyskeratotic acanthoma. If these histopathologic findings were seen in the setting of a rash, the differential diagnosis would include Darier disease, Grover disease, and Hailey-Hailey disease.

Acantholytic actinic keratosis demonstrates keratinocytic atypia, which is not seen here. Epidermolytic dyskeratosis may be seen in a solitary keratosis ("epidermolytic dyskeratotic acanthoma"), may occur as a histopathologic manifestation in ichthyosis (bullous congenital ichthyosiform erythroderma), or may be seen as an incidental finding in other lesions. Skin biopsies from lesions of herpes will show some acantholysis; however, the lesions are vesicular or ulcerated and often involve the folliculosebaceous units. Herpetic viral cytopathic changes (multinucleated cells, with ground glass nuclei and peripheral margination of nuclear chromatin) are typically present.

Bolognia J, Schaffer J, Cerroni L, eds. *Dermatology.* [Philadelphia]: Elsevier, 2018 (ch. 119).

57. **B.** Digital mucous cyst

The photomicrograph shows acral skin with a pseudocystic space within the dermis, without any lining epithelium. These findings are characteristic of a digital mucous cyst (also known as myxoid pseudocyst) usually located on the proximal nail fold in middle-aged or elderly individuals.

Hidrocystoma is typically a unilocular cyst lined by a double layer of cuboidal epithelium and occurs on the face, especially periorbital areas (small vellus hair follicles and superficial skeletal muscle are often clues for this body site). Pilar/trichilemmal cysts most commonly occur on the scalp and histologically show abrupt dense pink keratinization without a granular cell layer. Branchial cysts are located on the neck or angle of the jaw and are lined by squamous or ciliated columnar epithelium with prominent lymphoid tissue within the walls.

Bolognia J, Schaffer J, Cerroni L, eds. *Dermatology.* [Philadelphia]: Elsevier, 2018 (ch. 110).

58. **B.** *GNAQ* mutation

The characteristic histologic features of a blue nevus include pigmented dendritic melanocytes and melanophages interspersed between collagen bundles within the dermis. Blue nevi are most commonly associated with *GNAQ* mutations. In addition, these mutations may be found in uveal melanoma and Sturge-Weber. Genetic aberrations involving *BRAF*, most commonly the V600E

mutation, can be seen in benign nevi as well as melanomas. *c-KIT* mutations are seen in a subset of mucosal and acral melanomas, whereas the *PDGFB* translocation is associated with dermatofibrosarcoma protuberans.

Bolognia J, Schaffer J, Cerroni L, eds. *Dermatology.* [Philadelphia]: Elsevier, 2018 (ch. 112).

59. **A.** Bullous pemphigoid

The figure shows a subepidermal split with a mixed inflammatory infiltrate containing eosinophils. These features are characteristic of bullous pemphigoid (BP). The urticarial phase of BP may show eosinophilic spongiosis with dermal inflammation, including eosinophils, without an obvious blister. Direct immunofluorescence studies in BP demonstrate linear deposition of C3 and IgG at the dermal-epidermal junction.

Bullous lupus erythematosus often shows a subepidermal split but is most commonly associated with a neutrophilic infiltrate (eosinophils would be unusual). Pemphigus vulgaris demonstrates suprabasal acantholysis with intact basal keratinocytes forming a "tombstone" appearance. Skin biopsies from lesions of dermatitis herpetiformis typically demonstrate neutrophilic microabscesses within the dermal papillae.

Bolognia J, Schaffer J, Cerroni L, eds. *Dermatology.* [Philadelphia]: Elsevier, 2018 (ch. 30).

60. **C.** Mycosis fungoides/cutaneous T-cell lymphoma (CTCL)

The figure illustrates an atypical lymphoid infiltrate with prominent epidermotropism, findings characteristic of mycosis fungoides or cutaneous T-cell lymphoma. The intraepidermal lymphocytes have irregular nuclear contours and are larger than the dermal lymphocytes.

Squamous cell carcinoma in situ demonstrates atypical keratinocytes throughout the full thickness of the epidermis, sparing the basal keratinocytes ("eyeliner sign"). Extramammary Paget disease may also show sparing of the basal keratinocytes; however, the cells are large, with abundant pale eosinophilic cytoplasm, and may show intracytoplasmic lumina or glandular differentiation. Intraepidermal Merkel cell carcinoma will show Merkel cells with hyperchromatic nuclei and high nuclear to cytoplasmic ratio.

Bolognia J, Schaffer J, Cerroni L, eds. *Dermatology.* [Philadelphia]: Elsevier, 2018 (ch. 120).

PROCEDURAL DERMATOLOGY

61. **C.** Nasolacrimal duct

The nasolacrimal duct runs along the nasofacial sulcus inferior to the medial canthus. The nasolacrimal duct drains tears into the nasal passage. Injury to the proximal portion of the duct can produce symptoms of watery eyes and excessive tearing. However, in older patients that have dry eyes at baseline, injury to this structure can go unnoticed.

Bolognia J, Schaffer J, Cerroni L, eds. *Dermatology.* [Philadelphia]: Elsevier, 2018 (ch. 142).

62. **A.** *PTCH*

This patient has basal cell nevus syndrome (BCNS), an autosomal dominant condition caused by constitutive activating mutations in the hedgehog pathway genes, most commonly PTCH1 but also PTCH2 and SUFU. This occurs in approximately 1/60,000 live births. Major criteria for BCNS includes:

1. More than two basal cell carcinomas (BCCs) or one BCC before the age of 20 years

2. Odontogenic keratocysts of the jaw (proven by histology)
3. Three or more palmar or plantar pits
4. Bilamellar calcification of the falx cerebri
5. Bifid, fused, or markedly splayed ribs
6. First-degree relative with BCNS
Early onset medulloblastoma may be the presenting sign of BCNS, thus in children who are diagnosed with this tumor, BCNS should be suspected and a careful examination for other signs and symptoms should be performed. Radiation therapy for medulloblastoma can induce invasive BCCs in the radiation field, as described in the question stem. Mutations in PTEN are found in PTEN hamartoma syndromes (i.e., Cowden), TSC1 mutations in tuberous sclerosis, and P53 mutations in xeroderma pigmentosa.
Bolognia J, Schaffer J, Cerroni L, eds. *Dermatology.* [Philadelphia]: Elsevier, 2018 (ch. 108).

63. C. Clindamycin 300 mg PO x 1
Clindamycin prophylactic dosing is 600 mg PO x 1. In patients with increased risk of MRSA, the surgeon should consider prophylaxis with clindamycin or Trimethoprim-sulfamethoxazole DS. The single dose should be given 30–60 minutes prior to surgery. The other listed choices are appropriate choices for antibiotic prophylaxis.
Bolognia J, Schaffer J, Cerroni L, eds. *Dermatology.* [Philadelphia]: Elsevier, 2018 (ch. 151).

64. B. Protoporphyrin IX
Photodynamic therapy relies on the cellular mechanisms for porphyrin metabolism. While only red blood cells have the ability to convert the final step from protoporphyrin IX to heme, all cells in the body contain the enzymes necessary to complete the initial steps. Therefore when applied to the skin, aminolevulinic acid is absorbed by keratinocytes, preferentially those that are damaged by precancerous changes, and then undergoes the subsequent enzymatic conversion of the porphyrin pathway. The metabolites, specifically protoporphyrin IX, accumulate in the cell given that the keratinocyte lacks the ability to convert this metabolite to heme due to lack of ferrochelatase. Upon exposure to blue light, the porphyrin metabolites generate reactive oxygen species that cause cell death, preferentially affecting the damaged keratinocytes. Photodynamic therapy is a field treatment for broad areas of actinic damage in patients that have numerous actinic keratoses.
Bolognia J, Schaffer J, Cerroni L, eds. *Dermatology.* [Philadelphia]: Elsevier, 2018 (ch. 135).

65. E. B and C
When a patient presents with severe pain 1 week after surgery on the ear, infection must be suspected. The wound should be cultured, and the patient should be started on empiric antibiotics with coverage for pseudomonas. In addition, wounds of the external auditory meatus that are near circumferential are at risk of stenosis of the ear canal, especially if edema is present in the setting of infection. For patients at risk of stenosis, referral to otolaryngology should be considered for visualization of canal patency and consideration of placement of wick or stent to prevent permanent stenosis.
Bolognia J, Schaffer J, Cerroni L, eds. *Dermatology.* [Philadelphia]: Elsevier, 2018 (ch. 151).

66. C. 10 ms
Pulsed-dye laser is a 595-nm laser that has a peak absorption by hemoglobin and causes selective photothermolysis of blood vessels. The pulse duration is the characteristic of laser treatment that controls the duration of time the laser energy is delivered to the skin. The desired pulse duration is dependent on the diameter of the target. The optimal pulse duration is roughly the same as the thermal relation time (TRT) or the time required for heated tissue to lose 50% of its heat through diffusion. For facial vessels with diameter of 30–100 microns, the TRT is approximately 1–10 ms, and typical laser pulse durations range from 0.4–20 ms. With pulse durations of 10 ms or greater, there is little to no immediate purpura because cavitation and vessel rupture is avoided. However, delayed purpura can still occur secondary to vasculitis that can occur a few days after treatment. Pulse durations of 3 ms and below are at risk of generating immediate purpura; 10 ms pulse duration will have very low risk of purpura but still within the therapeutic treatment window.
Bolognia J, Schaffer J, Cerroni L, eds. *Dermatology.* [Philadelphia]: Elsevier, 2018 (chs. 136 and 137).

67. A. Oral acitretin
In a trial of renal transplant recipients at high risk for squamous cell carcinoma (SCC), oral acitretin 30 mg daily led to an 88% reduction in future SCC. Niacinamide has not been studied directly in organ transplant recipients but has shown an approximately 25%–30% reduction in SCC in immunocompetent patients. Topical 5-fluorouracil and imiquimod are effective field treatments for the precursors of SCC (actinic keratosis and preclinical lesions) and are expected to lead to partial reductions in future SCC, but this has not been adequately studied in organ transplant recipients. Change of immunosuppression from a calcineurin inhibitor such as tacrolimus to an mammalian target of rapamycin (mTOR) inhibitor such as sirolimus has been shown in clinical trials to cause an approximately 50% reduction in future SCC, although this reduction appears to be most pronounced for those patients with a lower burden of prior SCC.
Bolognia J, Schaffer J, Cerroni L, eds. *Dermatology.* [Philadelphia]: Elsevier, 2018 (ch. 108).

68. C. Glabella and perinasal area
While rare, soft tissue filler injections can result in intravascular and perivascular injections that induce vascular compression and tamponade, leading to soft tissue necrosis. The abundant superficial vasculature in the glabella and perinasal regions make these areas more susceptible to filler-associated vascular occlusion. Very rarely, intravascular filler injection can cause retrograde movement in the retinal artery and unilateral blindness. This most frequently occurs in the watershed area of internal and external carotid artery circulation in the central upper face in the glabella region.
Bolognia J, Schaffer J, Cerroni L, eds. *Dermatology.* [Philadelphia]: Elsevier, 2018 (ch. 158).

69. A. Cold compresses
Inadvertent injection of soft tissue filler into or around a vessel causing a tamponade effect can lead to vascular occlusion and tissue necrosis. Early signs of impending necrosis include severe unrelenting pain and reticular erythema that develops anytime from immediately after injection to 1–2 days later. Treatment should be initiated immediately to minimize tissue necrosis. The mainstay of treatment is flushing the area with hyaluronidase. Serial injections of >100 U are often required. Treatment with hyaluronidase may also be beneficial when non-HA fillers are used, as the hyaluronidase can act on the native extracellular matrix, relieving pressure by dissolving native hyaluronan. Additional treatments include warm compresses, massage, application of nitroglycerin paste to

promote vasodilation, hyperbaric oxygen, and anticoagulant therapy, including aspirin and occasionally low-molecular weight heparin.
Bolognia J, Schaffer J, Cerroni L, eds. *Dermatology*. [Philadelphia]: Elsevier, 2018 (ch. 158).

70. B. Croton oil
The Baker-Gordon peel has four components: phenol (88%), septisol liquid soap (eight drops), Croton oil (three drops), and distilled water. The efficacy of the peel is determined by the depth of penetration. Croton oil is the key ingredient for controlling the depth of the peel. Cutaneous complications including scarring (marbled scarring depicted in the figure), alabaster appearance with effacement of normal skin texture, hypopigmentation (darker skin types and men are more at risk), and persistent postoperative erythema are usually a result of an overly aggressive peel. Patients treated with Baker-Gordon peel must have cardiac monitoring during the procedure as cardiotoxicity is a risk of systemic absorption of phenol. Limiting the Croton oil helps minimize these risks.
Bolognia J, Schaffer J, Cerroni L, eds. *Dermatology*. [Philadelphia]: Elsevier, 2018 (ch. 154).

BASIC SCIENCE

71. D. Negatively regulate mTOR signaling
Tuberous sclerosis (TS) is an autosomal dominant disorder with cutaneous and systemic manifestations. TS is caused by a mutation in either *TSC1* or *TSC2*, which encode hamartin or tuberin, respectively. These proteins function together to negatively regulate mTOR signaling. Cutaneous manifestations of TS include hypomelanotic "ash leaf" macules, facial angiofibromas and fibrous cephalic plaques (pictured), shagreen patches (pictured), periungual fibromas, and café au lait macules. Systemic manifestations can involve nearly any organ system, but the most common manifestations are neurologic (cortical tubers, subependymal nodules, seizures, infantile spasms, intellectual impairment), cardiovascular (myocardial rhabdomyoma, Wolff-Parkinson-White syndrome), renal (angiomyolipomas, cysts), pulmonary (lymphangioleiomyomatosis in females), and ocular (retinal hamartomas, achromatic retinal patches).
Neurofibromatosis type 1 is due to mutations in *NF1*, which encodes neurofibromin, a protein that negatively regulates Ras signaling by catalyzing GTP hydrolysis to GDP. Muir-Torre syndrome is due to mutations in one of three DNA mismatch repair genes (*MSH2, MLH1, MSH6*). Gardner syndrome, or familial polyposis of the colon, is caused by mutations in the *APC* gene, which encodes a protein that negatively regulates the *Wnt/β-catenin* signaling pathway. Fabry disease is caused by a defect in glycosphingolipid metabolism due to mutations in the *GLA* gene, which encodes the enzyme α-galactosidase A.
Bolognia J, Schaffer J, Cerroni L, eds. *Dermatology*. [Philadelphia]: Elsevier, 2018 (ch. 61).

72. E. Defective nucleotide excision repair
The vignette and clinical image suggest a diagnosis of xeroderma pigmentosum (XP), caused by various mutations in the nucleotide excision repair pathway (NER). Patients present with extreme photosensitivity, significantly increased risk of cutaneous malignancy, and ophthalmologic complications. Neurologic complications are seen in a minority of patients. Defective transcription-coupled NER is seen in Cockayne syndrome, in which patients have no

increased risk of skin cancer and lack pigmentary changes. Rothmund-Thomson syndrome results from defective DNA replication and repair of UV damage, but patients typically possess additional features such as short stature and skeletal dysplasia. Mutations in *LMNA* gene result in defective structure and function of the nuclear envelope, which causes Hutchinson-Gilford progeria.
Bolognia J, Schaffer J, Cerroni L, eds. *Dermatology*. [Philadelphia]: Elsevier, 2018 (ch. 87).

73. D. AIRE
The above vignette describes a patient with chronic mucocutaneous candidiasis, autoimmune endocrinopathy, and ectodermal dysplasia. These features are characteristic of APECED (autoimmune polyendocrinopathy-candidiasis–ectodermal dystrophy) syndrome, which is due to mutations in the autoimmune regulator (*AIRE*) gene. Hypoparathyroidism and hypoadrenocorticism are the most common endocrinopathies but may not be apparent until teenage years or adulthood. Alopecia areata and vitiligo may also be seen.
STAT1 amplification is found in the most common form of chronic mucocutaneous candidiasis. While autoimmunity is seen in this condition, polyendocrinopathies are less common. Further, severe systemic infections are common. *STAT3* and *DOCK8* mutations are seen in patients with hyper IgE syndrome. *CARD14* mutations have been identified in pustular psoriasis and pityriasis rubra pilaris.
Bolognia J, Schaffer J, Cerroni L, eds. *Dermatology*. [Philadelphia]: Elsevier, 2018 (ch. 60).

74. C. Defective migration of melanoblasts
Piebaldism is an autosomal dominant disorder characterized by congenital patches of irregularly shaped (e.g., triangular) leukoderma that are stable and permanent but otherwise benign. These leukodermic patches often contain normally pigmented and hyperpigmented macules and patches, and a white forelock with underlying depigmented skin is found in 80%–90% of affected individuals. Most cases of piebaldism are due to a mutation in the *KIT* proto-oncogene, which is required for normal development and migration of melanocytes from the neural crest. A similar white forelock can also be found in Waardenburg syndrome (WS), a primarily autosomal dominant disorder of neural crest development due to mutations in *PAX3, MITF, EDNRB, EDN3*, or *SOX10*. Four clinical types have been described, and unlike piebaldism, WS patients may have additional findings, such as deafness, heterochromia, irides, and dystopia canthorum.
Vitiligo is characterized by an absence of functional melanocytes in affected skin. While the pathogenesis of vitiligo is multifactorial, evidence suggests that autoimmune destruction contributes to the loss of melanocytes. Oculocutaneous albinism is caused by defects in melanin synthesis. Overgrowth of the hyphal form of *Malassezia furfur* causes pityriasis (tinea) versicolor. Exposure to phenols/catechols, sulfhydryls, and other substances may result in chemical leukoderma.
Bolognia J, Schaffer J, Cerroni L, eds. *Dermatology*. [Philadelphia]: Elsevier, 2018 (ch. 65).

75. A. Type V collagen
The clinical image and vignette suggest a diagnosis of Ehlers-Danlos syndrome (EDS), of which there are several types. Hyperextensibility, abnormal scarring, and molluscoid pseudotumors (described previously) are characteristic of the classical subtype. This type is the most common and is associated with mutations in type V collagen

(COL5A1, COL5A2). Tenascin X is deficient in hypermobile EDS. Type III collagen (COL3A1) is most often mutated in the vascular subtype of EDS. Fibrillin 1 mutation is seen in Marfan syndrome, and ABCC6 mutation is seen in pseudoxanthoma elasticum.
Bolognia J, Schaffer J, Cerroni L, eds. *Dermatology*. [Philadelphia]: Elsevier, 2018 (ch. 97).

76. **B.** Mast cells
The clinical image depicts Darier sign, in which erythema and wheal formation develop in the setting of rubbing. This is characteristic of mastocytosis, a condition that can present in young children and can be vesiculobullous. The condition is most commonly caused by activating mutations in c-KIT, and a skin biopsy shows infiltration of mast cells in the dermis.
Bolognia J, Schaffer J, Cerroni L, eds. *Dermatology*. [Philadelphia]: Elsevier, 2018 (ch. 118).

77. **A.** Mismatch repair
This vignette describes a patient with multiple sebaceous neoplasms and family history of colon cancer, suggesting the diagnosis of Muir-Torre syndrome (MTS). This autosomal dominant disorder is associated with adenocarcinomas of the colon and genitourinary tract and less commonly malignancy of the breast, head and neck, gastrointestinal tract, and blood. Cutaneous manifestations include sebaceous neoplasms (adenomas more commonly than carcinomas), which can develop before, concurrently, or after the diagnosis of a visceral cancer, and keratoacanthomas. Multiple sebaceous neoplasms located outside the head and neck area should raise concern for MTS. MTS is caused by heterozygous germline mutations in DNA mismatch repair genes (*MSH2, MLH1, MSH6*).
Basal cell nevus syndrome results from mutation of *PTCH* gene, which functions to inhibit the sonic hedgehog/smoothened pathway. When inactivating mutation occurs, smoothened is constitutively activated with downstream *Gli* expression. Gap junction/connexin genes are involved in various disorders, including hidrotic ectodermal dysplasia, PPK + deafness, KID syndrome, and Vohwinkel syndrome. Fabry disease is an example of a lysosomal storage disorder, while Chediak-Higashi and Hermansky-Pudlak syndrome involve lysosomal trafficking/transport. Darier and Hailey-Hailey diseases involve calcium signaling/ATPase.
Bolognia J, Schaffer J, Cerroni L, eds. *Dermatology*. [Philadelphia]: Elsevier, 2018 (ch. 63).

78. **E.** 1A and 2B domains
According to the Human Intermediate Filament Database, ~78% of all the missense mutations associated with keratinopathies occur in the 1A and 2B domains. These domains harbor the helix initiation motif (1A) and the helix termination motif (2B) thought to play a key role in intermediate filament assembly.
Bolognia J, Schaffer J, Cerroni L, eds. *Dermatology*. [Philadelphia]: Elsevier, 2018 (ch. 56).

79. **E.** Connexin 26
Connexin 26 (*GJB2*) is mutated in keratitis-ichthyosis-deafness syndrome (KID Syndrome), which is pictured here. This autosomal dominant disorder manifests with hyperkeratotic erythematous skin lesions, which classically present on the face and acral sites, keratitis, and sensorineural deafness or severe hearing impairment (depicted by the hearing aide in the left ear). Connexin 43 is associated with oculodentodigital dysplasia. The other answer choices are not elements of gap junctions.
Bolognia J, Schaffer J, Cerroni L, eds. *Dermatology*. [Philadelphia]: Elsevier, 2018 (ch. 57).

80. **C.** 30S ribosomal subunit
The prescribed drug is doxycycline for Lyme disease. Tetracyclines inhibit protein synthesis by targeting the 30S ribosomal subunit. Macrolides target the 50S ribosomal subunit. Quinolones target DNA gyrase, and rifampin targets RNA polymerase. Penicillins and cephalosporins target cell wall synthesis, while trimethoprim and sulfonamides target folic acid metabolism.
Bolognia J, Schaffer J, Cerroni L, eds. *Dermatology*. [Philadelphia]: Elsevier, 2018 (ch. 127).

1. A 21-year-old man presents with the following pruritic eruption on his legs. He reports that he recently returned from a trip up to his family's lake house in Michigan. He denies any contact with pets or others with similar symptoms. What is the most likely diagnosis?

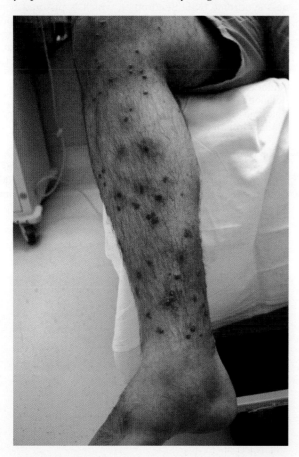

A. Herpes zoster
B. Arthropod assault
C. Cercarial dermatitis
D. Hot tub folliculitis
E. Seabather's eruption

2. A 60-year-old man presents with the following on the tongue. He reports left-sided ear pain and dizziness starting about 4 days prior. What is the most likely diagnosis?

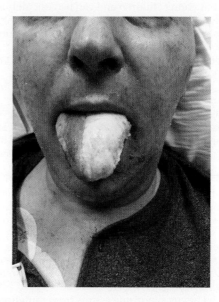

A. Giant cell arteritis
B. Chemotherapy-induced mucositis
C. Oral candidiasis
D. Herpes zoster

3. The patient started allopurinol 8 weeks ago and developed fevers, lymphadenopathy, and severe facial swelling with the following eruption. What is a possible long-term sequela from this reaction?

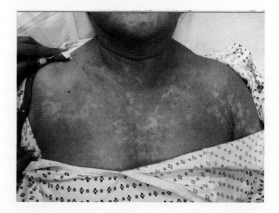

A. Stroke
B. Corneal scarring
C. Thyroiditis
D. Epistaxis

4. You are consulted on a 75-year-old man who presents with a necrotic ulcer on the face. He reports headaches, fevers, and a history of diabetes. He denies any recent travel. Hematoxylin and eosin reveals the following histopathology. What is the treatment of choice?

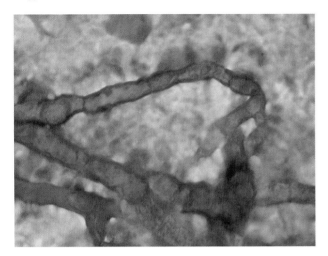

A. Aggressive surgical resection
B. Anidulafungin
C. Amphotericin B
D. Itraconazole
E. Both A and C

5. A 40-year-old patient presents with the following asymptomatic lesions on the nose and cheeks. He has a history of kidney transplant and has remained on oral tacrolimus for 3 years. What is the most likely association?

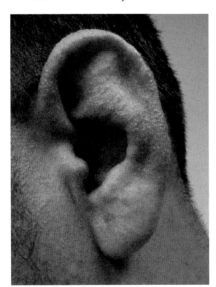

With permission from DeCrescenzo AJ, Philips RC, and Wilkerson MG, in *American Academy of Dermatology, Inc.*, 2016 (fig. 1).

A. Polyomavirus infection
B. Demodex overgrowth
C. Acantholytic disorder
D. Vitamin deficiency

6. A 47-year-old patient presents with annular plaques with scale located on the chest, arms, and back. The patient notes that this eruption flares after exposure to the sun. Which of the following will most likely be positive?

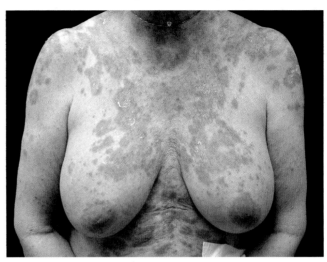

With permission from Pappas Taffer L, Callen JP, *Treatment of Skin Disease: Comprehensive Therapeutic Strategies*, 2018, Elsevier, 797–801.

A. Anti-Jo 1
B. Anti-Ro
C. Anti-Scl 70
D. Anti-La

7. In the same patient above, upon further questioning, she recalls starting a new medication for a fungal rash. Which of the following medications is most likely the culprit?
A. Fluconazole
B. Terbinafine
C. Voriconazole
D. Nystatin oral suspension

8. What is the best diagnosis of this single lesion?

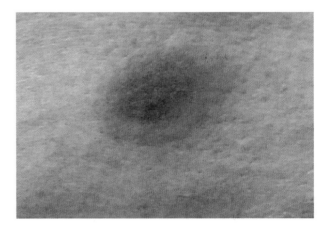

A. Erythema chronicum migrans
B. Fixed drug eruption
C. Allergic contact dermatitis
D. Erythema multiforme

9. A young man presents with this cutaneous eruption along with generalized malaise. He notes the rash and symptoms worsen after spending time outside. At the time of

presentation to your clinic, this patient is also most likely to complain of which of the following?

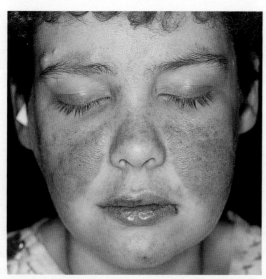

With permission from Hansen CB and Jeffrey PC, in *Dermatological Signs of Systemic Disease*, 5th edition, 2017, 1–12 (fig. 1-13).

A. Joint pains
B. No symptoms
C. Blood in the stool
D. Visual disturbance

10. In the patient above, hydroxychloroquine is started at 200 mg by mouth twice daily. After 6 months of therapy, the patient still has a persistent malar rash, proteinuria, joint aches, and generalized malaise. Which of the following are potential therapeutic options?
A. Switching to chloroquine
B. Adding quinacrine
C. Addition of topical steroids
D. Counseling on sun avoidance behavior
E. All of the above

11. Your new patient with chronic kidney disease presents with inflammatory papules and pustules on the face that did not respond to prior treatment with a topical retinoid and topical clindamycin-benzoyl peroxide combination. Which of these medications can be used without dose adjustment?
A. Trimethoprim/sulfamethoxazole
B. Minocycline
C. Cephalexin
D. Doxycycline

12. A 21-year-old female presents with malar rash, joint pains, proteinuria, thrombocytopenia on laboratory evaluation, and positive serology for antinuclear antibody and anti-double stranded DNA antibody (anti-dsDNA). This patient meets criteria for systemic lupus erythematosus and was started on hydroxychloroquine. You remind the patient that evaluation by which specialist is recommended for monitoring medication-associated toxicity?
A. Nephrologist
B. Urologist
C. Hepatologist
D. Ophthalmologist

13. The patient presented with these findings along with hair loss and oral ulcers. Antibody testing reveals positive anti-melanoma differentiation-associated gene 5 (MDA-5) antibody. The patient is most at risk for rapidly progressive:

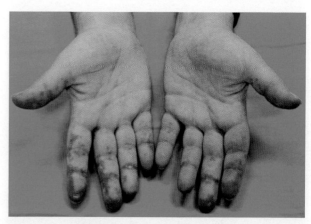

With permission from Barrientos N, Sicilia JJ, Moreno de Vega MJ, and Dominguez JD, in Anti-MDA5–positive dermatomyositis: A description of the cutaneous and systemic manifestations in 2 cases, *Actas Dermo-Sifiliográficas* [English Edition], 2018, 109(2):188–190.

A. Interstitial lung disease
B. Myositis
C. Malignancy
D. Cardiomyopathy

14. In addition to the nail findings shown, the patient may also have:

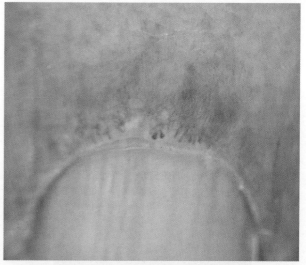

Photo courtesy of Curtis Asbury, MD, Selbyville, DE.

A. Proximal muscle weakness
B. Malar rash
C. Glomerulonephritis
D. Rash in the conchal bowl

15. This patient is diagnosed with systemic sclerosis. Which of the following treatments would NOT be appropriate for this associated symptom?

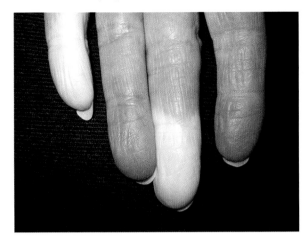

With permission from Le ST, Fett N, Haemel A in *Raynaud's Phenomenon*, 2017, 22–30 (fig. 3-10).

  A. Cold avoidance
  B. Discontinuation of cigarette smoking
  C. Addition of calcium channel blockers
  D. Addition of propranolol

16. The patient above complains of her wedding band feeling tight on her fingers. She also presents with mat telangiectasias, Raynaud phenomenon, and calcinosis cutis. She is started on methotrexate and prednisone 1 mg/kg. The addition of prednisone to the therapeutic regimen has placed which organ system at a higher risk of crisis?
  A. Heart
  B. Kidney
  C. Brain
  D. Muscle

17. This 35-year-old patient is at risk for which of the following?

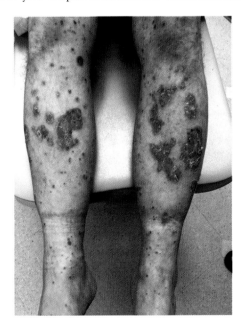

  A. Elevated triglycerides
  B. Elevated blood pressure

  C. Elevated fasting blood glucose
  D. All of the above

18. Discontinuation of the following would most likely impact her disease?

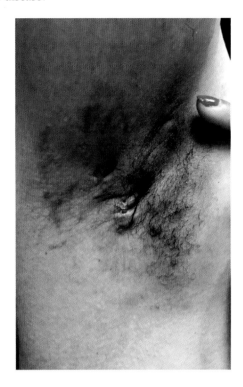

  A. Cocaine use
  B. Alcohol abuse
  C. Phencyclidine (PCP) use
  D. Cigarette smoking

19. Which of the following malignancies is the patient above most at risk for within areas of chronic disease?
  A. Melanoma
  B. Basal cell carcinoma
  C. Squamous cell carcinoma
  D. Merkel Cell Carcinoma

20. A 36-year-old female presents with acute erythroderma. Her primary lesions are illustrated in the figure. Which of the following diseases is most associated with this dermatosis?

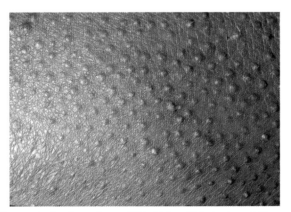

With permission from James WD, Elston DM, *Andrews' Diseases of the Skin Clinical Atlas*, Elsevier, 2018, 139–151.

A. Diabetes
B. HIV
C. Renal failure
D. Cardiovascular disease

21. Which of the following can be used in the treatment of this disorder? (More than one choice may be correct.)

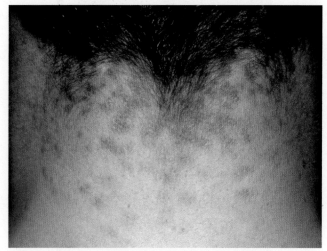

With permission from James WD, *Andrews' Diseases of the Skin Clinical Atlas*, 2018, Elsevier, chapter 11, 139–151.

A. Clarithromycin
B. Topical mupirocin
C. Isotretinoin
D. Topical ketoconazole
E. Minocycline
F. All of the above

22. Biopsy of a papule would demonstrate:

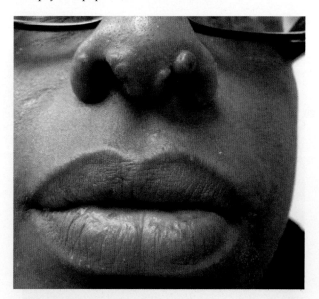

A. Tuberculoid granulomas with central caseation necrosis and peripheral lymphocytes
B. Hyaline deposits in the superficial and mid-dermis
C. Diffuse dermal infiltration with parasitized macrophages
D. Superficial and deep epithelioid granulomas lacking significant inflammatory infiltrate

23. A 17-year-old otherwise healthy girl presents for evaluation of the following. Lymphangiography reveals:

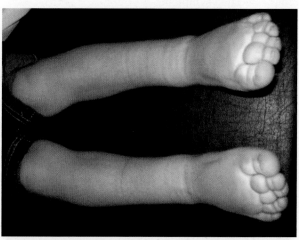

With permission from Del Pozo J, Gómez-Tellado M, López-Gutiérrez JC. Vascular malformations in childhood. Actas Dermosifiliogr. 2012;103(8):661-678.

A. Normal lymphatic vessels
B. Lymphatic hyperplasia with varicose dilation of lymphatics
C. Hypoplastic lymphatic vessels
D. Microfilaria emboli

24. The risk of which complication of chronic corticosteroid use is reduced by every-other-day dosing?
A. Opportunistic infection
B. Osteoporosis
C. Cataract formation
D. Osteonecrosis

25. The dosing of corticosteroids should be increased for maximum effect in which of the following scenarios?
A. A patient who is taking rifampin for hidradenitis suppurativa
B. A patient who is on oral contraceptives
C. A patient with stage IV chronic kidney disease
D. A patient who is on erythromycin for acne

26. Which of the following would NOT be a finding indicating possible Addison's disease?
A. Hypopigmentation around scars
B. Hyperpigmentation of the nipples
C. Palmar crease darkening
D. Longitudinal melanonychia
E. Decreased axillary and pubic hair

27. Which topical antifungal agent inhibits squalene epoxidase?
A. Terbinafine
B. Ciclopirox olamine
C. Nystatin
D. Oxiconazole

28. This patient presents with the following findings. Which of the following studies would most likely show an abnormality?

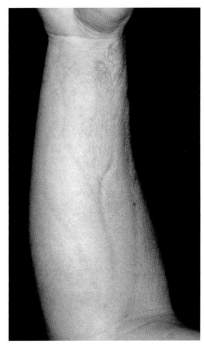

With permission from James WD, Berger TG, Elston DM, *Andrews' Diseases of the Skin*. 2016 Elsevier, 153–178.e7.

   A. Thyroid function test
   B. Complete blood count with differential
   C. Kidney function tests
   D. Chest radiography

29. The patient presents with new ulcerative lesions. Screening for which of the following diseases is appropriate?

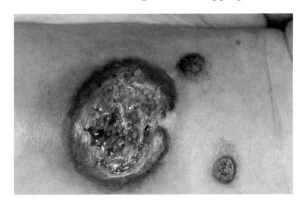

With permission from Najem CE, *Ferri's Clinical Advisor 2019*, Elsevier, 2019, 1177.e2–1177.e3.

   A. Crohn disease
   B. Ulcerative colitis
   C. Rheumatoid arthritis
   D. Hematologic disease
   E. All of the above

30. A 44-year-old female presents with this eruption. A biopsy sent for direct immunofluorescence reveals deposition of IgA and C3 perivascularly. This patient is at risk for involvement of which of the following organ systems?

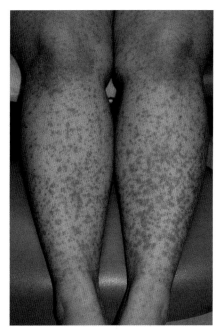

With permission from Nicole F, Callen JP, *Treatment of Skin Disease: Comprehensive Therapeutic Strategies*, 131, 429–432.

   A. Renal
   B. Gastrointestinal
   C. Rheumatologic
   D. All of the above

31. A 44-year-old female presents with xerosis, xerostomia, and difficulty wearing contact lenses. A laboratory evaluation revealed positive anti-SSA/Ro and anti-SSB/La antibody. In addition, she develops a new eruption on her lower legs. Which of the following diagnoses is most likely to explain her leg rash?
   A. Localized scleroderma
   B. Sarcoidosis
   C. Small vessel vasculitis
   D. Cutaneous T-cell lymphoma

32. This patient presents with nodules on her fingers. She has no prior history of skin disease. What other associated findings may be seen?

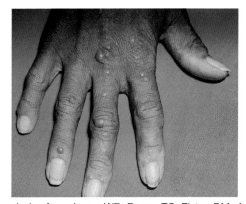

With permission from James WD, Berger TG, Elston DM, *Andrews' Diseases of the Skin*, 2016, Elsevier, chapter 31, 699–725.e1.

   A. Arthritis
   B. Malignancy
   C. Thyroid disease
   D. A and B
   E. All of the above

33. A 40-year-old male patient presents with the following findings. Which of the following systemic conditions should be considered given the cutaneous findings?

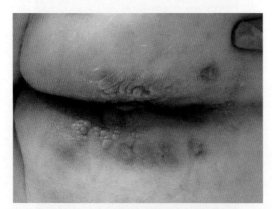

With permission from Rosenbach MA, Wanat KA, in *Dermatology*, 4th edition. 2017, 1644–1663 (fig. 93.17© 2018), Elsevier.

   A. Hepatitis C
   B. Irritable bowel syndrome
   C. Crohn's disease
   D. All of the above

34. The emergency room resident calls you with a consult of 47-year-old female with history of sarcoidosis who presents with fevers, joint pains, and lower extremity rash. The teledermatology platform is down. You expect the patient to have:
   A. Erythema nodosum
   B. Urticarial vasculitis
   C. Bullous pemphigoid
   D. Erythema induratum

35. The 45-year-old male patient with GI lymphoma presents with the skin findings shown. He reported a feeling of "sand in the eyes" and sores in the mouth along with subjective fevers. A review of medications revealed that allopurinol was started approximately 2 weeks ago for gout. Which of the following are known poor prognostic factors associated with this condition?

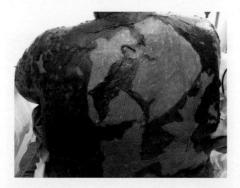

With permission from Craven NM and Creamer D. Toxic epidermal necrolysis and Stevens–Johnson syndrome, in *Treatment of Skin Disease: Comprehensive Therapeutic Strategies*, 5th edition, 2018, 830–833 (U fig. 245-1).

   A. Thyroid disease
   B. Age
   C. Malignancy
   D. B and C
   E. All of the above

36. The family of the patient above would like to know what steps can be taken to treat the condition. You highlight that the following is the single most important initial step in management:
   A. Starting systemic steroids
   B. Initiating treatment with Intravenous Immune Globulin (IVIG)
   C. Stopping allopurinol
   D. Starting cyclosporine

37. The patient complains of a recurrent blistering reaction along the penis. He has been treated with valacyclovir without improvement. When he returns to the office, polymerase chain reaction (PCR) for herpes simplex virus is negative. A biopsy is obtained that demonstrates interface dermatitis. Which of the following is the likely culprit?

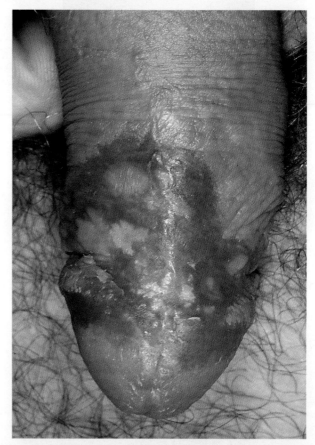

With permission from Habif TP, Exanthems and drug eruptions, in *Clinical Dermatology*, 6th edition, 2016, Elsevier (fig. 14.53).

   A. Ibuprofen
   B. Captopril
   C. Propranolol
   D. Nifedipine

38. A patient with advanced non-Hodgkin lymphoma presents with the following findings. HSV PCR is obtained and is negative. Which of the following may be associated with the entity?

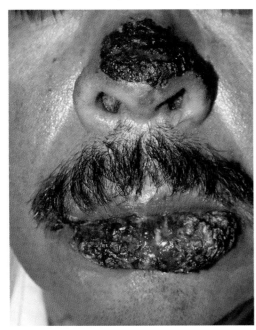

With permission from Tirado-Sánchez A and Bonifaz A, in Paraneoplastic pemphigus. A life-threatening autoimmune blistering disease., *Academia Española de Dermatología y Sifiliografía*, 2017, 108(10): 902–910, doi: 10.1016/j.ad.2017.04.024, Epub Aug 8, 2017.

A. Thyroid disease
B. Bronchiolitis obliterans
C. Renal disease
D. Arthritis

39. A male patient presents with the following lesions on the elbows, buttocks, and scalp. Which of the following autoimmune disorders is most commonly associated with the systemic disease causing the eruption?

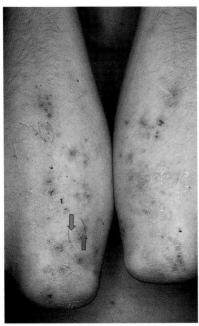

With permission from Kárpáti S, in An exception within the group of autoimmune blistering diseases: Dermatitis herpetiformis, the gluten-sensitive dermopathy, *Dermatologic Clinics*, 2011, 29(3):463–468.

A. Hashimoto thyroiditis
B. Sarcoidosis
C. Systemic lupus erythematosus
D. Addison disease

40. A male patient presents for an urgent visit with painful lower legs. You note redness, edema, and tenderness to the touch that is more pronounced on the left lower extremity but also present on the right medial lower shin. He denies a history of trauma, fever, or chills. Your next step is to:

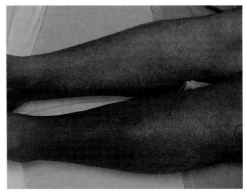

With permission from Hirschmann JV and Raugi GJ, in Lower limb cellulitis and its mimics: Part I. Lower limb cellulitis, *Journal of the American Academy of Dermatology*, 2012, 67(2):163.e1–163.e12.

A. Admit to the hospital for intravenous antibiotic treatment
B. Start outpatient oral antibiotics
C. Suggest leg elevation and compression therapy
D. Commence workup for deep fungal pathogen

PEDIATRIC DERMATOLOGY

41. A biopsy of the rash below would most likely show:

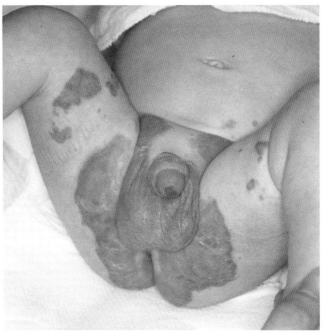

With permission from Herron, M (ed.), *Dermatological Signs of Systemic Disease*, 5th edition, 2017, Elsevier, 243–254 (fig. 29.6).

A. Ballooning degeneration of the spinous layer
B. Subcorneal pustules with PAS-positive organisms
C. Acanthotic epidermis with elongated rete ridges and diminished granular layer
D. Spongiosis with superficial perivascular lymphocytic infiltrate
E. Subcorneal pustules with neutrophils and gram-positive cocci

42. This neonate's skin findings may be explained by any of the following EXCEPT:

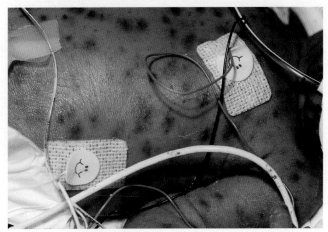

With permission from Paller AS, Cutaneous disorders of the newborn, in *Hurwitz Clinical Pediatric Dermatology*, Elsevier, 2016, chapter 2, 11–37.e4.

A. Congenital cytomegalovirus
B. Congenital rubella
C. Congenital leukemia
D. Congenital herpes simplex
E. Congenital toxoplasmosis

43. An otherwise healthy 16-year-old girl presents for evaluation of alopecia. She is distraught and asks about management options. Clinical and dermoscopic images are shown. What is the best treatment option?

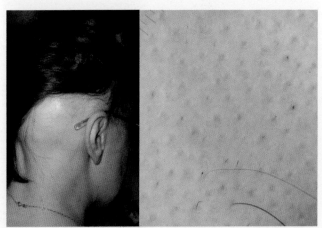

With permission from Bolognia J, Schaffer J, and Cerroni L, Basic principles of dermatology, in *Dermatology*, 4th edition, 2018, Elsevier, 1–43 (fig 0.43).

A. Reassurance and watchful waiting
B. Intralesional triamcinolone
C. Doxycycline
D. Griseofulvin at 10 mg/kg/day
E. Griseofulvin at 20 mg/kg/day

44. You are called to the newborn nursery to evaluate a scalp lesion on a 1-day-old, full-term infant. The baby was born via normal spontaneous vaginal delivery without complications. He is otherwise well and has no skin lesions elsewhere. A photograph is below. What is the most likely diagnosis?

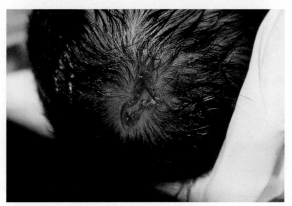

With permission from Paller AS, Mancini AJ (eds.), Cutaneous disorders of the newborn, in *Hurwitz Clinical Pediatric Dermatology*, 5th edition, 2016, Elsevier, 11–37 (fig. 2-34).

A. Aplasia cutis congenita
B. Trauma in the setting of forceps-assisted delivery
C. Herpes simplex virus
D. Adams-Oliver syndrome
E. Neonatal lupus

45. A 12-month-old boy is brought to your office for evaluation of recalcitrant diaper rash. He has been treated with zinc oxide barrier paste, topical steroids, and topical antifungals. Examination is shown. What is the next best step in management?

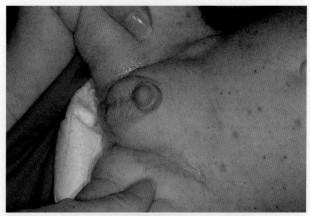

With permission from Paller AS, Mancini AJ (eds.), Cutaneous disorders of the newborn, in *Hurwitz Clinical Pediatric Dermatology*, 5th edition, 2016, Elsevier, 11–37 (fig 2-30).

A. Reassurance and more frequent diaper changes
B. Hydrocortisone and ketoconazole mixed together
C. Weekly oral fluconazole
D. Tacrolimus and calcipotriene
E. Skin biopsy

46. You are asked to evaluate a 1-month-old infant with several skin lesions. He is otherwise well and developing normally. Examination is shown. What is the most likely diagnosis?

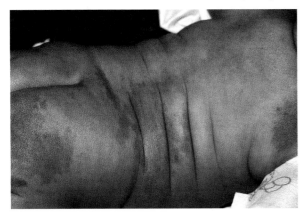

With permission from Paller AS, Mancini AJ (eds.), Vascular disorders of infancy and childhood, in *Hurwitz Clinical Pediatric Dermatology*, 5th edition, 2016, Elsevier, 279–316 (fig. 12-61).

A. Port wine stain
B. Capillary malformation–arteriovenous malformation syndrome
C. Phakomatosis pigmentovascularis type I
D. Phakomatosis pigmentovascularis type II
E. Phakomatosis pigmentovascularis type V

47. An 8-week-old baby boy is brought to the emergency department for a new eruption on the trunk; extremities, including palms and soles; and diaper area. The patient's mother had an uncomplicated pregnancy and term delivery. The patient is not febrile, with normal growth and development, but has been increasingly irritable and feeding poorly since the eruption began about 1 week ago. What is the preferred diagnostic test?

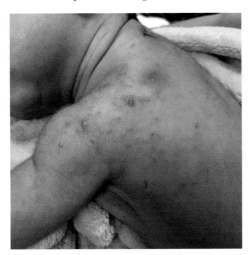

A. Skin biopsy
B. Sterile tissue culture
C. Tzanck smear
D. Mineral oil scraping
E. Nontreponemal serologic testing

48. A 14-month-old girl has been referred to you for evaluation of the recurrent, pruritic eruption shown. Her pediatrician empirically treated the whole family with topical permethrin with no improvement. What is the most likely diagnosis?

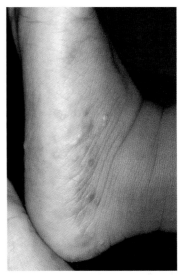

With permission from Paller AS, Mancini AJ (eds.), Cutaneous disorders of the newborn, in *Hurwitz Clinical Pediatric Dermatology*, 5th edition, 2016, Elsevier, 11–37 (fig. 2-20).

A. Dyshidrotic eczema
B. Scabies
C. Transient neonatal pustular melanosis
D. Acropustulosis of infancy
E. Impetigo

49. What are you most likely to see on dermoscopy when evaluating this patient?

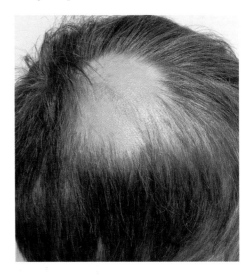

A. Black dots
B. Broken hairs
C. Follicular red dots
D. Exclamation point hairs
E. Comma hairs

50. A 6-year-old boy presents with his parents for evaluation of a lesion near his right ear. The lesion occasionally grows hair, and kids at school are starting to take notice. His parents would like to have the lesion removed. What is the most likely complication associated with surgical excision of this lesion?

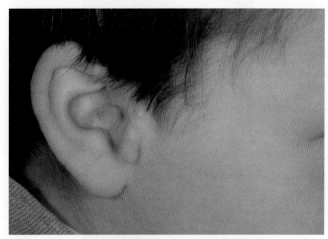

With permission from Paller AS, Mancini AJ, *Hurwitz Clinical Pediatric Dermatology*, Elsevier, 2015, 11–37.e4 (fig. 2-42© 2016).

A. Otitis externa
B. Otitis media
C. Chondritis
D. Recurrence
E. Hearing impairment

DERMATOPATHOLOGY

51. What would be the direct immunofluorescence findings associated with this lesion?

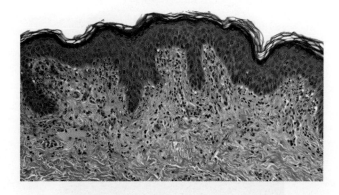

A. Linear IgA at the dermal-epidermal junction
B. Granular IgA at the tips of the dermal papillae
C. Linear IgG and C3 at the dermal-epidermal junction
D. Intercellular IgG and C3 within the epidermis

52. What is the best diagnosis?

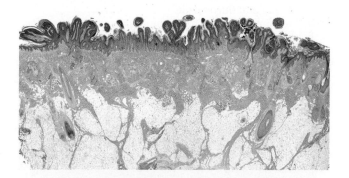

A. Nevus sebaceous
B. Verrucous carcinoma
C. Epidermal nevus
D. Lichen simplex chronicus

53. What is the best diagnosis?

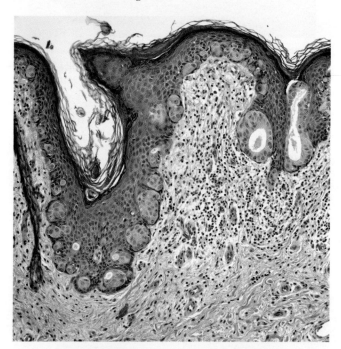

A. Melanoma in situ
B. Extramammary Paget disease
C. Bowen disease/squamous cell carcinoma in situ
D. Intraepidermal sebaceous carcinoma

54. What is the best diagnosis?

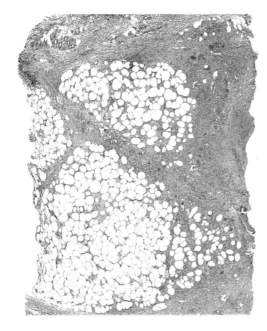

A. Erythema nodosum
B. Pancreatic panniculitis
C. Erythema induratum
D. Lupus panniculitis

55. The microscopic differential diagnosis for this lesion would NOT include which of the following?

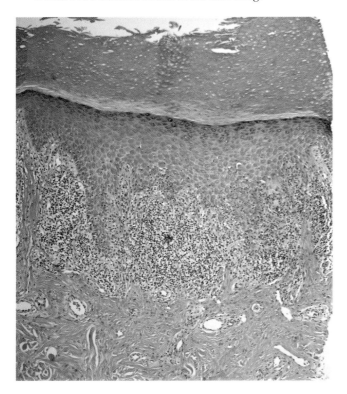

A. Lichen planus
B. Lichenoid drug reaction
C. Benign lichenoid keratosis
D. Psoriasis

56. What is the best diagnosis for this tumor?

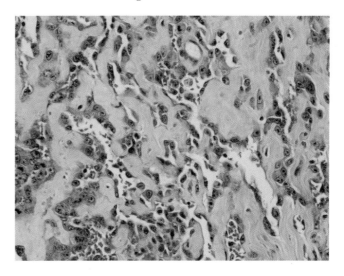

A. Angiosarcoma
B. Acquired tufted angioma
C. Cherry angioma
D. Glomus tumor

57. A 35-year-old man presents with a 1.5-cm pink-red crusted nodule on the left forearm. On examination, over a dozen umbilicated yellow papules are noted on the face and torso. The lesion on the arm is removed with a biopsy and sent for histopathologic evaluation (see figure). Based on the results of a subsequent genetic evaluation of the man's exome, another physician orders a screening colonoscopy. Two months later the patient calls back to your office to complain of a new, slightly painful lesion on the right forearm that grew rapidly. Without seeing the lesion, what is the most likely diagnosis?

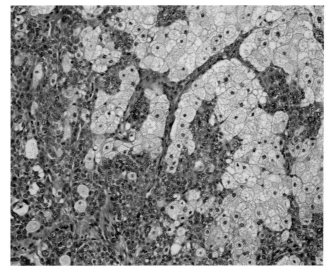

With permission from Rigel et al. *Cancer of the Skin*, Elsevier, 2011, chapter 13, 148 (fig. 13.25).

A. Sclerotic fibroma
B. Amelanotic melanoma
C. Merkel cell carcinoma
D. Keratoacanthoma
E. Desmoid tumor

58. What is the best diagnosis?

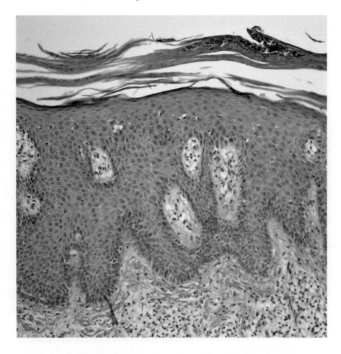

A. Mycosis fungoides/cutaneous T-cell lymphoma
B. Pityriasis lichenoides et varioliformis acuta (PLEVA)
C. Lichen simplex chronicus
D. Psoriasis

59. A patient presents with multiple lesions on the head and neck regions. A biopsy is performed and shown in the illustration. Mutation in which of the following genes might be involved in the pathogenesis?

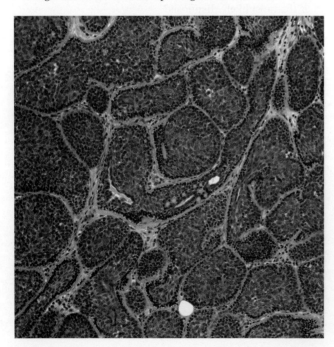

A. *PTCH1*
B. *CYLD*
C. *CTNNB1*
D. *FLCN*

60. What condition might be associated with these biopsy findings?

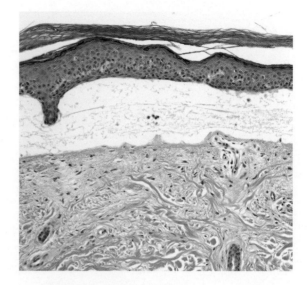

A. End-stage renal failure
B. Pregnancy
C. Osteoporosis
D. Tuberculosis

PROCEDURAL DERMATOLOGY

61. A patient presents for consideration of a medium-depth chemical peel for treatment of actinic damage. Her history is notable for past treatment with radiation to her face for recalcitrant acne over 30 years ago. What is your primary concern in treating this patient with a 35% trichloroacetic acid (TCA) peel in combination with Jessner's solution?
A. The peel might flare her acne.
B. Skin atrophy secondary to radiation treatment increases the risk of persistent erythema.
C. The radiation history makes her at increased risk of nonmelanoma skin cancers, and TCA peel is contraindicated in the field of active skin cancer.
D. Radiation decreases the number of pilosebaceous units in the skin and can affect healing time.

62. A patient presents for treatment of midfacial volume loss. You suggest treatment with a soft-tissue filler. In making your selection, you determine that you will select a filler with a high G'. The reason for this selection is:
A. A higher G' correlates with longer duration of filler.
B. You wish to select a filler with high elasticity and G' is proportional to elasticity.
C. G' is proportional to the thickness of the filler, and you wish to select a filler that will provide more lift.
D. A high G' indicates that filler is more easily dissolved with hyaluronidase, and you wish to choose a filler that can be rapidly reversed if complication arises.

63. A 68-year-old female presents for consideration of liposuction for her inner upper arms. What is the greatest risk in treating this area?
A. Compartment syndrome
B. Median nerve injury
C. Ulnar nerve injury
D. Necrosis

64. A patient presents for treatment with sclerotherapy for leg veins. You select a sclerosing agent that exerts its effects by causing dehydration of endothelial cells leading to endothelial destruction, fibrin deposition, and thrombus formation. The treatment is successfully completed. The patient later complains of intense muscle cramping. Which of the following sclerosing agents was most likely used?
    A. Sodium morrhuate
    B. Chromated glycerin
    C. Polidocanol
    D. Hypertonic saline

65. A patient presents for treatment of a basal cell carcinoma in the anterior right temple region. The cancer is removed in two stages, and the decision is made to proceed with a linear closure for repair of the wound. What is the appropriate plane of undermining, and what is the structure most at risk for injury in this location?
    A. Deep subcutaneous fat; temporal branch of cranial nerve VII
    B. Deep subcutaneous fat; superficial temporal artery
    C. Superficial subcutaneous fat; temporal branch of CN VII
    D. Superficial subcutaneous fat; superficial temporal artery

66. The following nail deformity occurred after biopsy of which part of the nail unit?

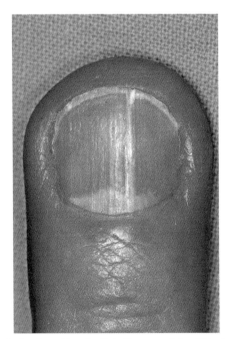

With permission from Haneke E, in *Surgery of the Skin*, 3rd edition, 2015, 755–780 (fig. 47.24).

    A. Proximal matrix
    B. Distal matrix
    C. Nail bed
    D. Proximal nail fold

67. All of the following muscles are innervated by the temporal branch of the cranial nerve VII EXCEPT:
    A. Frontalis
    B. Orbicularis oculi
    C. Corrugator
    D. Nasalis

68. This reconstruction following Mohs surgery for a basal cell carcinoma on the nose is best described as which of the following?

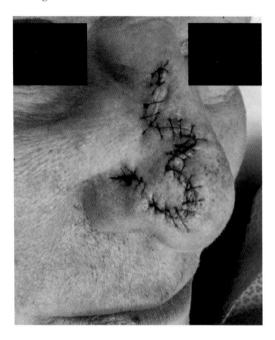

    A. Transposition flap
    B. Advancement flap
    C. Rotation flap
    D. Island pedicle flap
    E. Interpolation flap

69. A 73-year-old man with a remote history of basal cell carcinoma presents with the lesion shown on his nose. It is asymptomatic and has been gradually increasing in size over the last 6 months. A biopsy is performed that reveals spindle cells with high mitotic activity and anastomosing vascular channels. What is the patient's prognosis?

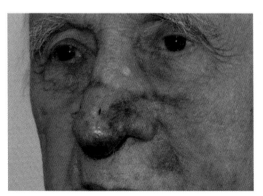

With permission from Mentzel T, *Clinics in Dermatology*, 2011, volume 29, issue 1 (80–90).

A. Expected stable disease with medical management
B. 95% cure rate after conservative excision, <5% risk of disease-specific death
C. 80% cure rate after wide excision, 10% risk of disease-specific death
D. 60% cure rate after wide excision and adjuvant radiation, 25% risk of disease-specific death
E. 30% cure rate after wide excision and adjuvant radiation with high rate of metastasis, at least 50% risk of disease-specific death

70. In what anatomical location would you select a nonabsorbable suture with the highest tissue reactivity and risk of infection?
A. Helical rim
B. Mucosal lip
C. Proximal nail fold
D. Scalp

BASIC SCIENCE

71. A 19-year-old patient with eight palmar pits is diagnosed with a basal cell carcinoma. When counseling him on the implications of his new diagnosis, he asks what the likelihood is of having a child affected with the same syndrome. Assuming an unaffected mate, which of the following is the correct answer?
A. 0% of any children
B. 25% of any children
C. 50% of any children
D. 100% of male children
E. The patient does not meet criteria for any syndrome

72. A patient presents to your office for skin "discoloration." On examination, you notice depigmented patches of skin and hair, as well as a broad nasal root and increased interpupillary distance. She has no other findings and her medical history is unremarkable. What genetic defect is the most likely explanation for these findings.

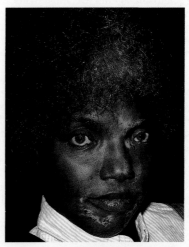

With permission from Paller AS, Mancini AJ (eds.), Disorders of pigmentation, in *Hurwitz Clinical Pediatric Dermatology*, 5th edition, 2016, Elsevier, 245–278 (fig. 11-19).

A. PAX3
B. MITF
C. SOX10
D. c-kit
E. TSC1

73. Match the epidermal proteins listed on the right with the letter (A–F) representing their most appropriate location in the epidermis.

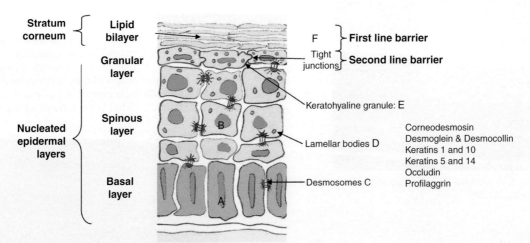

With permission from Baroni A, Structure and function of the epidermis related to barrier properties, *Clinics in Dermatology*, 2012, volume 30, issue 3, 257–262.

74. A patient presents with a diffuse thickening of the skin on the palms and soles. You perform a skin biopsy. What keratin genes are most likely responsible for this disease?

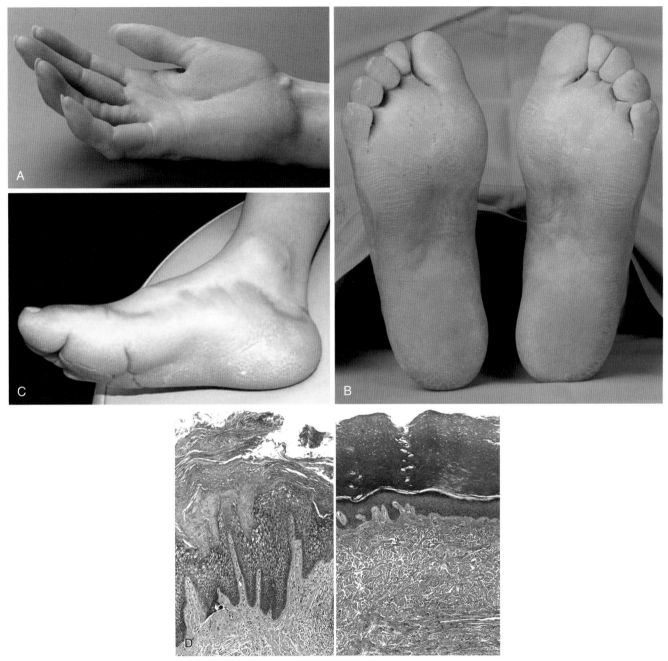

Courtesy Dieter Metze, MD. With permission from Metze D, in *Dermatology*, 2018, Elsevier, 58:924-943.e4. Courtesy Luis Requena, MD.

A. Keratins 5 and 14
B. Keratins 1 and 6c
C. Keratins 1 and 9

D. Keratins 1 and 10
E. Keratins 6 and 16

75. In the research lab you discover an epidermal protein that has several capabilities: inhibits transepidermal water loss, contributes to stratum corneum structure and function, acidifies the stratum corneum, and has an antistaphylococcal effect. You find through further research that the protein helps prevent the disease pictured. What protein have you most likely discovered?

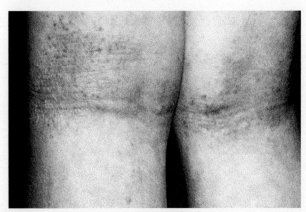

With permission from Beltrani VS, The clinical spectrum of atopic dermatitis. *J Allerg Clin Immunol.*, 1999, volume 104 (3 Suppl), S87–S98 (fig 3).

   A. Loricrin
   B. Transglutaminase-1
   C. BP180
   D. Filaggrin
   E. Cathelicidin

76. A teenager presents to your office complaining of black lesions on the face. What are they, and why are they black?

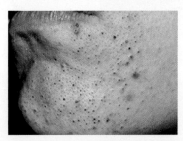

With permission from Benner N and Sammons D, in Overview of the treatment of acne vulgaris, *Osteopathic Family Physician*, 2013, 5(5):185–190.

   A. Multiple small nevi of the chin; color from melanin
   B. Closed comedones; color from normal lipids in the sebum
   C. Ingrown hairs; color from terminal hair growth
   D. Open comedones; color from topically applied acne product
   E. Open comedones; color from melanin and lipid oxidation

77. A patient presents to your clinic and asks for a therapy that can "cure" the cystic lesions on his torso and prevent further scarring of his skin. You prescribe an oral medication, but the patient is an astute premedicine student and wants to know more about the mechanism of action of the medication. Which answer is correct?

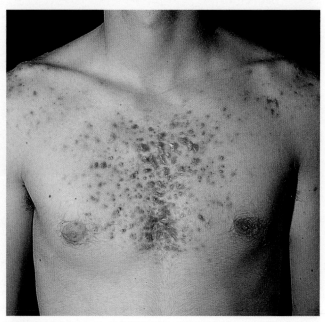

With permission from Habif T, *Clinical Dermatology*, 2016, Elsevier, chapter 7, 218–262.

   A. Affects DNA transcription, binds retinoic acid receptors (RAR) and retinoid X receptors (RXR), and receptor dimers bind DNA regulatory sequences in the nucleus called RAREs (retinoid hormone response elements)
   B. Affects mRNA translation, binds PPARα, and receptor dimers bind DNA regulatory sequences in the nucleus called PREs (peroxisome response elements)
   C. Affects DNA transcription, binds retinoic acid receptors (RAR) and retinoid X receptors (RXR), and monomeric receptors bind DNA regulatory sequences in the nucleus called RAREs (retinoid hormone response elements)
   D. Affects DNA transcription, binds retinoid Z receptors (RZR), and receptor dimers bind DNA regulatory sequences in the nucleus called RREs (retinoid response elements)
   E. Affects mRNA translation, binds androgen receptors (ARs), and monomeric receptors bind DNA regulatory sequences in the nucleus called AREs (androgen hormone response elements)

78. Vemurafenib's mechanism of action is:
   A. Immune checkpoint inhibitor
   B. MEK inhibitor
   C. Cytotoxic chemotherapy
   D. BRAF inhibitor

79. A child in your clinic has multiple crusted nodules on the scalp consistent with dermatophyte infection and tinea capitis. You prescribe oral griseofulvin. What is the mechanism of action of griseofulvin?

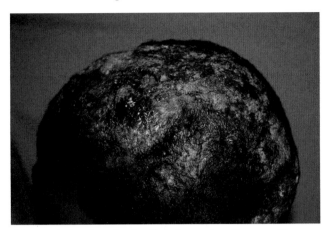

With permission from Isa-Isa R, Inflammatory tinea capitis: kerion, dermatophytic granuloma, and mycetoma, In *Clinics in Dermatology*, 2010, volume 28, issue 2, 133–136.

A. Interferes with DNA synthesis
B. Binds cell membrane sterols and increases membrane permeability
C. Inhibits fungal CYP450-dependent 14-α-demethylase to disrupt fungal cell membrane synthesis
D. Inhibits squalene epoxidase to disrupt fungal cell membrane synthesis
E. Interacts with polymerized microtubules to disrupt the mitotic spindle and inhibit mitosis

80. A patient from Alabama was performing yard work and suffered a spider bite on the thigh. The patient progressed to have renal insufficiency. What is the species of spider and its major toxin?

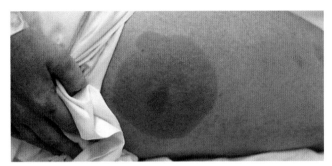

With permission from *Auerbach's Wilderness Medicine*, 2017, Elsevier, 993–1016.e6 (fig. 43-14).

A. Black widow spider; alpha-latrotoxin
B. Wolf spider; histamine
C. Jumping spider; hyaluronidase
D. Brown recluse spider; sphingomyelinase-D
E. Sac spider; lipase

GENERAL DERMATOLOGY

1. **C.** Cercarial dermatitis
   Swimmer's itch, or cercarial dermatitis, is caused by an allergic reaction to the cutaneous penetration of schistosomes. Humans can become exposed to these parasitic worms from freshwater sources containing infected snails. Cercarial dermatitis presents with pruritic papules on uncovered skin in contrast to seabather's eruption (E), which presents with pruritic papules under the bathing suit region. Seabather's eruption is caused by stinging jellyfish larvae present in saltwater areas. Herpes zoster (A) presents as vesicles with a red base clustered within a dermatomal distribution but may generalize or involve multiple dermatomes. Arthropod assault may present with pruritic edematous papules/plaques/vesicles (B). Hot tub folliculitis caused by pseudomonas often presents with follicular papules and pustules along sites of contact with a hot tub (usually most predominant on the trunk).
   Bolognia J, Schaffer J, Cerroni L, eds. *Dermatology*. [Philadelphia]: Elsevier, 2018 (ch. 83).

2. **D.** Herpes zoster
   While all the above diagnoses can cause diseases of the tongue, the sharp cutoff at the midline and prodromal symptoms are suggestive of herpes zoster (D). Herpes zoster is caused by the reactivation of latent varicella virus

and commonly seen in immunosuppressed and elderly patients, although young healthy adults can also be affected. Clinical presentation is preceded by prodromal symptoms (pruritus, tingling, pain) and manifests with grouped vesicles on an erythematous base in a dermatomal distribution. Ramsay Hunt syndrome presents with herpes zoster reactivation in the facial nerve causing facial palsy, otalgia, vesicles in a dermatomal distribution, and occasional hearing loss.

Giant cell arteritis (A) is a systemic granulomatous vasculitis of medium and large blood vessels usually affecting women over 50 years of age. Patients may present with temporal headaches, scalp tenderness and erythema, jaw claudication, and visual disturbances. Occasionally, patients may develop unilateral cutaneous and mucosal ulcerations. Systemic symptoms include polymyalgia rheumatica, fever, weight loss, and neurologic symptoms. Chemotherapy-induced mucositis (B) is often caused by cytotoxic chemotherapeutic agents. It clinically presents with single or multiple, round or irregular, gingival or oral mucosal ulcers, and would not have demarcation at the midline. Radiation therapy of the head and neck may also cause oral mucositis. Oral candidiasis (C) or thrush often presents with pseudomembranous changes with white plaques on the tongue and oral mucosa that wipes away, leaving behind normal or an erythematous underlying surface.

Bolognia J, Schaffer J, Cerroni L, eds. *Dermatology*. [Philadelphia]: Elsevier, 2018 (ch. 80).

3. **C.** Thyroiditis

Drug reaction with eosinophilia and systemic symptoms/drug-induced hypersensitivity syndrome (DRESS/DIHS) is a serious medication reaction that typically occurs 2–6 weeks after initiation of the culprit drug. The clinical presentation includes an exanthematous eruption, which can have bulla, pustules, purpura, or scaling in addition to facial swelling, fevers, and lymphadenopathy. Laboratory anomalies may include profound peripheral eosinophilia, atypical lymphocytosis, transaminitis, and renal dysfunction. Long-term sequelae may include cardiomyopathy and thyroiditis. High-dose steroids with a long taper and close monitoring for rebound are the preferred treatment. The patient should also be evaluated for signs and symptoms of heart failure and thyroid dysfunction during the steroid taper (usually 6–8 weeks). Some patients may require a second immunosuppressive agent such as cyclosporine or mycophenolate mofetil if DRESS is refractory to systemic steroids. Common drug culprits include aromatic anticonvulsants, allopurinol, minocycline, sulfonamides, and lamotrigine.

Stroke is not a direct sequela from DRESS. Corneal scarring can occur as sequela from Stevens Johnson syndrome/toxic epidermal necrolysis. This drug reaction is characterized by painful atypical targetoid papules that rapidly develop into vesicles and bulla with skin sloughing and mucosal involvement (eyes, mouth, nose, esophagus, anogenital). Corneal scarring and urethral/vaginal strictures may result. Epistaxis is not a direct sequela from DRESS.

Bolognia J, Schaffer J, Cerroni L, eds. *Dermatology*. [Philadelphia]: Elsevier, 2018 (ch. 21) (table 21.10).

4. **E.** Both A and C

Mucormycosis is an opportunistic fungal infection that typically affects immunocompromised hosts. Lesions are necrotic due to blood vessel invasion and thrombosis. The rhinocerebral subtype of infection often affects patients with diabetes. It presents with black necrotic eschars or ulcerations on the face and can be associated with headaches, facial pain, fevers, epistaxis, and ocular involvement. On H&E, hyphal structures present as broad, ribbonlike, nonseptate, and classically branch at 90 degrees. Infection is rapidly progressive and associated with high mortality. Aggressive surgical resection combined with amphotericin B or posaconazole provides the best chance of survival.

Anidulafungin (B) may be used for systemic candidiasis or aspergillosis. Amphotericin B (C) alone is a treatment option for mucocutaneous leishmaniasis. H&E or Giemsa stain will reveal parasitized histiocytes. Itraconazole (D) is the treatment of choice for paracoccidioidomycosis. This is a dimorphic fungal infection found predominantly in Central and South America. Clinically, patients present with painful pink-red ulcerated lesions on the face and oral/nasal mucosa. H&E will reveal the classic mariner's wheel yeast.

Bolognia J, Schaffer J, Cerroni L, eds. *Dermatology*. [Philadelphia]: Elsevier, 2018 (ch. 77).

5. **A.** Polyomavirus infection

Trichodysplasia spinulosa most commonly develops in solid organ transplant recipients on chronic immunosuppressive medications such as cyclosporine or tacrolimus. It is associated with polyomavirus infection (A). Clinically, it presents with skin-colored to pink follicular papules with keratinous spines on the central face. Rarely, it can spread to the trunk and extremities. There are case reports

of successful treatment with oral and topical antiviral medications as well as retinoids.

Demodex overgrowth (B) has been associated with rosacea as well as Demodex folliculorum, which presents with inflammatory papules and pustules that favor the face, often with a background of diffuse erythema. Demodicosis may be associated with immunosuppression.

Acantholytic disorders (C) such as Darier disease may present with skin-colored to brown papules in a seborrheic distribution or intertriginous distribution as seen in Hailey-Hailey. Lesions may be crusted, eroded, or fissured. Patients typically have other manifestations of this genetic condition, including nail and oral findings. Phrynoderma is a vitamin A deficiency (D) and can present with follicular keratoses classically described as "toad skin."

Bolognia J, Schaffer J, Cerroni L, eds. *Dermatology*. [Philadelphia]: Elsevier, 2018 (ch. 81).

6. **B.** Anti-Ro

This is a patient with subacute cutaneous lupus erythematosus (SCLE). Patients with SCLE are photosensitive, and eruptions commonly involve the upper extremities, lateral face, and superior aspects of the trunk. The lesions are often psoriasiform or annular. SCLE is associated with anti-SSA/Ro autoantibody positivity. Anti-Jo 1 is an autoantibody that can be positive in a subset of dermatomyositis patients. The anti-Scl 70 antibody may be positive in patients with systemic sclerosis. The anti-SSB/La antibody may be positive in patients with Sjögren disease. These patients may express anti-SSA/Ro positivity as well.

Bolognia J, Schaffer J, Cerroni L, eds. *Dermatology*. [Philadelphia]: Elsevier, 2018 (ch. 41).

7. **B.** Terbinafine

In patients with SCLE it is important to consider drug-induced presentations. Common potential culprits include terbinafine, thiazide diuretics, tumor necrosis factor-alpha inhibitors, proton pump inhibitors, calcium channel blockers, antiepileptics, taxanes, and thrombocyte inhibitors. Voriconazole is associated with photosensitivity and the development of squamous cell carcinomas. Fluconazole is uncommonly associated with cutaneous hypersensitivity reactions.

Bolognia J, Schaffer J, Cerroni L, eds. *Dermatology*. [Philadelphia]: Elsevier, 2018 (ch. 41).

8. **B.** Fixed drug eruption

Fixed drug eruptions (FDE) present as oval or round well-demarcated red plaques, sometimes with a dusky or bullous center. There may be one or few lesions, and mucosal involvement may occur. The initial eruption generally develops 1–2 weeks after the culprit medication, but upon reexposure the lesions may recur in the same location within 24 hours. Typically, lesions resolve with hyperpigmentation (although pseudoephedrine may cause nonpigmenting FDE). The most common causes of FDE include antibiotics (sulfa), NSAIDs, acetaminophen, aspirin, and barbiturates. Erythema chronicum migrans is the eruption of Lyme disease, which is often caused by *Borrelia burgdorferi* infection transmitted by *ixodes* ticks. It is characterized by an expanding red patch with central clearing and a central macule or papule (bull's eye) that may occasionally vesiculate. The eruption resolves spontaneously even without treatment.

Acute allergic contact dermatitis is characterized by pruritic, inflammatory papules and plaques, which may vesiculate. There is often a geometric configuration depending on the contactant.

Erythema multiforme is a reactive dermatosis that can be idiopathic in nature or triggered by infections or medications. It is often associated with herpes simplex virus or mycoplasma pneumoniae infection. The lesions are classically targetoid (may be atypical), with a predilection for acral and mucosal surfaces, and usually smaller than that of fixed drug eruption. Histology between fixed drug eruption and erythema multiforme is similar, and history as well as clinical examination is important in distinguishing these conditions. Bolognia J, Schaffer J, Cerroni L, eds. *Dermatology*. [Philadelphia]: Elsevier, 2018 (ch. 21).

9. **A.** Joint pains
The patient above is presenting with a classic butterfly rash of acute cutaneous lupus erythematosus (ACLE). The rash tends to occur after sun exposure and typically involves the malar cheeks and bridge of the nose but often spares the nasolabial folds. ACLE is often associated with active systemic lupus erythematosus (SLE), which most often involves multiple organ systems. Aside from the skin, other commonly involved systems include the joints, central nervous system (CNS), kidneys, and hematologic system. Other diagnoses to consider in a pediatric patient with photosensitive eruption include PMLE (no systemic symptoms), erythropoietic protoporphyria (burning skin with exposure to the sun), and Hydroa vacciniforme (a photodistributed vesiculobullous eruption that heals with scarring). Bolognia J, Schaffer J, Cerroni L, eds. *Dermatology*. [Philadelphia]: Elsevier, 2018 (ch. 41).

10. **E.** All of the above
All of the above are appropriate. Treatment of cutaneous lupus includes topical agents such as topical steroids and calcineurin inhibitors. Systemic therapy is often initiated with antimalarial medication, usually hydroxychloroquine. Quinacrine can be added to hydroxychloroquine to optimize therapy (without increasing the risk of ocular toxicity). In addition, hydroxychloroquine can be switched to chloroquine if there is an inadequate response to therapy. Reviewing sun protection and sun avoidance behavior can help reduce flares. In addition, smoking cessation is important for patients on antimalarials, as smoking may impair their therapeutic effect. Bolognia J, Schaffer J, Cerroni L, eds. *Dermatology*. [Philadelphia]: Elsevier, 2018 (ch. 41).

11. **D.** Doxycycline
Doxycycline does not require a dose adjustment for renal dysfunction. The other antibiotics require a dose adjustment based on creatinine clearance.

12. **D.** Ophthalmologist
The patient above with systemic lupus erythematosus has started hydroxychloroquine. This medication can be dosed up to 6.5 mg/kg/day. An alternative to this medication is chloroquine, which has been dosed between 3.5–4 mg/kg ideal body weight/day. Recent recommendations from the American Academy of Ophthalmology suggests using less than 5 mg/kg real weight/day of hydroxychloroquine and less than 2.3 mg/kg of real weight/day of chloroquine. It is suggested that patients on these medications see an ophthalmologist for monitoring of retinal toxicity. The patient with SLE should certainly see a nephrologist when renal disease is present, but ocular toxicity is most strongly associated with antimalarial medications. Bolognia J, Schaffer J, Cerroni L, eds. *Dermatology*. [Philadelphia]: Elsevier, 2018 (ch. 41).

13. **A.** Interstitial lung disease
Patients with anti-MDA5 (or CADM-140) positivity can present with a form of dermatomyositis that includes periungual skin ulceration, oral ulceration, Gottron papules, Gottron sign, alopecia, joint pains, and amyopathic disease. These patients are at risk of developing a rapidly progressive form of interstitial lung disease. Panniculitis may also be present in MDA-5-associated dermatomyositis Bolognia J, Schaffer J, Cerroni L, eds. *Dermatology*. [Philadelphia]: Elsevier, 2018 (ch. 42).

14. **A.** Proximal muscle weakness
The Kodachrome shows classic nailfold findings in dermatomyositis with dilatation of capillary loops alternating with drop-out of vessels. Periungual erythema and nailfold dystrophy are often present. Nailfold findings in SLE classically show wandering glomeruloid loops. Proximal muscle weakness is a cardinal feature of dermatomyositis. Malar rash, glomerulonephritis, and discoid lesions in the conchal bowl are all features of SLE. Bolognia J, Schaffer J, Cerroni L, eds. *Dermatology*. [Philadelphia]: Elsevier, 2018 (chs. 41 and 42).

15. **D.** Addition of propranolol
This patient has systemic sclerosis with Raynaud phenomenon, characterized by episodic vasospasm secondary to cold exposure, resulting in white, blue, and red discoloration of the fingers secondary to cold stimuli. Persistent Raynaud phenomenon may result in digital ulceration of the distal pulp. General principles for management include avoidance of cold exposure and keeping the extremities warm. In addition, smoking can aggravate the disease. Calcium channel blockers are the most frequently used medication for treatment of Raynaud phenomenon. Propranolol is not an appropriate treatment, as betablockers can aggravate Raynaud. Bolognia J, Schaffer J, Cerroni L, eds. *Dermatology*. [Philadelphia]: Elsevier, 2018 (ch. 43).

16. **B.** Kidney
The patient above has systemic sclerosis. As such she is at risk of developing renal crisis on high-dose systemic corticosteroids. In addition, these patients should be screened for interstitial lung disease prior to starting methotrexate. Bolognia J, Schaffer J, Cerroni L, eds. *Dermatology*. [Philadelphia]: Elsevier, 2018 (ch. 43).

17. **D.** All of the above
This patient has psoriasis vulgaris, presenting with well-demarcated pink-red plaques with silvery scale. Importantly, patients with psoriasis should be counseled on their increased risk for cardiovascular complications and metabolic syndrome, which requires meeting three of the following five criteria: increased waist circumference; increased triglycerides (>150 mg/dl); reduced High-density lipoprotein (HDL) (<40mg/dl in males; <50 mg/dl in females); increased blood pressure (systolic ≥ 130 and/or diastolic ≥85); and elevated fasting glucose ≥100 mg/dl. Recent studies have shown that systemic therapy with biologic agents may improve cardiovascular outcomes. Bolognia J, Schaffer J, Cerroni L, eds. *Dermatology*. [Philadelphia]: Elsevier, 2018 (ch. 53).

18. **D.** Cigarette smoking
This patient has hidradenitis suppurativa, or acne inversus, which presents with acneiform papules, nodules,

cysts, abscesses, comedones, sinus tract formation, and scarring, which manifests predominantly in flexural zones (intertriginous skin) and anogenital mucosae. Smoking cessation, weight reduction in patients that are overweight or obese, antiseptic soaps, and decreasing friction/moisture at areas of involvement are general interventions that can improve hidradenitis suppurativa.
Bolognia J, Schaffer J, Cerroni L, eds. *Dermatology.* [Philadelphia]: Elsevier, 2018 (ch. 38).

19. C. Squamous cell carcinoma
Patients with HS are at risk for multiple complications, including lymphedema, the formation of fistulae, anemia, and secondary amyloidosis. Additionally, those with long-standing scarring disease may be at risk for the development of squamous cell carcinoma.
Bolognia J, Schaffer J, Cerroni L, eds. *Dermatology.* [Philadelphia]: Elsevier, 2018 (ch. 38).

20. B. HIV
The patient has pityriasis rubra pilaris (PRP). Clinically, patients present with a generalized papulosquamous eruption with generalized lesions or erythroderma. Primary lesions are often pink-orange papules coalescing into plaques with notable islands of sparing. Folliculocentric keratotic papules likened to a "nutmeg grater" are classic. Additionally, palms and soles may show a waxy keratoderma. An association with HIV is noted in PRP type VI. In addition, acne conglobata and hidradenitis suppurativa may occur in type VI PRP. This type of PRP may not respond to classic therapeutic options but may benefit from antiretroviral treatment. Diabetes, renal failure, and cardiovascular disease are not typically associated with PRP.
Bolognia J, Schaffer J, Cerroni L, eds. *Dermatology.* [Philadelphia]: Elsevier, 2018 (ch. 9).

21. F. All of the above
Confluent and reticulated papillomatosis of Gougerot-Carteaud (CARP) is characterized by the presence of asymptomatic small hyperpigmented verrucous papules coalescing into reticulated thin plaques that can become confluent. Less commonly it may present as a hypopigmented variant. The differential diagnosis of CARP includes tinea versicolor, acanthosis nigricans, or prurigo pigmentosa in the right clinical setting. The etiology is unknown, but some have proposed that *Malassezia furfur* is implicated in the pathogenesis. Although tetracycline antibiotics, especially minocycline, are often first-line therapy, other antibiotics may also be used (e.g., azithromycin, clarithromycin, amoxicillin). Additionally, topical and oral retinoids, fusidic acid, topical mupirocin, lactic acid or urea, and topical antifungals have been used with varying degrees of success.
Bolognia J, Schaffer J, Cerroni L, eds. *Dermatology.* [Philadelphia]: Elsevier, 2018 (ch. 67).

22. D. Superficial and deep epithelioid granulomas lacking significant inflammatory infiltrate
This Kodachrome depicts papular lesions of cutaneous sarcoidosis, which characteristically manifest along the alar rim and periorificial surfaces. The patient also has infiltrative lesions of the nose, referred to as "lupus pernio," which is clinically relevant given the association with pulmonary disease. "Naked granulomas," or epithelioid histiocyte granulomas with a relative paucity of lymphocytic inflammatory infiltrate, are classically seen in sarcoidosis. Lupus vulgaris, or cutaneous tuberculosis, can be difficult to differentiate histologically from sarcoidosis, but characteristic features include central caseating necrosis within the granulomas and a lymphocytic infiltrate peripherally oriented around the granulomas. Lipoid proteinosis exhibits hyaline eosinophilic deposits in the dermis, and patients can present with skin-colored papules especially along the upper eyelid margin. Cutaneous leishmaniasis may present as papules or plaque on the nose but is often ulcerative or locally destructive, and biopsy of this entity would show diffuse histiocytes with internalized amastigotes.
Bolognia J, Schaffer J, Cerroni L, eds. *Dermatology.* [Philadelphia]: Elsevier, 2018 (ch. 93).

23. C. Hypoplastic lymphatic vessels
Primary lymphedema may be classified according to its age of onset into congenital (Milroy disease), peripubertal (praecox, aka Meige disease), and late-onset (tarda; >35 years of age). Multiple genes have been implicated in isolated and syndromic forms of lymphedema of which the encoded proteins often act in the vascular endothelial growth factor receptor-3 (VEGFR3) signaling pathway. Lymphedema praecox is the most common primary form of lymphedema commonly affecting young females (ages 9–25). This condition presents as severe lymphedema with no other identifiable proximal cause. The primary defect is due to congenital lymphatic hypoplasia. Lymphatic hyperplasia with dilatation of lymphatics may occur in secondary lymphedema, which may result from recurrent infections. Microfilaria emboli occur in filariasis, in which lymphedema is a complication.
Bolognia J, Schaffer J, Cerroni L, eds. *Dermatology.* [Philadelphia]: Elsevier, 2018 (ch. 105).

24. A. Opportunistic infection
There are numerous adverse effects of chronic corticosteroid use. Most are dose-related and may therefore be reduced with alternate-day dosing. However, cataracts, osteoporosis, and osteonecrosis are not dose-related. Myopathy, peptic ulcer disease, Gastroesophageal reflux disease, pancreatitis, hyperglycemia, weight gain, immunosuppression, mood disturbance, cutaneous atrophy, striae, purpura, acne, and hypothalamic-pituitary-adrenal axis suppression are reduced with alternate-day dosing or reduced dosing.
Bolognia J, Schaffer J, Cerroni L, eds. *Dermatology.* [Philadelphia]: Elsevier, 2018 (ch. 125).

25. A. Patient taking rifampin for hidradenitis suppurativa
Glucocorticosteroids are metabolized in the liver by CYP450. Prednisone is an intermediate-acting glucocorticoid that is converted to prednisolone. Drug interactions must be considered when prescribing glucocorticosteroids in order to prevent adverse effects from misdosing due to drug metabolism alterations. Rifampin is a P450 inducer, which requires an increased dosing of corticosteroid, as it would be metabolized quicker. Other inducers include phenytoin, phenobarbital, antiretrovirals, antituberculosis agents, bexarotene, griseofulvin, and St. John's wort. Erythromycin is a P450 inhibitor. Oral contraceptives alter protein binding and decrease hepatic metabolism of steroids. Patients with renal disease and chronic liver disease also have impaired metabolism of glucocorticosteroids, and dose reductions may be considered.
Bolognia J, Schaffer J, Cerroni L, eds. *Dermatology.* [Philadelphia]: Elsevier, 2018 (ch. 125).

26. A. Hypopigmented halo around scars

Addison disease is an endocrinopathy in which the adrenal glands are unable to produce sufficient mineralocorticoids and glucocorticoids. The cutaneous manifestation most characteristic of Addison disease is hyperpigmentation of the skin. The hyperpigmentation favors sun-exposed sites, sites of recurrent trauma or pressure, recent scars, nevi, mucous membranes, hair, nails, the axillae, areolae, or perineum. Decreased axillary and pubic hair may be seen in women, because their androgen production is largely in the adrenals. Hypopigmentation around scars is not a feature of Addison disease.

Bolognia J, Schaffer J, Cerroni L, eds. *Dermatology.* [Philadelphia]: Elsevier, 2018 (ch. 53).

27. A. Terbinafine

Allylamine antifungal agents act to inhibit squalene epoxidase in the ergosterol synthesis pathway. Allylamines include terbinafine and naftifine. Azoles (miconazole, clotrimazole, ketoconazole, oxiconazole, econazole) inhibit lanosterol 14a-demethylase. Ciclopirox olamine, a hydroxypyridone, interferes with membrane transport by binding to trivalent cations, thereby inhibiting cell membrane integrity and inhibiting enzymes essential for respiratory processes, cell wall structure, and other aspects of cell growth and metabolism. Nystatin exerts its antifungal activity by binding to ergosterol on fungal cell membranes, leading to pore formation.

Bolognia J, Schaffer J, Cerroni L, eds. *Dermatology.* [Philadelphia]: Elsevier, 2018 (ch. 127).

28. B. Complete blood count with differential

This patient has eosinophilic fasciitis with the "groove sign" or "dry riverbed sign" depicted in the Kodachrome. This finding highlights linear veins that appear depressed within thickened connective tissues. In patients with eosinophilic fasciitis, laboratory evaluation may demonstrate peripheral eosinophilia. In addition, some patients may have associated myeloproliferative disorders and aplastic anemia with associated thrombocytopenia, anemia, or pancytopenia.

Bolognia J, Schaffer J, Cerroni L, eds. *Dermatology.* [Philadelphia]: Elsevier, 2018 (ch. 43).

29. E. All of the above

The patient above has pyoderma gangrenosum (PG), which manifests with inflammatory ulcers with an active violaceous rim and undermined border. Pathergy may occur in this neutrophilic dermatosis. PG can be associated with various conditions, including hematologic disease (e.g., acute myeloid leukemia, monoclonal gammopathy), rheumatoid arthritis, and inflammatory bowel disease.

Bolognia J, Schaffer J, Cerroni L, eds. *Dermatology.* [Philadelphia]: Elsevier, 2018 (ch. 26).

30. D. All of the above

The patient above has an IgA small vessel vasculitis (some refer to this as adult-onset Henoch-Schönlein purpura); however, the presentation and prognosis differ from that in children. Adult-onset IgA vasculitis is more likely to present with skin necrosis and increased likelihood of associated chronic renal insufficiency (up to 30%), especially if purpura is above the waistline. In addition, neoplasm-associated IgA vasculitis may occur in the setting of solid organ cancer, in particular lung cancer. Adults are also more likely than children to have gastrointestinal involvement (abdominal pain, diarrhea), arthritis (more commonly affecting the lower extremity joints), and leukocytosis.

Bolognia J, Schaffer J, Cerroni L, eds. *Dermatology.* [Philadelphia]: Elsevier, 2018 (ch. 24).

31. C. Small vessel vasculitis

The patient above has Sjögren syndrome, presenting with xerosis, xerostomia, and xerophthalmia. Patients with Sjögren syndrome may have associated small vessel vasculitis, which can present with palpable purpura or urticarial vasculitis. Other serious systemic complications may include B-cell lymphomas—in particular, extranodal marginal zone lymphomas of the mucosa-associated lymphoid tissue (MALT) type, peripheral neuropathy, and systemic vasculitis. Small vessel vasculitis may occur in connective tissue disorders, most commonly rheumatoid arthritis, systemic lupus erythematosus, and Sjögren syndrome.

Bolognia J, Schaffer J, Cerroni L, eds. *Dermatology.* [Philadelphia]: Elsevier, 2018 (ch. 45).

32. E. All of the above

This patient has multicentric reticulohistiocytosis (MRH), which often presents around age 50 and is seen more commonly in women. Patients present with red-orange papules and nodules along the fingers and hands. MRH is associated with joint disease and autoimmune disease, including thyroiditis, Sjögren syndrome, vitiligo, and ulcerative colitis. Patient may also have an associated malignancy (e.g., lung cancer).

Bolognia J, Schaffer J, Cerroni L, eds. *Dermatology.* [Philadelphia]: Elsevier, 2018 (chs. 53 and 91).

33. C. Crohn's disease

The patient above has perianal tags and plaques. This finding can be seen in up to 40% of patients with Crohn's disease. Other associated skin findings of cutaneous Crohn's may include labial or scrotal erythema and edema, knife-like genital ulcers, and erythematous plaques that may be vegetative or ulcerative with draining sinuses, fistulas, and scarring. Patients with hepatitis C may have various associated cutaneous findings, including leukocytoclastic vasculitis, mixed cryoglobulinemic vasculitis, necrolytic acral erythema, or lichen planus (classically oral erosive).

Bolognia J, Schaffer J, Cerroni L, eds. *Dermatology.* [Philadelphia]: Elsevier, 2018 (chs. 53 and 93).

34. A. Erythema nodosum

The patient above has the constellation of findings seen in Lofgren syndrome and therefore would be expected to have associated erythema nodosum. The findings seen in Lofgren syndrome include erythema nodosum, joint pains, hilar adenopathy, and fevers. These patients may need supportive measures and possible systemic steroids. There may be spontaneous resolution between 1 and 2 years. Urticarial vasculitis may be associated with systemic lupus erythematosus. Bullous pemphigoid typically occurs in elderly and may be associated with neurologic disease (e.g., dementia, Parkinson disease). Erythema induratum is a panniculitis that typically occurs in young women or infection with mycobacterial tuberculosis.

Bolognia J, Schaffer J, Cerroni L, eds. *Dermatology.* [Philadelphia]: Elsevier, 2018 (ch. 93).

35. D. B and C

The patient has toxic epidermal necrolysis (TEN). The SCORTEN system may be used to evaluate prognosis and

includes the following: age >40 years, malignancy, initial body surface area greater than 10%, tachycardia greater than 120 beats per minute, serum glucose level elevated more than 14 mmol/L, serum urea level greater than 10 mmol/L, and serum bicarbonate level less than 20 mmol/l. For patients scoring between 0 and 1 point, the mortality rate is 3.2%; 2 points has an associated mortality rate of 12.1%; 3 points has an associated mortality rate of 35.8%; 4 points has an associated mortality rate of 58.3%; and 5 or more points has an associated mortality rate of 90%.
Bolognia J, Schaffer J, Cerroni L, eds. *Dermatology*. [Philadelphia]: Elsevier, 2018 (ch. 20).

36. C. Stopping allopurinol
Reviewing patient medications and identifying the likely offending medication is critical in treating SJS/TEN. This includes reviewing when medications were initiated and reviewing the likelihood that a given drug could cause the reaction. Delay in removal of the culprit medication can result in higher mortality. Supportive care is also very important: attention to wound care, eye examination, and oral care are all necessary. Systemic steroids, intravenous immune globulin (IVIG), cyclosporine, and TNF-alpha inhibitors have been used as treatment once the offending medication is stopped.
Bolognia J, Schaffer J, Cerroni L, eds. *Dermatology*. [Philadelphia]: Elsevier, 2018 (ch. 20).

37. A. Ibuprofen
The patient above is presenting with a fixed drug eruption (commonly develops in the oral or anogenital mucosae). In this location, the eruption can be confused with recurrent herpes simplex virus. Common culprits include: tetracyclines, sulfonamides, beta-lactam antibiotics, macrolides, fluoroquinolones, acetaminophen, NSAIDs, aspirin, dapsone, barbiturates, proton pump inhibitors, and azole medications.
Bolognia J, Schaffer J, Cerroni L, eds. *Dermatology*. [Philadelphia]: Elsevier, 2018 (ch. 21).

38. B. Bronchiolitis obliterans
The clinical scenario and picture above are consistent with paraneoplastic pemphigus. An associated complication includes bronchiolitis obliterans, resulting in respiratory failure. This can be detected with pulmonary function tests early in the disease. Bronchiolitis obliterans may also occur in the setting of chronic graft-versus-host disease.
Bolognia J, Schaffer J, Cerroni L, eds. *Dermatology*. [Philadelphia]: Elsevier, 2018 (ch. 29).

39. A. Hashimoto thyroiditis
This patient has dermatitis herpetiformis, a skin manifestation of Celiac disease presenting with intensely pruritic papules and vesicles along extensor surfaces. Other commonly associated autoimmune conditions include Hashimoto thyroiditis and insulin-dependent diabetes mellitus. Treatment including a gluten-free diet and dapsone therapy may result in prompt improvement of the skin disease.
Bolognia J, Schaffer J, Cerroni L, eds. *Dermatology*. [Philadelphia]: Elsevier, 2018 (ch. 31).

40. C. Suggest leg elevation and compression therapy
This patient has acute lipodermatosclerosis (LDS). The patient is presenting with bilateral erythema, edema, and tenderness, which is more pronounced on the lower medial shins. This panniculitis results in the setting of venous hypertension. Other findings that point toward LDS may include bound-down fibrotic plaques and thickening of the skin. In the chronic phase, hyperpigmentation and sclerosis of the skin likened to an "inverted Champaign bottle" appearance may develop. The differential diagnosis includes cellulitis; however, bilateral lower leg cellulitis is uncommon, and the patient denies fevers or prior history of trauma. The differential diagnosis for "red legs" also includes allergic contact dermatitis. Treatment with leg elevation and compression is recommended. High-potency topical steroids, intralesional topical steroids, pentoxifylline, and stanozolol may also be useful in the treatment of LDS.
Bolognia J, Schaffer J, Cerroni L, eds. *Dermatology*. [Philadelphia]: Elsevier, 2018 (ch. 100).

PEDIATRIC DERMATOLOGY

41. A. Ballooning degeneration of the spinous layer
Acrodermatitis enteropathica is an autosomal recessive disorder caused by mutations in the gene *SLC39A4*, which encodes the zinc transporter ZIP4. Affected infants develop periorificial and acral erythema, scale, and erosions and may also develop diarrhea and alopecia, which together are considered the triad of acrodermatitis enteropathica. Manifestations typically appear soon after weaning from breast milk to formula for breastfed babies, or within weeks of birth for formula-fed infants. Infants may also develop stomatitis, glossitis, nail dystrophy, irritability, photophobia, candida infection, and failure to thrive. Histopathology is notable for ballooning degeneration of the spinous layer, and treatment consists of lifelong zinc supplementation.
Spongiosis with superficial perivascular lymphocytic infiltrate describes the histopathologic findings of allergic and irritant contact dermatitis. A biopsy of candidiasis would show subcorneal pustules with PAS-positive organisms. Acanthotic epidermis with elongated rete ridges and diminished granular layer describes the histopathologic findings of psoriasis. Subcorneal pustules with neutrophils and gram-positive cocci would be seen in a biopsy of impetigo.
Bolognia J, Schaffer J, Cerroni L, eds. *Dermatology*. [Philadelphia]: Elsevier, 2018 (ch. 13).

42. D. Congenital herpes simplex
Extramedullary hematopoiesis (EMH), also referred to as a "blueberry muffin baby," is an indication of bone marrow dysfunction. EMH is characterized by red to violaceous papules and nodules, which may be widely disseminated in neonates. Biopsy of these lesions shows a diffuse dermal infiltrate of immature erythrocytes, leukocytes, and megakaryocytes.

43. B. Intralesional triamcinolone
The clinical figure depicts alopecia areata in an ophiasis pattern. The patient is distraught, so reassurance and watchful waiting is not a practical option. Further, this pattern is often recalcitrant, and self-resolution is uncommon. While exclamation point hairs are the classic dermoscopic finding, small perifollicular yellow dots are another characteristic finding. Intralesional triamcinolone is classically the first-line treatment option. The other choices are not known to be effective in alopecia areata. Griseofulvin at high doses (20 mg/kg/day) is used for the treatment of tinea capitis, which also presents with alopecia, scale, crusting, and short broken hairs.
Bolognia J, Schaffer J, Cerroni L, eds. *Dermatology*. [Philadelphia]: Elsevier, 2018 (ch. 69).

44. A. Aplasia cutis congenita

The clinical image depicts a sharply demarcated ulceration on the vertex scalp and is most consistent with aplasia cutis congenita (ACC). While ACC can be seen in association with several syndromes, including Adams-Oliver (ACC and limb malformation), the vignette does not describe any other associated findings. The ulceration does not appear to be punched out or grouped, as would be expected for herpes simplex virus. The vignette describes a spontaneous vaginal delivery without intervention, making trauma unlikely. While neonatal lupus is considered for rashes or lesions on the scalp and face, the morphology and location here are classic for ACC.

Bolognia J, Schaffer J, Cerroni L, eds. *Dermatology.* [Philadelphia]: Elsevier, 2018 (ch. 64).

45. E. Skin biopsy

Langerhans cell histiocytosis should be suspected in an infant with recalcitrant dermatitis in a flexural distribution with erosions and purpura. A skin biopsy is diagnostic. It may mimic seborrheic dermatitis, but clues for diagnosis include the presence of erosions and purpura. Erosive irritant contact dermatitis is also in the differential but typically spares the folds. Other entities on the differential for diaper dermatitis include cutaneous candidiasis and psoriasis.

Bolognia J, Schaffer J, Cerroni L, eds. *Dermatology.* [Philadelphia]: Elsevier, 2018 (ch. 91).

46. D. Phakomatosis pigmentovascularis type II

The clinical image depicts port wine stains in conjunction with dermal melanocytosis, suggesting a diagnosis of phakomatosis pigmentovascularis, of which there are five types:

1. nevus flammeus + epidermal nevus
2. nevus flammeus + dermal melanocytosis +/- nevus anemicus
3. nevus flammeus + nevus spilus +/- nevus anemicus
4. nevus flammeus + dermal melanocytosis + nevus spilus +/- nevus anemicus
5. cutis marmorata telangiectatica congenita + dermal melanocytosis.

Types II and IV include nevus flammeus (port wine stain) and dermal melanocytosis.

Bolognia J, Schaffer J, Cerroni L, eds. *Dermatology.* [Philadelphia]: Elsevier, 2018 (ch. 104).

47. D. Mineral oil scraping

Scabies should be considered in an infant with vesicular, pustular, or nodular lesions, especially on the palmoplantar and diaper areas. Skin scraping using mineral oil (D) is a common and rapid tool for diagnosis. Treatment of choice for infants older than 2 months is permethrin 5% cream. Alternatively, sulfur ointment 5%–10% is considered safe in infants.

Bedside diagnostic tests should be considered prior to more invasive tests and are important in the evaluation of vesicular and pustular lesions in the newborn. Tzanck smear (C) is useful in the evaluation of erythema toxicum neonatorum (Etox), transient neonatal pustular melanosis (TNPM), and neonatal herpes simplex viral infection. These conditions, however, typically present within days of birth. Etox and TNPM are asymptomatic and self-resolving, while herpes infection may be associated with systemic illness, including internal organ and central nervous system involvement. Skin biopsy (A) and sterile tissue culture (B) may be performed in the correct clinical setting to evaluate for other entities in the differential diagnosis, such as disseminated candidiasis, bacterial sepsis, and Langerhans cell histiocytosis.

Nontreponemal serologic testing (E) of the newborn and mother should be performed if there is a concern for congenital syphilis. Although early congenital syphilis may present with bullous lesions on the palms and soles, they are likely to be associated with other findings such as snuffles, dactylitis, pseudoparalysis, epiphysitis, and hepatitis.

Bolognia J, Schaffer J, Cerroni L, eds. *Dermatology.* [Philadelphia]: Elsevier, 2018 (chs. 34 and 84).

48. D. Acropustulosis of infancy

The above vignette and clinical photograph support a diagnosis of acropustulosis of infancy, an idiopathic pustular disorder that presents in the first 2 years of life. The eruption tends to be pruritic, with recurrences every few weeks to months. While scabies is certainly in the differential diagnosis, the lack of affected family members and the lack of improvement with empiric treatment of the household make this diagnosis less likely. Transient neonatal pustular melanosis would not typically occur in a 14-month old. The lack of xerosis, deep-seated vesicles, scaling, and honey-colored crusting make dyshidrotic eczema and impetigo less likely.

Bolognia J, Schaffer J, Cerroni L, eds. *Dermatology.* [Philadelphia]: Elsevier, 2018 (ch. 34).

49. D. Exclamation point hairs

This photo depicts a round patch of smooth alopecia, which is highly characteristic of alopecia areata. Dermatoscopic evaluation of alopecia areata often shows so-called "exclamation point hairs," which are short hairs in which the distal end is broader than the proximal end; yellow dots may also be seen. Black dots and broken hairs are seen in trichotillomania (A, B); follicular red dots are characteristic of discoid lupus erythematosus (C); and comma hairs are seen in tinea capitis (D).

Bolognia J, Schaffer J, Cerroni L, eds. *Dermatology.* [Philadelphia]: Elsevier, 2018 (ch. 69).

50. C. Chondritis

The clinical image depicts an exophytic papule in the preauricular region consistent with an accessory tragus. These lesions represent faulty development of the first branchial arch and can occur anywhere from the preauricular region to the angle of the mouth. Multiple lesions can be seen in Goldenhar syndrome (unilateral facial asymmetry, ocular and otorhinolaryngological abnormalities, deafness, macrosomia, skeletal defects, and cardiac or renal abnormalities). Careful surgical excision is required in order to remove any protruding portion of underlying cartilage that can be contiguous with the cartilage of the external ear.

Bolognia J, Schaffer J, Cerroni L, eds. *Dermatology.* [Philadelphia]: Elsevier, 2018 (ch. 64).

DERMATOPATHOLOGY

51. B. Granular IgA at the tips of the dermal papillae

There are collections of neutrophils within the tips of the papillary dermis. These subepidermal neutrophilic microabscesses are characteristic of dermatitis herpetiformis (DH). Direct immunofluorescence (DIF) will usually show granular deposition of IgA at the tips of the dermal papillae. A fibrillar pattern of IgA may also be seen in DH. Linear IgA deposition at the dermal-epidermal junction

(DEJ) is a feature of linear IgA disease, whereas IgG and C3 at the DEJ is typical of bullous pemphigoid and pemphigoid gestationis. Intercellular IgG and C3 deposition is seen in pemphigus.

Bolognia J, Schaffer J, Cerroni L, eds. *Dermatology*. [Philadelphia]: Elsevier, 2018 (ch. 31).

52. **A.** Nevus sebaceous

The figure shows a broad excision with epidermal acanthosis, papillomatosis, and hyperorthokeratosis with underlying atrophic sebaceous glands (directly connected to the epidermis) and absence of mature hair follicles. The normal skin at the periphery (on either side) shows well-developed hair follicles extending into the fat with hair shafts. This is an example of nevus sebaceous. During adolescence these lesions tend to show markedly enlarged sebaceous lobules.

Verrucous carcinoma is a well-differentiated squamous cell carcinoma, most commonly seen on acral or mucosal surfaces that characteristically show a pushing border. Epidermal nevi demonstrate acanthosis, papillomatosis, and hyperkeratosis, and may resemble seborrheic keratosis or acanthosis nigricans. Lichen simplex chronicus shows acanthosis, hypergranulosis, and hyperkeratosis with stratum lucidum on hair-bearing skin ("hairy-palm" sign).

Bolognia J, Schaffer J, Cerroni L, eds. *Dermatology*. [Philadelphia]: Elsevier, 2018 (ch. 111).

53. **B.** Extramammary Paget disease

The photomicrograph shows single and clustered large cells with abundant pale eosinophilic cytoplasm within the epidermis. Glandular differentiation is apparent. These features are characteristic of extramammary Paget disease (EMPD). All of the answer choices are in the histological differential diagnosis of EMPD. Melanoma in situ (MIS) typically shows atypical melanocytes within the basal layer of the epidermis whereas squamous cell carcinoma in situ (SCCIS) will involve the entire thickness of the epidermis. Glandular differentiation is not seen in MIS or SCCIS. Intraepidermal sebaceous carcinoma will show cells with scalloped nuclei and clear cytoplasm containing microvesicles. Immunohistochemical stain for cytokeratins such as Cam5.2, CK7, and EMA are positive in EMPD and may be helpful in distinguishing this entity from its histologic mimics.

Bolognia J, Schaffer J, Cerroni L, eds. *Dermatology*. [Philadelphia]: Elsevier, 2018 (ch. 73).

54. **A.** Erythema nodosum

The figure illustrates a predominantly septal panniculitis with thickened fibrous septae, histiocytic infiltrate, and multinucleated giant cells between the fat lobules. Erythema nodosum (EN) is the prototype of septal panniculitis. Histiocytes surrounding cleftlike spaces (Miescher granuloma) are often seen. The inflammation in EN is predominantly septal, with only focal involvement of the periphery of the fat lobule. Early lesions typically show acute inflammation, while later lesions show chronic and granulomatous inflammation. Erythema induratum shows prominent involvement of the fat lobules with presence of vasculitis in well-established lesions. Pancreatic panniculitis demonstrates enzymatic fat necrosis within the fat lobules with "ghost cells" (anucleate adipocytes with granular debris and an eosinophilic rim) with a neutrophilic infiltrate and stippled calcifications. Lupus panniculitis typically shows lymphoid aggregates with plasma cells and fibrinoid degeneration

within the septae, giving a hyalinized appearance of the subcutaneous fat.

Bolognia J, Schaffer J, Cerroni L, eds. *Dermatology*. [Philadelphia]: Elsevier, 2018 (ch. 100).

55. **D.** Psoriasis

The photomicrograph demonstrates lichenoid interface dermatitis (bandlike lymphocytic infiltrate with necrotic keratinocytes). The differential diagnosis of this pattern includes lichen planus, lichenoid drug reaction, and benign lichenoid keratosis (in the setting of a single lesion). Presence of eosinophils, superficial as well as deep inflammatory infiltrate, and parakeratosis are some features that favor a lichenoid drug reaction over lichen planus.

Psoriasis demonstrates acanthosis, parakeratosis with collections of neutrophils, and dilated capillaries within the papillary dermis.

Bolognia J, Schaffer J, Cerroni L, eds. *Dermatology*. [Philadelphia]: Elsevier, 2018 (ch. 11).

56. **A.** Angiosarcoma

The figure illustrates irregular vascular channels lined by atypical, hyperchromatic endothelial cells. These features are characteristic of an angiosarcoma. Angiosarcoma is most commonly seen on sun-damaged skin (head & neck areas) of elderly individuals.

Acquired tufted angioma demonstrates nodules composed of densely packed capillaries lined by typical endothelial cells. Cherry angiomas will show dilated vascular spaces lined by cytologically bland endothelial cells. Glomus tumors may show vascular spaces but are composed of uniform and round glomus cells without any cytologic atypia.

Bolognia J, Schaffer J, Cerroni L, eds. *Dermatology*. [Philadelphia]: Elsevier, 2018 (ch. 114).

57. **D.** Keratoacanthoma

The initial biopsy shows a sebaceous carcinoma. A sebaceous carcinoma outside the head and neck region in an individual less than 60 years old should raise concern for Muir-Torre syndrome (MTS). MTS is due to mutations in *MSH2, MLH1,* and *MLH6.* One of these mutations was presumably found in this patient upon exome sequencing, given the screening colonoscopy that was ordered. However, it would also be reasonable to order a colonoscopy in this patient even without genetic data. Patients with MTS have an increased risk of colon cancer, as well as a variety of other solid tumors. MTS patients classically present with one of two types of lesions: either sebaceous neoplasms or keratoacanthomas. Keratoacanthomas can grow quickly as in this patient. Sebaceous adenomas, hyperplasia, and sebaceomas (sebaceous epitheliomas) are also found in patients with MTS.

Sclerotic fibromas are found in Cowden syndrome and are usually skin-colored nodules. Desmoid tumors are soft tissue tumors associated with Gardner syndrome. Increased risk of Merkel cell carcinoma and melanoma are not typically attributed to MTS and would be the less likely diagnoses in this case.

Bolognia J, Schaffer J, Cerroni L, eds. *Dermatology*. [Philadelphia]: Elsevier, 2018 (ch. 11).

58. **D.** Psoriasis

The figure demonstrates characteristic features of psoriasis, including acanthosis, parakeratosis with collections of neutrophils, and increased capillaries within the papillary dermis.

Prominent epidermotropism of lymphocytes with atypical forms would be expected in biopsies from lesions of

mycosis fungoides. PLEVA typically shows confluent parakeratosis with prominent necrotic keratinocytes and/or superficial epidermal necrosis. Lichen simplex chronicus typically demonstrates acanthosis, hyperkeratosis, and presence of the pale blue "stratum lucidum" on hair-bearing skin.
Bolognia J, Schaffer J, Cerroni L, eds. *Dermatology*. [Philadelphia]: Elsevier, 2018 (ch. 8).

59. **B.** *CYLD*
The lesion demonstrates multiple tumor islands arranged in a "jigsaw puzzle" appearance, with an outer layer of cells with small hyperchromatic nuclei and an inner zone composed of cells with oval and vesicular nuclei. This is consistent with a cylindroma. Deposits of hyaline droplets and a lining of basement membrane around individual lobules are often present in cylindromas. Patients affected with Brooke-Spiegler syndrome demonstrate mutations affecting the tumor suppressor gene *CYLD* and may have multiple cylindromas, spiradenomas, and trichoepitheliomas on the scalp and face.
Defects in the *PTCH1* lead to basal cell carcinomas as seen in Gorlin syndrome. Mutations in the *beta-catenin* pathway have been demonstrated in some cases of pilomatricoma. Birt-Hogg-Dube syndrome is caused by germline mutations in the folliculin (*FLCN*) gene, and the affected individuals may have fibrofolliculomas, trichodiscomas, perifollicular fibromas, and acrochordons on the skin.
Bolognia J, Schaffer J, Cerroni L, eds. *Dermatology*. [Philadelphia]: Elsevier, 2018 (ch. 111).

60. **A.** End-stage renal failure
The figure illustrates a pauci-inflammatory subepidermal blister consistent with porphyria or pseudoporphyria (in the absence of serum, urine, or stool porphyrin abnormalities). Pseudoporphyria can be seen in the setting of end-stage renal disease (aka bullous dermatosis in end-stage renal failure), hemodialysis (aka bullous dermatosis of hemodialysis), or secondary to numerous drugs, including furosemide, tetracyclines, ciprofloxacin, nalidixic acid, and NSAIDs.
Pemphigoid gestationis demonstrates histopathologic features similar to bullous pemphigoid, including a prominent eosinophilic infiltrate. Pauci-inflammatory subepidermal blisters are not associated with tuberculosis or osteoporosis.
Bolognia J, Schaffer J, Cerroni L, eds. *Dermatology*. [Philadelphia]: Elsevier, 2018 (ch. 49).

PROCEDURAL DERMATOLOGY

61. **D.** Radiation decreases the number of pilosebaceous units in the skin and can affect healing time.
Similar to isotretinoin, radiation treatment leads to a decreased number of pilosebaceous units in the skin, which is the mechanism by which it improves acne. This is similar to the mechanism of efficacy of isotretinoin and also why use of an oral retinoid in the preceding 6 months is a contraindication for medium to deep chemical peels. Given the risk of subsequent nonmelanoma skin cancers, thyroid cancer, and salivary carcinomas arising in patients treated with x-ray radiation for the treatment of acne, this therapy has largely been abandoned.
Bolognia J, Schaffer J, Cerroni L, eds. *Dermatology*. [Philadelphia]: Elsevier, 2018 (ch. 154).

62. **B.** You wish to select a filler with high elasticity and G' is proportional to elasticity.
G' is a measure of elasticity, which is the ability of a filler to resist deformation under pressure. This means that the filler has a great ability to provide lift and support. This is an important property for midfacial volume restoration, as soft-tissue fillers in this region provide support to the soft tissue of the lower face. High G' fillers are less deformable and cannot be easily spread in the skin.
Bolognia J, Schaffer J, Cerroni L, eds. *Dermatology*. [Philadelphia]: Elsevier, 2018 (ch. 158).

63. **A.** Compartment syndrome
Post-liposuction edema is a common side effect from the procedure. When treating the extremities, especially circumferential treatment of the arms and thighs, prolonged postoperative edema may result in mild compartment syndrome and local capillary ischemia. True necrosis is rare. Use of compression garments after treatment helps mitigate this side effect.
Bolognia J, Schaffer J, Cerroni L, eds. *Dermatology*. [Philadelphia]: Elsevier, 2018 (ch. 156).

64. **D.** Hypertonic saline
Hyperosmotic agents such as hypertonic saline exert their effect by inducing endothelial cell damage via dehydration. This is in contrast to chemical irritants, such as chromated glycerin and polyiodide iodide that act as corrosives, and detergent sclerosants that cause vascular injury by altering the surface tension around endothelial cells. Osmotic agents are more likely to cause muscle cramping than agents in the other classes.
Bolognia J, Schaffer J, Cerroni L, eds. *Dermatology*. [Philadelphia]: Elsevier, 2018 (ch. 155).

65. **C.** Superficial subcutaneous fat; temporal branch of CN VII
The superficial subcutaneous fat above the superficial musculo-aponeurotic system (SMAS) is the appropriate plane of undermining in this region. In the anterior aspect of the temple region adjacent to the lateral brow, the temporal branch of the facial nerve is in its most superficial location within or immediately deep to the SMAS.
Bolognia J, Schaffer J, Cerroni L, eds. *Dermatology*. [Philadelphia]: Elsevier, 2018 (ch. 142).

66. **A.** Proximal matrix
Split nails or longitudinal ridging may occur due to biopsy of the proximal nail matrix. The proximal matrix produces the superior surface of the nail plate while the distal nail matrix produces the inferior surface of the plate. Therefore surgery involving the distal matrix has a lower risk of producing nail dystrophy, as the upper layers of the nail plate will cover the defect.
Bolognia J, Schaffer J, Cerroni L, eds. *Dermatology*. [Philadelphia]: Elsevier, 2018 (ch. 149).

67. **D.** Nasalis
The temporal branch of the facial nerve innervates the muscles of the upper face, including the frontalis, corrugator, and superior portion of the orbicularis oculi. The procerus is occasionally innervated by the temporal branch of the facial nerve but more often by the zygomatic branch. The nasalis muscle is innervated by the zygomatic branch. Injury to the temporal branch of the facial nerve leads to ptosis of the ipsilateral brow.
Bolognia J, Schaffer J, Cerroni L, eds. *Dermatology*. [Philadelphia]: Elsevier, 2018 (ch. 142).

68. **A.** Transposition flap

The image depicts a bilobe transposition flap on the nose, which is accomplished by transposition of the primary lobe of the flap into Mohs surgery defect, transposition of the secondary lobe of the flap into the defect left by the primary lobe, and primary closure of the defect left by the secondary lobe. By definition, transposition flaps involve transposing skin over and around projections or peninsulas of the normal surrounding skin, creating the appearance of multiple broken lines and angles when repaired. This appearance of broken rather than continuous suture lines often helps to camouflage the final scar. Advancement and rotation flaps are sliding flaps that do not lift over or around intervening skin; thus, these flaps generally have long straight or curved suture lines when repaired. An island pedicle flap, or V-to-Y advancement flap, is a variant of an advancement flap that is advanced on a subcutaneous pedicle, and the dermal connections to the surrounding skin are completely severed. Island pedicle flaps usually leave a triangular-shaped scar with a straight line "tail" coming off of one corner. Interpolation flaps are staged flaps in which distant skin is transposed into the surgical defect, leaving a vascular pedicle attached to site of origin of the flap for a period of time between 2–6 weeks. In a second-stage procedure, the pedicle is then excised and the base of the flap is inset. A classic example of an interpolation flap is the paramedian forehead flap.
Bolognia J, Schaffer J, Cerroni L, eds. *Dermatology.* [Philadelphia]: Elsevier, 2018 (ch. 147).

69. **E.** 30% cure rate after wide excision and adjuvant radiation with high rate of metastasis, at least 50% risk of disease specific death

This presentation is typical of angiosarcoma, which has a high potential for both local recurrence and distant metastasis. A nonhealing bruiselike lesion on the face of an elderly patient should raise suspicion and prompt biopsy. Recommended treatment after initial workup for metastatic disease is wide local excision and adjuvant radiation. Even with appropriate treatment, 5-year survival is only 10%–30%.
Bolognia J, Schaffer J, Cerroni L, eds. *Dermatology.* [Philadelphia]: Elsevier, 2018 (ch. 114).

70. **B.** Mucosal lip

The nonabsorbable suture with the highest tissue reactivity and highest risk of infection is silk. Silk sutures are chosen in locations where minimizing irritation and discomfort are paramount, such as the eyelid margin or mucosal lip. Polyester is another nonabsorbable suture used on mucosal surfaces. Polypropylene is a nonabsorbable suture used as a running subcuticular suture, while ethilon is a nonabsorbable suture with low tissue reactivity commonly used to close the epidermis.
Bolognia J, Schaffer J, Cerroni L, eds. *Dermatology.* [Philadelphia]: Elsevier, 2018 (ch. 144).

BASIC SCIENCE

71. **C.** 50% of any children

Basal cell nevus syndrome (BCNS, Gorlin syndrome) is an autosomal dominant disorder caused by an inactivating mutation in the tumor suppressor gene *PTCH1* or rarely *PTCH2*. Autosomal dominant disorders have a 50% chance of affecting any offspring, male or female.

The diagnosis of BCNS requires either two major or one major and two minor criteria. Major criteria for the diagnosis of BCNS include more than two basal cell carcinomas (BCCs) or one BCC diagnosed before age twenty; odontogenic keratocysts of the jaw; three or more palmar or plantar pits; calcification of the falx cerebri; bifid ribs; or a first-degree relative with BCNS. Minor criteria include macrocephaly; congenital malformations including frontal bossing or cleft palate; certain other skeletal abnormalities; radiographic abnormalities; bilateral ovarian fibromas; and medulloblastoma. The patient in this vignette meets criteria for BCNS with three or more palmar pits and a BCC diagnosed before the age of 20 years.
Bolognia J, Schaffer J, Cerroni L, eds. *Dermatology.* [Philadelphia]: Elsevier, 2018 (ch. 108).

72. **A.** PAX3

The vignette and clinical image suggest a diagnosis of Waardenburg syndrome given the white forelock and cutaneous depigmentation. Her examination is also notable for dystopia canthorum, supporting a diagnosis of Waardenburg syndrome, type 1, which is caused by mutations in *PAX3*. There are 4 types of Waardenburg syndrome, a rare autosomal dominant or autosomal recessive disorder characterized by a combination of achromia of the skin, hair, or both; congenital deafness; partial or total heterochromia irides; hyperplasia of the medial eyebrow; broad nasal root; and dystopia canthorum (increased distance between medial canthi but normal interpupillary distance). Waardenburg type 2 lacks facial dysmorphism, has iris heterochromia, and, often, sensorineural deafness. Waardenburg type 3 has associated limb abnormalities, and type 4 has aganglionic megacolon. Mutations in *MITF* and *SOX10* are associated with Waardenburg syndrome types 2 and 4, respectively. *C-kit* is mutated in piebaldism, which features hair and skin depigmentation but lacks characteristic facial features of Waardenburg syndrome and has no internal sequelae. *TSC1* is mutated in tuberous sclerosis.
Bolognia J, Schaffer J, Cerroni L, eds. *Dermatology.* [Philadelphia]: Elsevier, 2018 (ch. 66).

73. **A—Keratins** 5 and 14
B—Keratins 1 and 10
C —Desmoglein & Desmocollin and Corneodesmosin
D—Corneodesmosin
E—Profilaggrin
F—Occludin
Keratins 5 and 14 are the main keratins expressed in the basal layer of the epidermis. Keratins 1 and 10 are the main keratins expressed in the spinous layer of the epidermis. Profilaggrin is packaged in keratohyalin granules in the granular layer and ultimately forms filaggrin in the stratum corneum. Lamellar bodies are largely composed of lipids but also contain proteins, such as corneodesmosin. Desmosomes contain desmoglein and desmocollin, as well as corneodesmosin. Occludin is found in tight junctions.
Bolognia J, Schaffer J, Cerroni L, eds. *Dermatology.* [Philadelphia]: Elsevier, 2018 (ch. 56).

74. **C.** Keratins 1 and 9

The two most common types of diffuse palmoplantar keratoderma are epidermolytic (Vorner) and nonepidermolytic (Unna-Thost) palmoplantar keratoderma (PPK). The clue to the correct answer is the histology, which demonstrates vacuolization and epidermolysis of the

granular layer—therefore the patient has epidermolytic PPK (EPPK). Diffuse EPPK is caused by mutations in keratins 1 or 9. Keratin 9 is expressed in palmoplantar epidermis, unlike keratins 5 and 14 (basal layer) and keratins 6 and 16 (spinous layer), and its mutation has been linked to EPPK (unlike keratin 10). Keratin 6c mutation is associated with diffuse nonepidermolytic PPK.
Bolognia J, Schaffer J, Cerroni L, eds. *Dermatology.* [Philadelphia]: Elsevier, 2018 (chs. 56 and 58).

75. **D.** Filaggrin
Filaggrin, best known for its ability to aggregate keratin intermediate filaments, has multiple beneficial effects for the human skin barrier. Filaggrin breakdown products are collectively known as "natural moisturizing factor" or "NMF." This helps hydrate the stratum corneum. Filaggrin is an intrinsically unstructured protein. Mutations in filaggrin gene (*FLG*) have been associated with skin barrier disorders, such as ichthyosis vulgaris, atopic dermatitis, or contact sensitization in individuals with eczema.
Bolognia J, Schaffer J, Cerroni L, eds. *Dermatology.* [Philadelphia]: Elsevier, 2018 (ch. 56).

76. **E.** Open comedones; color from melanin and lipid oxidation
The patient has multiple open comedones on the chin. The exposure of sebum to the air leads to oxidation of lipids and melanin, creating a black color.
Bolognia J, Schaffer J, Cerroni L, eds. *Dermatology.* [Philadelphia]: Elsevier, 2018 (ch. 36).

77. **A.** Affects DNA transcription, binds retinoic acid receptors (RAR) and retinoid X receptors (RXR), and receptor dimers bind DNA regulatory sequences in the nucleus called RAREs (retinoid hormone response elements)
The prescribed medication, oral isotretinoin, is a retinoid. Retinoids exert their effects on DNA transcription by binding to two distinct families of nuclear receptors: retinoic acid receptors (RARs) and retinoid X receptors (RXRs). Dimers of retinoid receptors (either RAR/RXR or RXR/RXR) bind to DNA regulatory sequences in the nucleus called retinoid hormone response elements (RAREs). Each

retinoid receptor family has three isotypes, RAR α, β, and γ and RXR α, β, and γ.
Bolognia J, Schaffer J, Cerroni L, eds. *Dermatology.* [Philadelphia]: Elsevier, 2018 (ch. 126).

78. **D.** BRAF inhibitor
Melanomas that harbor a V600E mutation in BRAF (where valine is replaced by glutamic acid at the 600th codon) can be treated with vemurafenib, which disrupts the RAF-MEK-ERK pathway. Immune checkpoint inhibitors include anti-CTLA-4 antibodies (ipilimumab, tremelimumab), anti-PD-1 antibodies (nivolumab, pembrolizumab), and anti-PD-L1 antibodies (atezolizumab, durvalumab, avelumab). MEK inhibitors include cobimetinib and trametinib. The addition of MEK inhibitors to BRAF inhibitor therapy in melanoma increases efficacy and reduces BRAF-related adverse events (such as squamous cell carcinomas). Dacarbazine, carboplatin, and cisplatin are examples of cytotoxic chemotherapies.
Bolognia J, Schaffer J, Cerroni L, eds. *Dermatology.* [Philadelphia]: Elsevier, 2018 (ch. 113).

79. **E.** Interacts with polymerized microtubules to disrupt the mitotic spindle and inhibit mitosis
Antifungals have different mechanisms of action. Griseofulvin inhibits dermatophyte mitosis by disrupting the mitotic spindle. Flucytosine interferes with DNA synthesis. Imidazoles and triazoles inhibit 14-α-demethylase to disrupt fungal cell membrane synthesis. Allylamines and benzylamines inhibit squalene epoxidase to disrupt fungal cell membrane synthesis. Polyenes and ciclopirox olamine increase cell membrane permeability.
Bolognia J, Schaffer J, Cerroni L, eds. *Dermatology.* [Philadelphia]: Elsevier, 2018 (ch. 127).

80. **D.** Brown recluse spider; sphingomyelinase-D
The brown recluse spider (*Loxosceles reclusa*) is primarily found in the south-central United States and can cause dermonecrotic reactions. Patients can have systemic reactions, including shock, hemolysis, renal insufficiency, and disseminated intravascular coagulation.
Bolognia J, Schaffer J, Cerroni L, eds. *Dermatology.* [Philadelphia]: Elsevier, 2018 (ch. 85).